A Practical Approach to Cardiovascular Medicine

To my mother, Masoumeh Toti, for her continuous support and love.

and

To my mentor, Irv Weissman, for being a true role model and
a source of inspiration. [R.A.]

To my wife Mabel, for bringing so much love and joy to my life. [M.P.]

To my wonderful wife Gloria and to my beautiful daughters
Catherine and Margaret.

and

To the memory of my loving parents Lillian and Samuel. [P.W.]

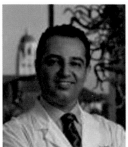 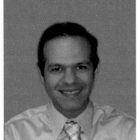 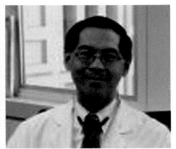

Reza Ardehali   **Marco Perez**   **Paul Wang**

A Practical Approach to Cardiovascular Medicine

EDITED BY

Reza Ardehali MD PhD
Department of Internal Medicine
Division of Cardiology
Stanford University School of Medicine
Stanford, CA, USA

Marco Perez MD
Department of Internal Medicine
Division of Cardiology
Stanford University School of Medicine
Stanford, CA, USA

Paul Wang PhD
Department of Internal Medicine
Division of Cardiology
Stanford University School of Medicine
Stanford, CA, USA

WILEY-BLACKWELL

A John Wiley & Sons, Ltd., Publication

Library of Congress Cataloging-in-Publication Data

A practical approach to cardiovascular medicine / edited by Reza Ardehali, Marco Perez, Paul Wang.
    p. ; cm.
   Includes bibliographical references and index.
   ISBN 978-1-4051-8039-9 (pbk. : alk. paper)   1. Heart–Diseases–Handbooks, manuals, etc.   2. Cardiology–Handbooks, manuals, etc.   I. Ardehali, Reza.
II. Perez, Marco, M.D.   III. Wang, Paul, Ph.D.
   [DNLM: 1. Cardiovascular Diseases–diagnosis.   2. Cardiovascular Diseases–therapy.
3. Cardiology–methods.   WG 120]
   RC669.15.P727 2011
   616.1'2–dc22

                                                                              2010047389

A catalogue record for this book is available from the British Library.

This book is published in the following electronic formats: ePDF 9781444393873; Wiley Online Library 9781444393897; ePub 9781444393880

Set in 9.5 on 12 pt Palatino by Toppan Best-set Premedia Limited

Printed and bound in Malaysia by Vivar Printing Sdn Bhd

1   2011

Contents

Section III Heart Failure

Section IV Valvular and Vascular Disease

Section V Arrhythmias and Sudden Cardiac Death

Section VI Cardiovascular Disease in Special Populations

Contributors

Amin Al-Ahmad MD
Department of Internal Medicine
Division of Cardiology
Stanford University School of Medicine
Stanford, CA, USA

Jesus Almendral MD
Department of Internal Medicine
Division of Cardiology
Stanford University School of Medicine
Stanford, CA, USA

Reza Ardehali MD PhD
Department of Internal Medicine
Division of Cardiology
Stanford University School of Medicine
Stanford, CA, USA

Euan Ashley MRCP DPhil
Department of Internal Medicine
Division of Cardiology
Stanford University School of Medicine
Stanford, CA, USA

Ramin Beygui MD
Department of Internal Medicine
Division of Cardiology
Stanford University School of Medicine
Stanford, CA, USA

John Cooke MD PhD
Department of Internal Medicine
Division of Cardiology
Stanford University School of Medicine
Stanford, CA, USA

William F. Fearon MD
Department of Internal Medicine
Division of Cardiology
Stanford University School of Medicine
Stanford, CA, USA

Michael Fowler MB FRCP
Department of Internal Medicine
Division of Cardiology
Stanford University School of Medicine
Stanford, CA, USA

Karen Friday MD
Department of Internal Medicine
Division of Cardiology
Stanford University School of Medicine
Stanford, CA, USA

Victor F. Froelicher MD
Department of Internal Medicine
Division of Cardiology
Stanford University School of Medicine
Stanford, CA, USA

Anurag Gupta MD
Department of Internal Medicine
Division of Cardiology
Stanford University School of Medicine
Stanford, CA, USA

Mohammad Haghdoost MD
Department of General Surgery
Stanford University School of Medicine
Stanford, CA, USA

Shahriar Heidary MD
Department of Internal Medicine
Division of Cardiology
Stanford University School of Medicine
Stanford, CA, USA

Micheal Ho MD
Department of Internal Medicine
Division of Cardiology
Stanford University School of Medicine
Stanford, CA, USA

Henry Hsia MD
Department of Internal Medicine
Division of Cardiology
Stanford University School of Medicine
Stanford, CA, USA

Jeffrey Hsing MD
Department of Internal Medicine
Division of Cardiology
Stanford University School of Medicine
Stanford, CA, USA

Sharon Hunt MD
Department of Internal Medicine
Division of Cardiology
Stanford University School of Medicine
Stanford, CA, USA

Arvindh Kanagasundram MD
Department of Internal Medicine
Division of Cardiology
Stanford University School of Medicine
Stanford, CA, USA

Chandra Katikireddy MD
Department of Internal Medicine
Division of Cardiology
Stanford University School of Medicine
Stanford, CA, USA

Richard Lafayette MD
Department of Internal Medicine
Division of Nephrology
Stanford University School of Medicine
Stanford, CA, USA

David P. Lee MD
Department of Internal Medicine
Division of Cardiology
Stanford University School of Medicine
Stanford, CA, USA

Nicholas J. Leeper MD
Department of Internal Medicine
Division of Cardiology
Stanford University School of Medicine
Stanford, CA, USA

Joshua Lehrer MD
Department of Internal Medicine
Division of Cardiology
Stanford University School of Medicine
Stanford, CA, USA

David Liang MD PhD
Department of Internal Medicine
Division of Cardiology
Stanford University School of Medicine
Stanford, CA, USA

Ronald Lo MD
Department of Internal Medicine
Division of Cardiology
Stanford University School of Medicine
Stanford, CA, USA

Robert Maranda MD
Department of Internal Medicine
Division of Cardiology
Stanford University School of Medicine
Stanford, CA, USA

Michael V. McConnell MD
Department of Internal Medicine
Division of Cardiology
Stanford University School of Medicine
Stanford, CA, USA

Azar Mehdizadeh MD
Department of Internal Medicine
Division of Cardiology
Stanford University School of Medicine
Stanford, CA, USA

Aiden O'Loughlin MBBS
Department of Internal Medicine
Division of Cardiology
Stanford University School of Medicine
Stanford, CA, USA

Shirley Park MD
Department of Internal Medicine
Division of Cardiology
Stanford University School of Medicine
Stanford, CA, USA

Marco Perez MD
Department of Internal Medicine
Division of Cardiology
Stanford University School of Medicine
Stanford, CA, USA

Stanley G. Rockson MD
Department of Internal Medicine
Division of Cardiology
Stanford University School of Medicine
Stanford, CA, USA

Karim Sallam MD
Department of Internal Medicine
Stanford University School of Medicine
Stanford, CA, USA

Ingela Schnittger MD
Department of Internal Medicine
Division of Cardiology
Stanford University School of Medicine
Stanford, CA, USA

Maulik Shah MD
Department of Internal Medicine
Division of Cardiology
Stanford University School of Medicine
Stanford, CA, USA

Farheen Shirazi MD
Department of Internal Medicine
Division of Cardiology
Stanford University School of Medicine
Stanford, CA, USA

Yen Tibayan MD
Department of Internal Medicine
Division of Cardiology
Stanford University School of Medicine
Stanford, CA, USA

Paul Wang PhD
Department of Internal Medicine
Division of Cardiology
Stanford University School of Medicine
Stanford, CA, USA

Matthew T. Wheeler MD PhD
Department of Internal Medicine
Division of Cardiology
Stanford University School of Medicine
Stanford, CA, USA

Andrew Wilson MBBS PhD
Department of Internal Medicine
Division of Cardiology
Stanford University School of Medicine
Stanford, CA, USA

Christopher Woods MD PhD
Department of Internal Medicine
Division of Cardiology
Stanford University School of Medicine
Stanford, CA, USA

Alan Yeung MD
Department of Internal Medicine
Division of Cardiology
Stanford University School of Medicine
Stanford, CA, USA

Patrick Yue MD
Department of Internal Medicine
Division of Cardiology
Stanford University School of Medicine
Stanford, CA, USA

Roham T. Zamanian MD
Department of Internal Medicine
Division of Pulmonary and Critical Care
Stanford University School of Medicine
Stanford, CA, USA

Paul Zei MD PhD
Department of Internal Medicine
Division of Cardiology
Stanford University School of Medicine
Stanford, CA, USA

List of Abbreviations

6MWT	6-min walk test	AS	aortic stenosis
AAA	abdominal aortic aneurysm	ASA	aspirin
		ASD	atrial septal defect
ABG	arterial blood gases	AV	atrioventricular
ABI	ankle brachial index	AVRT	atrioventricular re-entrant tachycardia
ABPM	ambulatory blood pressure monitoring	AVNRT	atrioventricular nodal re-entrant tachycardia
ACC	American College of Cardiology	AVR	atrial valve replacement
ACE-I	angiotensin-converting enzyme inhibitor	BBB	bundle branch block
ACR	acute cellular rejection	BMI	body mass index
ACS	acute coronary syndromes	BMP	basic metabolic panel
		BMS	bare metal stent
ADA	American Diabetes Association	BNP	brain natriuretic protein
		BP	blood pressure
AF	atrial fibrillation		
AHA	American Heart Association	CABG	coronary artery bypass graft
AI	aortic insufficiency	CAD	coronary artery disease
AIVR	accelerated idioventricular rhythm	CAV	cardiac allograft vasculopathy
AMR	antibody-mediated rejection	CBC	complete blood count
		CCA	common carotid artery
AR	aortic regurgitation	CCB	calcium channel blocker
ARB	angiotensin receptor II blocker	CCU	coronary care unit
		CHB	complete heart block
ARVC	arrhythmogenic right ventricular cardiomyopathy	CHD	coronary heart disease
		CHF	congestive heart failure
		CMV	cytomegalovirus
ARVD	arrhythmogenic right ventricular dysplasia	CNI	calcineurin inhibitor
		CNS	central nervous system

COPD	chronic obstructive pulmonary disease	HE	hypertensive emergency
CPB	cardiopulmonary bypass	HJR	hepatojugular reflex
CPR	cardiopulmonary resuscitation	HIV	human immunodeficiency virus
CRI	chronic renal insufficiency	HOCM	hypertrophic obstructive cardiomyopathy
CRP	C-reactive protein	HR	heart rate
CRT	cardiac resynchronization therapy	HSVC	high superior vena cava
CT	computed tomography	HTN	hypertension
CVA	cerebrovascular accident	HU	hypertensive urgency
CVD	cardiovascular disease		
CVP	central venous pressure	IABP	intra-aortic balloon pump
CVVH	continuous venovenous hemofiltration	ICD	implantable cardioverter defibrillator
CXR	chest X-ray	ICU	intensive care unit
		IE	infective endocarditis
DBP	dystolic blood pressure	IL	interleukin
DCC	direct current cardioversion	IVC	inferior vena cava
		IVCD	intraventricular conduction defect
DES	drug-eluting stent	IVUS	intravascular ultrasound
DM	diabetes mellitus		
		JVP	jugular venous pressure
EBCT	electron beam computed tomography		
		LA	left atrium
ECG	electrocardiography	LAD	left anterior descending artery
ECMO	extracorporeal membrane oxygenation	LAP	left atrial pressure
EF	ejection fraction	LBBB	left bundle branch block
ESD	end-systolic diameter	LDL	low-density lipoprotein
ESR	erythrocyte sedimentation ratio	LFT	liver function test
		LHF	left heart failure
ETT	exercise treadmill test	LIMA	left internal mammary artery
FT4	free thyroxine	LMWH	low-molecular-weight heparin
FVC	forced vital capacity		
FEV1	forced expiratory volume in 1 s	lp(a)	lipoprotein a
		LPA	left pulmonary artery
		LSVC	low superior vena cava
GFR	glomerular filtration rate	LV	left ventricular
GI	gastrointestinal	LVD	left ventricular dysfunction
GP	glycoprotein		
		LVEDP	left ventricular end-diastolic pressure
HCM	hypertrophic cardiomyopathy	LVEDV	left ventricular end-diastolic volume
HDL	high-density lipoprotein		

LVEF	left ventricular ejection fraction	PCA	patient-controlled anesthesia
LVH	left ventricular hypertrophy	PCH	pulmonary capillary hemangiomatosis
LVOT	left ventricular outflow tract	PCI	percutaneous coronary intervention
		PCN	penicillin
MAOI	monoamine oxidase inhibitor	PCP	phenylcyclidine
		PCWP	pulmonary capillary wedge pressure
MAP	mean arterial pressure		
MET	metabolic equivalent	PDA	patent ductus arteriosus
MI	myocardial infarction	PE	pulmonary embolism
MMF	mycophenolate mofetil	PEA	pulseless electrical activity
MPA	main pulmonary artery	PEEP	positive end-expiratory pressure
MR	mitral regurgitation		
MRI	magnetic resonance imaging	PFO	patent foramen ovale
		PFT	pulmonary function test
MRSA	methicillin-resistant *Staphylococcus aureus*	PHT	pressure half-time
		PHTN	portal hypertension
MV	mitral valve	PMBV	percutaneous mitral balloon valvotomy
MVP	mitral valve prolapse		
MVR	mitral valve replacement	PND	paroxysmal nocturnal dyspnea
NRT	nicotine replacement therapy	PPAR	peroxisome proliferator-activated receptor
NSAID	nonsteroidal anti-inflammatory drug	PPM	permanent pacemaker
		PRA	panel reactive antibody
NSVT	nonsustained ventricular tachycardia	PS	pulmonic stenosis
		PTCA	percutaneous transluminal coronary angioplasty
NTG	nitroglycerin		
NYHA	New York Heart Association	PTLD	post-transplant lymphoproliferative disorder
OTC	over the counter	PVC	premature ventricular contraction
PAC	premature atrial contraction	PVD	premature ventricular depolarization
PAD	peripheral artery disease	PVOD	pulmonary veno-occlusive disease
PAH	pulmonary artery hypertension		
		PVR	pulmonary vascular resistance
PAP	pulmonary artery pressure		
PASP	pulmonary artery systolic pressure	RA	right atrium
		RAD	right axis deviation
PAWP	pulmonary artery wedge pressure	RAE	right atrial enlargement
		RAP	right atrial pressure

RCA	right coronary artery	TEE	transesophageal echocardiogram
RCT	randomized controlled trial	TFT	thyroid function test
RF	regurgitant fraction	TG	triglyceride
RHF	right heart failure	TGA	transposition of great arteries
RPA	right pulmonary artery		
RV	right ventricular	TIMI	thrombolysis in myocardial infarction
RVAD	right ventricular assist device		
		TLI	total lymphoid irradiation
RVEDP	right ventricular end-diastolic pressure	TnI	troponin I
		TOF	tetralogy of Fallot
RVH	right ventricular hypertrophy	TR	tricuspid regurgitation
		TSH	thyroid stimulating hormone
RVOT	right ventricular outflow tract		
		TTE	transthoracic echocardiography
RVSP	right ventricular systolic pressure		
		TV	tricuspid valve
		TVR	target vessel revascularization
SAM	systolic anterior motion		
SBP	systolic blood pressure	TWI	T-wave inversion
SCD	sudden cardiac death		
SLE	systemic lupus erythematosus	UFH	unfractionated heparin
		UPEP	urine protein electrophoretic pattern
SOB	shortness of breath		
SPEP	serum protein electrophoretic pattern		
		VAD	ventricular assist device
STEMI	ST elevation myocardial infarction	VLDL	very-low-density lipoprotein
SVC	superior vena cava	VPB	ventricular premature beat
SVG	saphenous vein graft		
SVR	systemic vascular resistance	VSD	ventricular septal defect
		VT	ventricular tachycardia
SVT	supraventricular tachycardia		
		WBC	white blood cell
		WHO	World Health Organization
TB	tuberculosis		
TC	total cholesterol	WPW	Wolff–Parkinson–White

Foreword

Medical knowledge is increasing at an unprecedented rate and physicians in training are expected to master a large body of knowledge that can seem overwhelming. While many refer to textbooks and the Internet for updates in diagnostic methods, new therapies, and clinical trials addressing medical issues, a practical handbook that can be used even at the bedside is what prompted the design of this book. This cardiology handbook emphasizes evidence-based medicine in an up-to-date, practical, reader-friendly context, and addresses an unmet need in an era of information overload.

This book was originally designed with the need of a cardiology fellow trainee in mind. A major strength of this handbook relates to its editors and authors: it was primarily written and edited by cardiology fellows who know both about how busy the service can be and what information is needed for effective patient care. We believe that this book can serve as practical guide not only to cardiology fellows in training, but also to a wider audience that includes other trainees in medicine, surgery, and anesthesiology, as well as practicing internists and cardiologists. The practical format of this book includes boxes and flowcharts (for diagnosis and treatment), evidence-based practice (landscape trials) and clinical pearls (succinct advice from master clinicians). The dedication and commitment to patient care of the authors and editors are evident in the quality of the final product. We are confident that this book can be used by many physicians with the goal of improved patient care.

For more than five decades, Stanford has been a leader in cardiovascular care, research and education. From the first heart-lung transplant to innovative intracoronary devices to basic research on cardiac development, Stanford has contributed enormously to the advancement of cardiovascular therapy. Its programs in cardiology and cardiothoracic surgery have trained hundreds of experts, who have gone on to become leaders in their fields. This book has grown out of the Stanford Cardiology tradition of giving its fellows a pivotal role in patient care and educating colleagues and peers. Each chapter is written by a fellow in training with direct supervision of a member of the

Stanford faculty. The book holds true to the core values of our institution: patient care, research, and education.

Alan C. Yeung, MD
Li Ka Shing Professor of Medicine
Chief, Cardiovascular Medicine
(Clinical)
Stanford University School of Medicine

Robert C. Robbins, MD
Professor and Chairman, Cardiothoracic Surgery
Director, Cardiovascular Institute
Stanford University School of Medicine

SECTION I

I Preventive Cardiology

1   Prevention of Cardiovascular Disease

Maulik Shah and Reza Ardehali
Department of Internal Medicine, Division of Cardiology, Stanford University School of Medicine, Stanford, CA, USA

Cardiovascular disease (CVD) remains the leading cause of death in industrialized nations and its incidence is increasing in developing countries. The lifetime risk for the development of coronary heart disease (CHD) for men at age 40 remains at nearly 50%. Given this large risk, clinical and public health approaches to combat the development of CVD are essential. CVD accounts for over 800 000 deaths each year in the United States alone, with the majority resulting from coronary artery disease (CAD). In addition, over 17 million Americans have known or asymptomatic CHD. As the annual economic costs associated with heart disease morbidity and mortality exceed $500 billion, strong efforts are required for adequate screening and prevention.

Prevention of Coronary Heart Disease

- As the prevalence of CHD is high worldwide, the prevention of even a small proportion of disease has an enormous effect.
- **Primary prevention** refers to risk reduction in a population *without* known heart disease.
- **Secondary prevention** refers to risk reduction in a population *with* known heart disease.
- Understanding CHD risk factors has allowed for better screening guidelines and preventive measures.
- There are four major categories of risk factors (Table 1.1):
  - Predisposing factors (e.g. age, sex)
  - Risk-modifying behaviors (e.g. smoking, exercise)
  - Metabolic risk factors (e.g. hyperlipidemia, diabetes)
  - Disease markers (e.g. coronary calcium score).

A Practical Approach to Cardiovascular Medicine, First Edition. Edited by Reza Ardehali, Marco Perez, Paul Wang.
© 2011 Blackwell Publishing Ltd. Published 2011 by Blackwell Publishing Ltd.

Table 1.1 Conventional risk factors for CHD

Risk factor	Modifiable	Notes
Smoking	Yes	Ischemic heart disease accounts for 35–40% of all smoking-related deaths
Hypertension	Yes	Each increment in systolic BP of 20 mmHg or in diastolic BP of 10 mmHg *doubles* the risk of CVD
Hyperlipidemia	Yes	A 10% increase in serum cholesterol is associated with a 20–30% increase in CHD incidence
Diabetes	Yes/no	Age-adjusted rates of CHD in diabetics are 2–3 times higher than in those without diabetes
Family history of premature coronary disease	No	

Smoking

Cigarette smoking accounts for nearly 400 000 deaths annually. There are nearly 1 billion smokers worldwide. Even one to four cigarettes a week can increase the risk of myocardial infarction (MI) and all-cause mortality. Smoking increases risk by several mechanisms including:

- Increasing blood pressure (BP)
- Increasing sympathetic tone
- Reducing myocardial oxygen supply
- Elevating the level of oxidized low-density lipoprotein (LDL) cholesterol
- Impairing endothelium-dependent coronary artery vasodilation
- Increasing inflammation, platelet aggregation, and thrombosis.

Smoking cessation is the single most important intervention in preventive cardiology. Reductions in smoking improve outcomes, including reducing risk of MI and cardiovascular mortality.

Physicians should assess smoking status in all patients, recommend quitting smoking to all smokers, and offer support and referral to smoking cessation programs.

Bupropion, varenicline, and nicotine replacement therapy (NRT) have all been shown to increase success rates for quitting.

EVIDENCE-BASED PRACTICE

Mortality risk reduction associated with smoking cessation in patients with CHD

Context: Health policy-makers need to understand where to focus resources in smoking cessation.

Goal: To conduct a systemic review to determine the magnitude of risk reduction achieved by smoking cessation in patients with CHD.

Method: Twenty studies were included for quantitative review of efficacy of smoking cessation in patients diagnosed with CHD.

Results: Despite many differences in patient characteristics, including age, sex, type of coronary disease, smoking cessation resulted in a 36% relative risk reduction in mortality for patients with CHD.

Take-home message: Smoking cessation is associated with a large reduction in risk of all-cause mortality for patients with CHD. The risk reduction is consistent regardless of age, sex, and other patient characteristics.

Hypertension

Hypertension (HTN) is an often-overlooked and silent risk factor for heart disease. Over 70 million Americans have HTN (see Chapter 3).

Most epidemiologic studies have indicated that both systolic and diastolic BP elevation contribute to an increased risk of heart disease. This risk is especially important in elderly patients and patients with a known history of CHD.

HTN, as defined by the Joint National Committee on Prevention, Detection, Evaluation and Treatment of Hypertension in its seventh report, is:
* Two or more BP readings above 140/90
* Readings must be done on two or more separate office visits.

Each increment in systolic BP of 20 mmHg or in diastolic BP of 10 mmHg *doubles* **the cardiovascular risk.**

Hyperlipidemia

Several clinical trials have established that lipid-lowering measures are effective in reducing cardiovascular morbidity and mortality (see Chapter 2).

The goals for lipid therapy (Table 1.2) are based on the presence or absence of CHD, as well as the number of risk factors present for the development of CHD.

Diabetes Mellitus

* Diabetic patients have a two- to eight-fold increased risk for cardiovascular events as compared to age-matched nondiabetic individuals.
* Diabetes leads to both macro- and micro-vascular complications in cardiovascular patients.

Table 1.2 Goals for lipid therapy

Risks	Ideal LDL goal (mg/dL)	Non-HDL goal (mg/dL)	Revised goal (mg/dL) for initiation of pharmacotherapy
CHD or equivalent	<100 (or <70)	<130	Regardless of LDL
2+ Risk factors	<130	<160	10-year risk 10–20% >130
			10-year risk <10% >160
0–1 risk factor	<160	<190	>190

- Insulin resistance and the metabolic syndrome are also associated with increased mortality and cardiovascular risk, even long before the onset of clinical diabetes.
- By age 40, CHD is the leading cause of death in both diabetic men and women.
- Data suggest that tight glycemic control can prevent microvascular complications in diabetics (i.e. diabetic retinopathy).
- However, there are very few data suggesting that glycemic control in diabetics can control macrovascular complications.
- Recommendations:
  - For diabetics a multifactorial approach involving diet, exercise, and medications is essential.
  - Target BP is <130/80 mmHg as per the American Diabetes Association (ADA) guidelines.
  - Favored medications for HTN include angiotensin-converting enzyme inhibitors (ACE-Is), beta-blockers, and diuretics.
  - Goal LDL is <100 mg/dL given that diabetes is considered a CHD equivalent.

EVIDENCE-BASED PRACTICE

Multifactorial intervention and cardiovascular disease in patients with type 2 diabetes – the Steno-2 Study

Context: The benefit of an integrated intensive behavior modification and an intensive targeted and tailored polypharmacy in high-risk patients with type 2 diabetes.

Goal: To assess whether a multifactorial treatment approach to diabetics results in lower rates of cardiovascular disease.

Method: Eighty patients with type 2 diabetes and microalbuminuria were randomly assigned to receive conventional treatment in accordance with national guidelines and 80 to receive intensive treatment, with a stepwise implementation of behavior modification and pharmacologic therapy that targeted hyperglycemia, HTN, dyslipidemia, and microalbuminuria, along with secondary prevention of cardiovascular disease with Aspirin (ASA). Intensive, multifactorial treatment resulted in an HbA_{1C} below 6.5%, total cholesterol <175 mg/dL, and BP <130/80 mmHg.

Results: The rates of cardiovascular disease as assessed by cardiovascular death, nonfatal MI, or stroke over the course of 8 years of follow-up in the intensive treatment arm were less than half those found in the conventional treatment arm.

Take home message: A target-driven, long-term, intensified intervention that addresses multiple risk factors in patients with type 2 diabetes and microalbuminuria reduces the risk of cardiovascular and microvascular events by about 50%.

Specific Medications

- **Aspirin:**
  - **Secondary prevention.** Meta-analyses demonstrate that ASA reduces the rate of cardiovascular events by 25% in patients with existing heart disease. This group includes those with a history of MI, coronary artery bypass graft (CABG), angina, stroke, percutaneous coronary intervention (PCI), and peripheral vascular disease.
    - All patients with known CHD should be on ASA
    - For patients with an ASA allergy, other antiplatelet agents should be used.
  - **Primary prevention.** The data for ASA in primary prevention are mixed. It is now thought that those patients without known heart disease, but with a 10-year risk of CHD estimated at >6%, should be on ASA.
- **Beta-blockers:**
  - A number of trials have shown that beta-blockers are effective at reducing cardiovascular events in patients with known CHD.
  - The more effective the beta-blocker is at reducing heart rate, the more effective it is at reducing cardiovascular events.
- **ACE-Is:**
  - ACE-Is reduce the risk of CHD events in patients with known heart disease.
  - This risk reduction is magnified in patients with known left ventricular (LV) dysfunction and in diabetics. In fact, in patients with LV dysfunction, ACE-I treatment reduces total mortality by 26% at 30 days.
- **Statins:**
  - Statin therapy is indicated in any patient with CVD regardless of LDL level.

EVIDENCE–BASED PRACTICE

The Heart Outcomes Prevention Evaluation Study

Context: Benefit of ACE-I on cardiovascular events in high-risk patients.

Goal: To evaluate the role of an ACE-I, ramipril, in patients who are at high risk for cardiovascular events but who do not have LV dysfunction or heart failure.

Method: A total of 9297 high-risk patients with evidence of vascular disease or diabetes plus one other cardiovascular risk factor without LV dysfunction were randomly assigned to receive ramipril (10 mg once per day orally) or matching placebo for a mean of 5 years. The primary outcome was a composite of MI, stroke, or death from cardiovascular causes.

Results: Treatment with ramipril reduced the rates of death from cardiovascular causes by 26%, from stroke by 32%, and from MI by 20%.

Take home message: ACE-Is significantly reduce the rates of death, MI, and stroke in a broad range of high-risk patients who are not known to have a low ejection fraction or heart failure.

Physical Activity

- One of the most modifiable risk factors for CHD.
- The importance of physical activity should be addressed in clinic visits, for both primary and secondary prevention purposes.
- Energy expenditure of 1000 kcal/week is associated with a nearly 30% reduction in all-cause mortality.
- Exercise improves CHD risk by:
  - Increasing HDL
  - Decreasing LDL
  - Reducing BP
  - Decreasing triglycerides
  - Increasing insulin sensitivity
  - Improving endothelial function.
- **Primary prevention.** The United States Surgeon General recommends at least 30 min/day of moderate-intensity exercise on "most" days (150 min/week).
- **Secondary prevention.** American College of Cardiology (ACC)/AHA guidelines recommend at least 30–60 min of moderate-intensity aerobic exercise on most days.
- Walking is sufficient exercise for most patients and has the fewest barriers to successful adoption.
- Cardiac rehabilitation program use is associated with significant lowering of recurrent event rates and can be a critical resource for practitioners.

Weight Loss

- Obesity continues to be an epidemic in the United States, with a growing proportion of the population now considered to be overweight (BMI 25–29.9) or obese (BMI 30 or higher).
- Obesity may have a small independent association with cardiovascular risk over many years but contributes to risk most strongly by influencing other risk factors.
- Weight loss of only 5–10% can result in significant improvements in BP and lipid profiles.
- Weight loss recommendations should be given to any patient with a BMI >25 according to the North American Association for the Study of Obesity. These involve:
  - Caloric restriction
  - Behavioral therapy
  - Physical activity.

Alcohol Consumption

- Moderate alcohol consumption is associated with reduced risk of MI, stroke, sudden cardiac death, and cardiac death (relative risk reduction of 20% according to meta-analyses of several studies).

- No clinical trial has established that alcohol use causes this association.
- Excess alcohol consumption is related to increased mortality and morbidity.
- Alcohol also has effects, often deleterious, on several other organ systems, including increased BP in some and increased breast cancer risk in women.
- Therefore, recommendations on alcohol use should be individualized to each patient; alcohol intake should not be recommended to non-users for medical purposes.
- Moderate alcohol consumption is classified as 1–2 drinks daily in men and 1 drink daily in women.
- In the absence of a history of alcohol problems, this level of intake can be acceptable in patients who report alcohol use.

Diet

- Six decades of observational and metabolic studies have found an association between diet and risk for CHD, either directly or, more often, through effects on risk factors.
- Dietary effects on CVD risk are complex and can depend on the metabolic context, particularly obesity and the amount of exercise.
- There are few large trials studying the impact of dietary changes and CHD, in part due to design challenges.
- The current consensus recommendation based on all these studies is to promote a diet that is rich in unprocessed foods, including greater intake of fresh fruits and vegetables, whole grains, and fish, with limited amounts of meat and high-fat dairy products.
- Though there are no large clinical trials studying *trans*-fat and the risk of heart disease, there is observational evidence that *trans*-fat intake is associated with higher rates of heart disease; *trans*-fats are found mainly in highly-processed convenience and snack foods.
- No diet program can be applied to all patients. An individualized approach, with possible involvement of a nutritionist, may prove most beneficial.

CLINICAL PEARLS

- CHD is the leading cause of morbidity and mortality in Western nations.
- Prevention of CHD revolves around recognition and modification of clinical risk factors.
- Aggressive lipid-lowering therapy has been shown to reduce CHD mortality and morbidity
- HTN is an often under-recognized clinical entity and requires vigilance on proper BP readings, especially in diabetics.

(Continued)

- Smoking cessation is the single most important intervention to reduce risk of CHD.
- There is a 50% reduction in cardiovascular events within the first 4 years after smoking cessation.
- Remember, buproprion is effective for smoking cessation, but must be avoided in patients at risk for seizures; nicotine replacement therapy, available without prescription, can be combined with bupropion.
- Weight loss, exercise, and diet can improve HTN and reduce cardiovascular risk.
- Obesity contributes to CAD risk factors. The distribution of fat is a more important factor than the total amount of fat.
- Exercise, diet and weight loss, and smoking cessation can increase HDL levels.
- Exercise, caloric restriction, and behavioral modification are the keys to effective weight loss.
- C-reactive protein (CRP), homocysteine, and lipoprotein (a) are novel risk factors associated with CAD. CRP is useful as a tool to identify patients who may benefit from earlier lipid therapy.

Recommended Reading

Clinical Trials and Meta-Analyses

Gaede P, Vedel P, Larsen N, Jensen JV, Parving HH, Pederson O. Multifactorial intervention and cardiovascular disease in patients with type 2 diabetes. *N Engl J Med* 2003;**348**:383–393.

Yusuf S, Sleight P, Pogue J et al. Effects of an angiotensin-converting-enzyme inhibitor, ramipril, on cardiovascular events in high-risk patients. The Heart Outcomes Prevention Evaluation Study Investigators. *N Engl J Med* 2000;**342**:145–153.

Guidelines

AHA Guidelines for Primary Prevention of Cardiovascular Disease and Stroke: 2002 Update. *Circulation* 2002;**106**:388–391.

Chobanian AV, Bakris GL, Black HR et al.; National Heart, Lung, and Blood Institute Joint National Committee on Prevention, Detection, Evaluation, and Treatment of High Blood Pressure; National High Blood Pressure Education Program Coordinating Committee. The Seventh Report of the Joint National Committee on Prevention, Detection, Evaluation, and Treatment of High Blood Pressure: the JNC 7 report. *JAMA* 2003;**289**:2560–2572.

Smith SC Jr, Allen J, Blair SN et al. AHA/ACC guidelines for secondary prevention for patients with coronary and other atherosclerotic vascular disease: 2006 update: endorsed by the National Heart, Lung, and Blood Institute. *Circulation* 2006;**113**(19):2363–2372.

The Clinical Practice Guideline Treating Tobacco Use and Dependence 2008 Update Panel and Staff. A Clinical Practice Guideline for Treating Tobacco Use and Dependence: 2008 Update A U.S. Public Health Service Report. *Am J Prev Med* 2008;**35**(2):158–176.

Review Articles

Bonow RO, Mann DL, Zipes DP, Libby P. *Braunwald's Heart Disease. A Textbook of Cardiovasclar Medicine*, 7th edn. Philadelphia, WB Saunders, 2011.

Lloyd-Jones D, Adams RJ, Brown TM et al. Heart disease and stroke statistics – 2010 update: A report from the American Heart Association. *Circulation* 2010;**121**(7):e46–215.

Thomson CC, Rigotti NA. Hospital and clinic-based smoking cessation interventions for smokers with cardiovascular disease. *Prog Cardiovasc Dis* 2003;**45**:459–479.

2 Dyslipidemia

Karim Sallam and Reza Ardehali

Department of Internal Medicine, Stanford University School of
Medicine, Stanford, CA, USA

Disorders of lipid metabolism contribute directly to the progression of atherosclerosis. Lipid-lowering therapy (pharmacologic or otherwise) has proven to
be effective in reducing the rate of atherosclerosis and vascular events, including coronary artery disease (CAD). Identification and treatment of patients
with abnormal lipid profiles is largely based on patients' risk profiles.

Diagnosis

- Screening for dyslipidemia in those with a normal lipid profile is recommended every 5 years from the age of 20.
- At least annual screening is recommended for those at risk, including those
with CAD.
- Fasting serum lipid profile is normally preferred.
- Metabolic causes of dyslipidemia should be screened for and treated if
suspected clinically, which is more effective than lipid-lowering therapy.
Such causes include diabetes, liver disease, hypothyroidism, and nephrotic
syndrome.
- Progestins, corticosteroids, or anabolic steroids can all lead to
dyslipidemia.

Risk Assessment

Patients who must be considered for lipid-lowering therapy include those
with established CHD and those with risk factors for CHD.
- **Coronary heart disease (CHD) or equivalent** (see Table 2.1):
  - >20% 10-year risk of CHD
  - Diabetes mellitus

A Practical Approach to Cardiovascular Medicine, First Edition. Edited by Reza Ardehali,
Marco Perez, Paul Wang.
© 2011 Blackwell Publishing Ltd. Published 2011 by Blackwell Publishing Ltd.

- • Peripheral vascular disease
- • Abdominal aortic aneurysm
- • CAD.
- • **CHD risk factors that modify low-density lipoprotein (LDL) goal** (Table 2.1):
  - • Family history of premature CAD (<55 men, <65 women)
  - • Low high-density lipoprotein (HDL) <45 men, <55 women
  - • Hypertension
  - • Smoking
  - • Age (>45 in men, >55 in women)
  - • HDL >60 removes one risk factor.

Table 2.1 CHD risk factors that modify low-density lipoprotein (LDL) goal

Risks	Ideal LDL goal	Non HDL goal	Revised goal for initiation of pharmacotherapy
CHD or equivalent	<100 (or <70)	<130	Regardless of LDL
2+ risk factors	<130	<160	10-year risk 10–20% >130 10-year risk <10% >160
0–1 risk factors	<160	<190	>190

EVIDENCE-BASED PRACTICE

Air Force/Texas Coronary Atherosclerosis Prevention Study

Context: Benefit of lipid reduction in patients with mild hyperlipidemia without CAD.

Goal: To evaluate if lovastatin reduces incidence of first coronary events and CAD mortality.

Method: Double-blind RCT in 6605 men and postmenoupasal women with average to elevated LDL and triglyceride (TG), and low HDL randomized to 20–40 mg of lovastatin or placebo.

Results: Lovastatin improved lipid profile and incidence of first coronary events by 42%.

Take-home message: Even patients without mild hypelipidemia benefit from (lova)statin therapy.

EVIDENCE-BASED PRACTICE

The West of Scotland Coronary Prevention Study (WOSCOPS)

Context: Benefit of lipid reduction in patients with hyperlipidemia without CHD.

Goal: To evaluate if pravastatin therapy can reduce coronary events and mortality.

Method: 6595 men without a history of myocardial infarction (MI) and high total cholesterol were randomized to pravastatin 40 mg/day or placebo.

Results: At 5 years, the incidence of nonfatal coronary events in the pravastatin arm was reduced by 31% and cardiovascular-related mortality by 32%.

Take-home message: Patients with hyperlipidemia and no CAD benefit from (prava)statin therapy.

Treatment

Therapeutic Lifestyle Changes

- In a significant number of patients, lifestyle modification may result in adequate lipid management.
- Maintain calories from saturated fat at <7%; total fat must account for no more than 25–35% of total calories.
- Increase percentage of monounsaturated fats up to 10% of total calories and polyunsaturated fats to 20% of caloric intake.
- Total daily cholesterol intake no more than 200 mg.
- Addition of plant sterols/stanols, omega-3-fatty acids, and viscous fiber to diet.
- Exercise and weight loss may achieve a modest improvement in lipid profile.
- At least 6 weeks of lifestyle modification may be considered before instituting pharmacotherapy.

Lipid-Lowering Therapies (Table 2.2)

- **HMG-CoA reductase inhibitors (statins):**
  - Competitive inhibitor of the rate-limiting step of cholesterol biosynthesis
  - May lower LDL by 18–55%, TGs by 7–30%
  - Some statins may increase HDL by up to 15%
  - Check LFTs at baseline, 3 months after starting therapy, and every 6 months. Discontinue if LFTs >3 times upper limit of normal
  - Efficacy and side effect profile of different agents vary.
- **Bile acid sequestrants:**
  - Bind bile salts in the small intestine, shunting cholesterol into bile salt synthesis

Table 2.2 Effect of lipid-lowering agents

Agent	LDL	TG	HDL
Statins	↓ 18–55%	↓ 7–30%	↑ 5–15%
Bile acids	↓ 15–30%	No significant effect	↑ 3–5%
Nicotinic acid	↓ 5–25%	↓ 20–50%	↑ 15–35%
Fibrates	↓ 5–20%	↓ 20–50%	↑ 10–35%
Ezetimibe	↓ 18–20%	↓ 5–11%	↑ 1–5%

- May lower LDL by 15–30%, increase HDL by 3–5%, and small rise or no change in TG
- GI upset is the main side effect; also can decrease absorption of other medications.
- **Nicotinic acid:**
  - Thought to participate in tissue respiration oxidation–reduction reactions, lowers hepatic LDL and very-low-density lipoprotein (VLDL) synthesis, and decreases hepatic TG esterification
  - May lower LDL by 5–25% and TG by 20–50%; increases HDL by 15–35%
  - Major side effects are hyperglycemia, hyperuricemia, and hepatotoxicity
  - Relative contraindication in patients with gout, chronic liver disease, or diabetics
  - Most benefit achieved at doses in excess of 500 mg.
- **Fibrates:**
  - Activate peroxisome proliferator-activated receptors (PPARs), a class of intracellular receptors that modulate carbohydrate, fat metabolism, and adipose tissue differentiation
  - May lower LDL by 5–20% and TG by 20–50%; increase HDL by 10–35%
  - Major side effects are dyspepsia and myopathy
  - WHO study showed increased non-CHD mortality but data have not been reproduced.
- **Ezetimibe:**
  - Thought to reduce the absorption of cholesterol from the intestine
  - May lower LDL by 20%, closer to 25% when used in combination with a statin (which is more than is achieved with a statin alone)
  - Contraindicated in liver disease; no need to monitor LFTs unless given with a statin.
- **Omega-3-fatty acids:**
  - Reduce hepatic production of TG
  - Reduce TG and have a modest effect on reducing LDL and raising HDL
  - Associated with increased risk of bleeding and decreased glucose control.

Complimentary and Alternative Therapies
- Plant stanols and sterols reduce LDL with no effect on TG or HDL.
- Soluble fiber has modest lowering effects on total cholesterol (TC) and LDL.
- Soy protein has modest lowering effects on TC, LDL, and TG.
- Guggul has also been shown to reduce TC, LDL, and TG.
- All of the above supplements can cause GI upset.
- Red yeast rice, both in capsule and extract form, reduces TC and LDL with no known significant adverse effects.

Approach to Treatment (Figure 2.1)
- LDL goal directs therapy (see Table 2.1).
- Patients with mild elevation in LDL should institute lifestyle modifications for 6 weeks before pharmacotherapy is attempted.

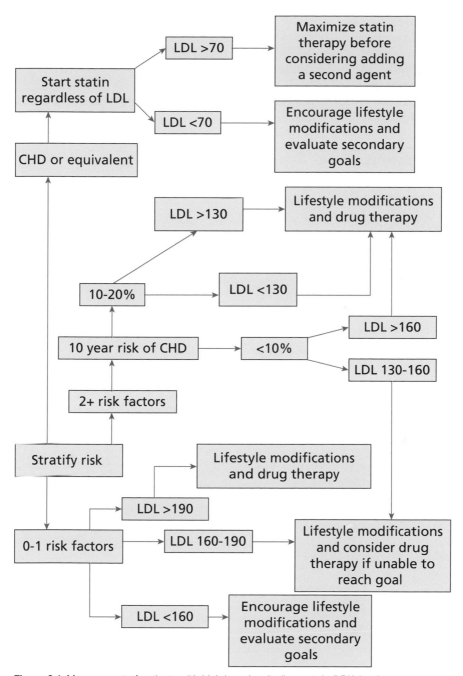

Figure 2.1 Management of patients with high low-density lipoprotein (LDL) levels

- Once LDL goal is achieved, HDL and TG levels can be considered.
- Statins are first-line therapy; start at a low dose (10–20 mg) to assess lipid-lowering effect and tolerability, and titrate up gradually.
- Second agent may be added if lipid goal not achieved even with maximum statin dose.
- Patients with CHD equivalent should be on a statin regardless of LDL and dose adjusted to reach LDL goal <70.

EVIDENCE-BASED PRACTICE

Scandinavian Simvastatin Survival Study (4S Study)
Context: Benefit of lipid lowering with a statin on secondary prevention of CAD.
Goal: To evaluate if simvastatin reduces coronary events in patients with CAD and hyperlipidemia.
Methods: 4444 individuals with a history of angina or MI, total cholesterol 213–309, and serum tryglycerides <222 randomized to simvastatin 20–40 mg/daily) or placebo. (Patients with MI within 6 months, CHF or planned coronary revascularization excluded.)
Results: At 5 years the simvastatin arm had a 30% lower rate of all-cause mortality and a 42% reduction in coronary-related mortality.
Take-home message: Patients with hyperlipidemia and a history of CAD benefit from lipid reduction with (simva)statin

---

EVIDENCE-BASED PRACTICE

Heart Protection Study
Context: Benefit of lipid reduction in patients with CHD and "goal" lipid profiles.
Goal: To evaluate if simvastatin reduces mortality and vascular events in high-risk patients.
Methods: Randomized, double blinded, 2 x 2 factorial placebo controlled; 20 536 patients with CHD or equivalent and low-to-average LDL. [Patients with end-stage renal disease, end-stage liver disease, or severe congestive heart failure (CHF) excluded.]
Results: Simvastatin reduced mortality and vascular events even in patients with low LDL.
Take-home message: Patients with CHD or equivalent benefit from aggressive lipid lowering with (simva)statin.

Approach to Low HDL
- No clear consensus on treating low-risk patients with isolated low HDL.
- Smoking cessation and routine exercise have been shown to increase HDL levels.

Box 2.1 Treatment goals for hypertriglyceridemia

TG level	High risk (CHD or high LDL)	Low risk
<150	Therapy guided by LDL goals, no TG targeted therapy	
150–199	Nonpharmcacologic therapy	
200–499	Therapy to achieve non-HDL >30+ LDL	Nonpharmacologic therapy, then consider pharmacologic therapy
>500	Pharmacologic therapy directed at TG independent of LDL	

- Patients with low HDL and elevated TG should have therapy directed at achieving non-HDL goal and instituting lifestyle modifications.
- Patients with a history of CHD or high-risk patients should have a goal HDL of >40.
- In those patients, a fibrate or a nictonic acid derivative should be considered if statin therapy does not achieve that goal.

Approach to Hypertriglyceridemia (Box 2.1)

- TG >1000 (and to a lesser extent >500) warrants immediate pharmacotherapy to prevent pancreatitis, regardless of lipid profile or risk factors.
- Elevated TGs are often markers for high LDL, metabolic syndrome, or a sedentary lifestyle, and current recommendation emphasizes treating those factors.
- Patients with elevated LDL and TG 200–499 have a goal of non-HDL cholesterol 30 points higher than LDL.
- Initial therapy is aimed at achieving LDL goal as per above guidelines.
- Lifestyle modifications include weight loss, smoking cessation, improving blood glucose control, and increasing physical activity.
- In high-risk patients, if above interventions are not sufficient, consider adding fibrates or nicotinic acid derivatives to regimen.

Hereditary Lipid Disorders

Familial Hypercholesterolemia

- Caused by defective LDL receptor mutation inherited in autosomal dominant fashion.
- Approx 1 in 500 individuals are heterozygous with LDL levels 2–3 times normal. Homozygotes have LDL levels 3–6 times normal
- In addition to premature atherosclerosis, those patients have tendon xanthomas and premature corneal arcus.
- Even at a young age, carriers will have elevated LDL and TC without elevated TG.
- Therapeutic lifestyle changes should be instituted once disease is identified at a young age.

- Decision when to start pharmacotherapy should be individualized based on lipid profile, responsiveness to lifestyle modifications, and coexisting risk factors.
- Usually patients will need combination pharmacotherapy to achieve goals.

Familial Hypertriglyceridemia
- Isolated overproduction of TG and VLDL with low–normal LDL and HDL.
- Inheritance pattern not clearly defined with TG levels between 200 and 500.
- Concomitant conditions such as alcoholism can exacerbate TG levels >1000.
- Lifestyle modifications should be instituted once disease is identified.
- Patients should be screened for hypothyroidism, advised to abstain from alcohol ingestion, and screened for medications that could be contributing to elevations.
- Therapy recommendations for TG <1000 are as per guidelines outlined above.

Familial Low HDL
- Group of disorders with low to absent HDL levels secondary to mutations in lipid transport proteins with variable presentations and inheritance patterns.
- Patients have low–normal LDL levels, which seem to confer survival advantage.
- Therapeutic interventions have no significant effect on lipid profile or survival.

Approach to Prevention of CAD

- **Primary prevention:**
  - Statins, cholestyramine, and gemfibrozil lower the incidence of CAD-related mortality in patients with dyslipidemia but no history of CAD
  - Their effect is thought to be related to changes in lipid profile, so it is hypothesized that lipid goals achieved with any combination therapy will lower the incidence of first coronary events or CAD-related mortality (see Chapter 1). However, recent studies indicate a potential pleotrophic effect of statins, independent of their lipid-lowering effect
  - Statins are first-line therapy, but any combination of lipid-lowering agents is considered acceptable to lower risk of CAD.
- **Secondary prevention:**
  - All patients with CHD equivalent should receive a statin (according to data from the Heart Protection Study)
  - Statins, bile acid sequestrants, and niacin lower the incidence of CAD-related mortality in patients with a history of CAD

- Risk of coronary events decreases proportionally with lower LDL, but with no clear cut-off; thus even CAD patients with "normal LDL" benefit from aggressive lipid-lowering therapy
- Combination therapy that raises HDL and lowers TG with fibrates or niacin has been shown to lower CAD-related mortality beyond that achievable with statins alone.

EVIDENCE-BASED PRACTICE

A Study to Evaluate the Effect of Rosuvastatin on Intravascular Ultrasound-Derived Coronary Atheroma Burden (ASTEROID)

Context: Benefit of aggressive lipid reduction on atheroma size.

Goal: To evaluate if rosuvastatin therapy can reduce atheroma measured by intravascular ultrasound (IVUS).

Method: Single-arm open label study involving 507 patients with baseline CAD as determined by IVUS who received rosuvastatin 40 mg/day for 2 years. Repeat IVUS measurements on 349 patients were performed 2 years later to evaluate atheroma size.

Results: Rosuvastatin lowered LDL by 53% and increased HDL by 15%. Atheroma size decreased in 63% of patients and increased in 37% of patients.

Take-home message: (Rosuva)statin therapy may decrease coronary atherosclerosis burden.

EVIDENCE-BASED PRACTICE

Ezetimibe and Simvastatin in Hypercholesterolemia Enhances Atherosclerosis Regression (ENHANCE) trial

Context: Comparison of ezetimibe plus simvastatin versus simvastatin monotherapy on atherosclerosis progression.

Goal: To evaluate if combination therapy with ezetimibe and simvastatin has a larger beneficial effect on carotid artery intima–media thickness than simvastatin monotherapy.

Method: Double-blind, randomized trial comparing the effects of daily therapy with 80 mg of simvastatin either with placebo or with 10 mg of ezetimibe in 720 patients with familial hypercholesterolemia. Ultrasonography used to assess the primary outcome; the intima–media thickness of the walls of the carotid artery.

Results: Combination therapy resulted in a greater reduction in the LDL levels, but the mean change in the carotid artery intima–media thickness was not significantly different in the two groups.

Take-home message: In patients with familial hypercholesterolemia, combination therapy with ezetimibe and simvastatin did not result in a significant difference in changes in intima–media thickness, as compared with simvastatin alone.

CLINICAL PEARLS

- Treat LDL goals before considering secondary goals.
- Patients with CHD benefit from a statin regardless of baseline lipid profile.
- Patients with acute MI benefit from early start of statin treatment regardless of LDL levels.
- Different statins should be tried before other agents are added/substituted for efficacy or side effect profile.
- When starting a statin, there is no need to measure creatinine phosphokinase unless patient experiences muscle pain.
- Niacin tolerability is improved by gradual titration of dose and premedication with Aspirin.
- Patients with TG >1000 need to be hospitalized and treated with a fibrate urgently.
- The Friedwald LDL calculation [LDL = total cholesterol – (HDL–TG/5)] yields an inaccurate estimate of LDL levels in patients with TG >400. Direct LDL measurement is an alternative.

Recommended Reading

Clinical Trials and Meta-Analyses

Heart Protection Study Collaborative Group. MRC/BHF Heart Protection Study of cholesterol lowering with simvastatin in 20536 high-risk individuals: a randomised placebo-controlled trial. *Lancet* 2002;**360**:7–22.

Rubens HB, Robins SJ, Collins D et al. Diabetes, plasma insulin, and cardiovascular disease: subgroup analysis from the Department of Veterans Affairs high-density lipoprotein intervention trial (VA-HIT). *Arch Intern Med* 2002;**162**:2597–2604.

Guidelines

McCrindle BW, Urbina EM, Dennison BA et al. Drug therapy of high-risk lipid abnormalities in children and adolescents: a scientific statement from the American Heart Association Atherosclerosis, Hypertension, and Obesity in Youth Committee, Council of Cardiovascular Disease in the Young, with the Council on Cardiovascular Nursing. *Circulation* 2007; **115**(14):1948–1967.

Review Articles

Rosenson RS. Low HDL-C: a secondary target of dyslipidemia therapy. *Am J Med* 2005; **118**(10):1067–1077.

3 Hypertension

Christopher Woods[1] and Richard Lafayette[2]
[1]Department of Internal Medicine, Division of Cardiology and
[2]Department of Internal Medicine, Division of Nephrology, Stanford
University School of Medicine, Stanford, CA, USA

Hypertension (HTN) is defined by the Joint National Committee on Prevention, Detection, Evaluation, and Treatment of Hypertension in its seventh report (JNC7) as a sustained BP established by two or more elevated (>140/90 mmHg) BP readings performed while seated on two or more separate office visits. HTN is a significant cardiovascular disease (CVD) risk factor, with the risk of myocardial infarction (MI), congestive heart failure (CHF), stroke, and kidney disease increasing linearly with HTN such that, on average, each increment in systolic BP (SBP) of 20 mmHg, or in diastolic BP (DBP) of 10 mmHg, *doubles* the CVD risk. Moreover, evidence from numerous placebo-controlled trials has demonstrated that appropriate BP control decreases these risks, including that of mortality from stroke or MI. Therefore, understanding and treating HTN is important.

A Practical Approach to Cardiovascular Medicine, First Edition. Edited by Reza Ardehali, Marco Perez, Paul Wang

EVIDENCE-BASED PRACTICE

Effects of ACE inhibitors, calcium antagonists, and other blood-pressure-lowering drugs: results of prospectively designed overviews of randomized trials

Context: Multiple regimens had been studied regarding the impact on CVD morbidity and mortality of treated versus untreated HTN.

Goal: To assess whether one initial treatment regimen is better than another.

Method: A quantitative review of nine trials assessing patients treated with an angiotensin-converting enzyme inhibitor (ACE-I) (four trials, 12 124 patients), calcium antagonists (two trials, 5520 patients with HTN), or other treatments (three trials, 20 408 patients with HTN) versus placebo in terms of stroke, coronary artery disease (CAD), and major CVD event. In addition, a quantitative review of eight trials with 37 872 patients with HTN compared different treatment regimens.

Results: There were significant decreases in the incidences of stroke and major CVD events in all studies. In both the ACE-I and other studies, there was also a significant decrease in the incidence of CAD. There were no major differences between treatment regimens.

Take-home message: Drug therapy is indicated in isolated systolic HTN to prevent mortality.

EVIDENCE-BASED PRACTICE

Risk of untreated isolated systolic hypertension in the elderly: meta-analysis of outcome trials

Context: Isolated systolic HTN in the elderly is a common entity that is treatable.

Goal: To assess the risk of untreated isolated systolic HTN on CVD mortality.

Method: A quantitative review of eight trials in older patients to assess the association between isolated systolic HTN and stroke or coronary events.

Results: A 10 mmHg elevation or higher initial SBP was significantly associated with an increase in total mortality, and treatment reduced this risk by 13%, with a number needed to treat of 18 for men and 38 for women.

Take-home message: Drug therapy is indicated in isolated systolic HTN to prevent mortality.

Classification

The classification according to the JNC7 (Table 3.1) applies to adults on no antihypertensive agents, who are not acutely ill and who have not been diagnosed with urgent or emergency HTN. Treatment of isolated HTN can significantly decrease CVD mortality. Once a diagnosis of persistent hypertension is established, evaluation should be carried out to determine the major cardiovascular risk status, to assess for end-organ damage, and to identify possible

Table 3.1 HTN classification according to JNC7

Classification	Systolic BP (mmHg)	Diastolic BP (mmHg)
Normal	<120	<80
Pre-HTN	120–139	80–89
Stage I HTN	140–159	90–99
Stage II HTN	>160	>100

secondary causes. It is worth considering ambulatory BP monitoring (ABPM) to evaluate for episodic HTN, autonomic dysfunction, or persistent HTN despite increasing medications.

The target BP is <140/90 mmHg in patients with fewer than three risk factors for CAD. For patients with more than three risk factors for CAD or CAD-equivalent disease (diabetes mellitus, chronic kidney disease, abdominal aortic aneurysms), or a Framingham risk score of ≥10%, the goal is <130/80 mmHg. These guidelines do not reflect recent findings suggesting that, in select populations, aggressive BP control to a systolic of less than 120 provides no benefit.

Work-Up

It is important to assess for the presence of hypertensive urgency or emergency. If present, proceed to immediate therapy as outlined below.

Assess for major cardiovascular risk factors:
- HTN
- Smoking
- Body mass index (BMI) >30
- Dyslipidemia
- Diabetes mellitus
- Chronic kidney disease
- Age (>55 in men; >65 in woman)
- Family history of premature cardiovascular disease (men <55 years; women <65 years).

Assess for chronic end-organ damage:
- Left ventricular hypertrophy (LVH), angina, or prior MI, CHF
- Stroke, transient ischemic attack, intracranial hemorrhage
- Chronic kidney disease (*reduced eGFR or elevated albumin excretion*)
- Peripheral vascular disease
- Retinopathy.

More than 90% of people with HTN have primary (essential) HTN, in which no single etiology can be identified. Nonetheless, secondary (identifiable) causes should be elicited, including certain endocrinopathies, renovascular disease, drug use, and sleep apnea (see secondary causes below). In such settings, further diagnostic tests are warranted to identify and treat the underlying cause. In particular, HTN occurring in patients younger than 40 years of age should prompt consideration of secondary causes.

Tests to Consider

- **Physical exam:**
  - Careful BP measurement in both upper and lower limbs
  - Auscultation over the cardiac apex with patient in left lateral decubitus to assess for presence of an S4 gallop, indicative of hypertensive heart disease
  - Complete eye exam to assess for retinal hemorrhages, exudates, or papilledema
  - Evaluate for signs of neurologic deficits.
- **Laboratory tests:**
  - Basic chemistry panel (including glucose, electrolytes, and creatinine level for evaluation of both chronic kidney disease and/or acute renal failure).
  - Complete blood count
  - TSH/FT4
  - Urinalysis
  - Urine spot microalbumin-to-creatinine ratio
  - Lipid profile.
- Other diagnostic tests:
  - Electrocardiography (ECG)
  - Transthoracic echocardiogram can be considered in patients with long-standing HTN and major cardiac risk factors to assess for LVH and diastolic dysfunction.

Controlling BP

EVIDENCE-BASED PRACTICE

ALLHAT (Antihypertensive and Lipid-Lowering Treatment to Prevent Heart Attack Trial)

Context: Assess whether choice of initial antihypertensive medical therapy influences long-term outcomes.

Goal: To compare whether an ACE-I or calcium channel blocker (CCB) is better at controlling CVD compared to a diuretic.

Method: Multicenter RCT involving 33 357 participants ≥55 years of age with HTN and ≥1 CHD risk factor assigned to chlorthalidone, amlodipine, or lisinopril.

Results: Equal efficacy in controlling BP among all agents in terms of preventing combined CVD morbidity and mortality. Possibly lower rates of incident heart failure with thiazide use.

Take-home message: Unless there is a compelling indication, first-line therapy with a thiazide diuretic is recommended.

All patients with pre-, stage I and II HTN must be counseled on lifestyle modifications when appropriate. Lifestyle modifications can result in significant BP decreases: weight loss: 5–20 mmHg/10 kg; DASH diet: ~10 mmHg; decreased sodium intake: ~7 mmHg; physical activity: ~5 mmHg; decreased alcohol intake: 3 mmHg. While such modifications in lifestyle are to be encouraged, it should also be noted, however, that lifestyle modifications alone have not been shown to systematically reduce CVD events, including mortality.

Patients with hypertensive emergency must be hospitalized to treat for end-organ damage. Admission to ICU is preferred for intravenous antihypertensive medication and close monitoring.

EVIDENCE-BASED PRACTICE

Anglo-Scandinavian Cardiac Outcomes Trial-Blood Pressure Lowering Arm (ASCOT-BPLA)

Context: Assess whether beta-blockers are useful in preventing cardiovascular events as compared to CCBs.

Goal: To compare whether atenolol or amlodipine is more effective in preventing fatal and nonfatal CVD events.

Method: Multicenter RCT involving 19 257 participants 40–79 years of age with HTN and ≥3 other CHD risk factors were assigned to either amlodipine (with ACE-I as required) versus atenolol (with thiazide as required).

Results: Study stopped prematurely because fewer individuals on the amlodipine regimen had primary endpoints of stroke and all-cause mortality.

Take-home message: Beta-blocker-based therapy is not a recommended as first-line therapy for isolated HTN.

Medications

- With Stage I HTN, only one antihypertensive should be started. For Stage II HTN, however, a two-drug combination is indicated.
- In patients with risk factors for CAD or CAD without diabetes, without other indications, American Heart Association (AHA) guidelines support any effective antihypertensive regimen, although beta-blockers should be considered less effective.
- Initial drug therapy and indications for specific drugs are summarized in Figure 3.1 and Table 3.2.
- If a patient remains persistently hypertensive despite treatment with a three-drug regimen (including a diuretic), assessment for secondary causes of HTN *should* be pursued (see below).

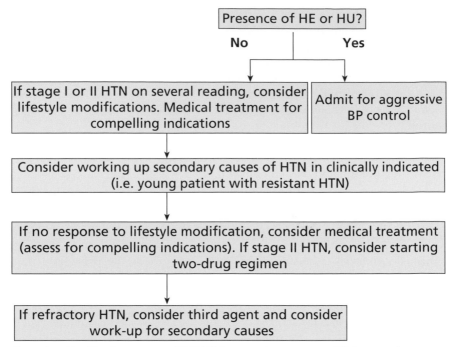

Figure 3.1 Algorithm for treatment of HTN. HE, hypertensive emergency; HU, hypertensive urgency

EVIDENCE-BASED PRACTICE

Benazepril plus Amlodipine or Hydrochlorothiazide for Hypertension in High-Risk Patients (ACCOMPLISH trial)

Context: Assess appropriate therapy when a two-drug regimen is needed to control BP.

Goal: To compare whether benazepril plus amlodipine or hydrochlorothiazide plus amlodipine is better in a population of patients with high cardiovascular risk.

Method: Multicenter RCT involving 11 506 participants with HTN and high cardiovascular risk. The primary endpoint was the composite of death from cardiovascular causes, nonfatal myocardial infarction, nonfatal stroke, hospitalization for angina, resuscitation after sudden cardiac arrest, and coronary revascularization.

Results: Study stopped prematurely after a mean follow-up of 36 months. Though BP goals were reached in both arms equally, the combination of benazepril–amlodipine was superior to benazepril–hydrochlorothiazide in terms of primary endpoint.

Take-home message: In patients with high cardiovascular risk and stage II HTN in whom combination therapy is necessary to reach goals, the combination of an ACE-I with a dihydropyridine calcium channel blocker may be beneficial.

Table 3.2 Indications for specific medication classes

	Thiazide–diuretic	Beta-blocker	ACE-I	ARB	CCB	Aldosterone antagonist
≥3 risk factors for CAD	Yes	Yes	Yes		Yes	
Diabetes mellitus	Yes	Yes	Yes*	Yes*	Yes	
Chronic renal insufficiency			Yes*	Yes*		
Stroke	Yes*		Yes*			
Post myocardial infarction/ stable angina		Yes^Δ	Yes^Δ			Yes
Left ventricular dysfunction	Yes	Yes^Δ	Yes^Δ	Yes		Yes^Δ

*First line.
^ΔAll should be used if clinically feasible.
ACE-I, angiotensin-converting enzyme inhibitor; ARB, angiotensin II receptor blocker; CCB, calcium channel blocker.

Causes of Resistant HTN

- Volume overload
- Excessive salt intake
- Nonadherence, inadequate dose
  - Drug induced:
  - NSAID use
  - Illicit or other sympathomimetic use (cocaine, anorectics, etc.)
  - Oral contraceptives
  - Chronic steroid therapy
  - Cyclosporine or tacrolimus
  - Licorice
- Secondary causes (identifiable diseases):
  - Sleep apnea
  - Chronic renal insufficiency
  - Primary aldosteronism from either multiple nodules or a single adrenal neoplasm:
    - Hallmarks: association of hypokalemia with normal to elevated sodium, suppression of plasma renin activity, and aldosterone over-production (elevated 24-h urine aldosterone). When these are present, CT/MRI of the adrenal gland is warranted. If a lesion cannot be found, aldosterone antagonism may be useful
  - Renovascular disease:
    - Not all stenotic lesions are alike, and therefore not all lesions should be bypassed empirically. In other words, the criteria listed above regarding assessing for secondary HTN must apply: poor HTN control, elevation in creatinine with angiotensin inhibition. When these are present, it is prudent to pursue this diagnosis in consultation with nephrology
  - Catecholamine-secreting tumors:
    - Plasma-free metanephrine concentrations are equivalent to 24-h urine catecholamine quantification

 – Pheochromocytoma is the most common of these rare disorders. CT is first line for localization in adrenal glands (most common location), while MRI is better for localizing to sympathetic chain if CT is unremarkable
- Cushing syndrome
- Thyroid or parathyroid disease
- Coarctation of the aorta.

Hypertensive Emergency and Urgency

Hypertensive urgency (HU) refers to a marked elevation in BP without end-organ damage, and can often be treated as resistant hypertension with close outpatient follow-up. Hypertensive emergency (HE) is characterized by HTN resulting in acute end-organ damage, as opposed to the more chronic effect of long-standing HTN. HE would be atypical with a SBP <150 mmHg, or DBP <100 mmHg, and most typically BP exceeds 180/100 mmHg. The goal of therapy is to target the BP to <180/100 mmHg, and to drop diastolic BP by 10–15%, and no more than 25% of the presenting value within 30–60 min, typically using IV therapy to eliminate the deleterious impact on end-organ perfusion. Once this is achieved, a transition to PO medications is made according to the particular end-organ involvement.

Clinical Presentations
- CNS: headache, altered mental status and/or encephalopathy, retinopathy, papilledema
- CVD: angina, dyspnea, cough, pulmonary edema
- Renal: renal failure with oliguria and/or hematuria
- Pre-eclampsia versus eclampsia: visual defects, headache and/or altered mental status, stroke, right upper quadrant pain

Tests to Consider
In addition to the tests mentioned above, consider:
- Cardiac biomarkers to evaluate for myocardial injury
- Chest X-ray to assess for pulmonary edema
- Echo to assess for CHF
- Head CT to rule out any intracranial injury.

Suggested Agents for Particular Emergencies (Box 3.1)
- **Cardiac:**
  - Acute pulmonary edema (systolic or diastolic dysfunction):
    – Consider nitrates plus loop diuretics (i.e. lasix)
    – Avoid cardiac depressants (beta-blockers), hydralazine, enalaprilat
  - Acute coronary syndrome:
    – Consider nitrates, cardioselective beta-blockers
    – Avoid hydralazine because of increased cardiac work and enalaprilat

---

Box 3.1 Dosing recommendations in hypertensive crisis

- **Nitroprusside:** Initial dose 0.25–0.5 µg/kg; max: 8–10 µg/kg/min for no more than 10 min. Do not use for longer than 3 days without checking for cyanide levels; employ extra caution with renal failure
- **Nitroglycerin:** Initial dose nitroglycerin sublingual 0.4 mg, then 5–100 µg/min
- **Labetalol:** Initial dose 20 mg; then 20–80 mg every 10 min to a total dose of 300 mg, or 0.5–2 mg/min
- **Metoprolol:** Start 5 mg IV q2min x 3 doses, and then start 50 mg PO q6h
- **Esmolol:** Start 100 µg IV over 1 min, then 150 µg/kg/min and increase q4min by 50 µg/kg/min to goal
- **Nicardipine:** 5 mg/h; maximum dose: 15 mg/h
- **Fenoldopam:** Initial dose 0.1 µg/kg/ min, titrate q15 min to goal
- **Phentolamine:** Start 1–5 mg IV bolus q30 min, max 15 mg
- **Hydralazine:** IV bolus: 10 mg given every 20–30 min; maximum dose: 20 mg
- **Phentolamine:** IV bolus: 5–10 mg every 5–15 min
- **Enalaprilat:** IV bolus: 1.25 mg every 6 h
- **Clonidine:** Initial dose: 0.1–0.3 PO bid

- Aortic dissection:
  - Consider beta-blocker/nitrates, or labetalol as sole agent to decrease cardiac impulse (dp/dt). Cardiac surgery consult is required. For type A dissection, surgical management is mandatory. Type B may be managed medically
  - Avoid hydralazine because of increased cardiac work.
- **Cerebrovascular:**
  - Hypertensive encephalopathy:
    - Consider labetalol, nicardipine, nitrates
    - Avoid central acting agents
  - Ischemic stroke:
    - Involve neurology early regarding permissive HTN
  - Hemorrhagic stroke:
    - Involve neurosurgery emergently
    - Consider CCB to limit spasm
- **Elevated circulating catecholamines:** pheochromocytoma, sympathomimetic (amphetamine, PCP, cocaine, MAOI + tyramine-containing foods):
  - Consider labetalol (alpha/beta) as first line, phentolamine (pure alpha), CCB, nitrates:
    - For illicit stimulant-induced hypertension, consider ativan/nicardipine as first line
  - Avoid pure beta-blocker out of concern for unopposed alpha effects, sudden withdrawal of antihypertensive agents such as clonidine
  - Readminister agent and/or treat with preferred agent.

- **Eclampsia/pregnancy:**
  - Consider nicardipine or labetalol for ICU. Classically hydralazine, but only appropriate in non-ICU settings
  - Avoid nitroprusside (fetal cyanide toxicity), ACE-I/ARB because of potential birth defects and impaired renal function in fetus.

CLINICAL PEARLS

- Thiazide diuretics are first-line therapy in HTN in patients without compelling indications.
- Stage I HTN typically can be controlled with a single agent; stage II HTN will likely require two (consider combination agents).
- Over 90% of HTN is primary. Evaluate for secondary causes when clinical signs suggest and when poor BP control despite three or more drug therapy (but make sure a diuretic has been tried).
- Long-term aerobic exercise is beneficial in the treatment of HTN and may reduce its incidence.
- In patients with diabetes mellitus or proteinuric chronic renal failure, therapy must be started if SBP is persistently above 130 mmHg and/or DBP is persistently above 80 mmHg.
- In patients with ostial atherosclerotic renal artery stenosis who are candidates for percutaneous intervention, stenting is recommended, whereas balloon angioplasty with bailout stent placement is recommended for lesions due to fibromuscular dysplasia.
- In acute aortic dissection, esmolol is normally used in combination with a vasodilator, typically nitroprusside, while labetalol may be used alone because of its predominant alpha properties.
- A sequala of ischemic stroke could be impaired cerebral blood flow as a direct result of vascular insult or elevated cerebral pressure due to edema. This may result in an elevated BP (Cushing's reflex: HTN, bradycardia, respiratory depression). Some degree of HTN after ischemic stroke is believed to be beneficial (permissive HTN) to promote cerebral blood flow to areas that are metabolically active but ischemic.
- In both ischemic and hemorrhagic stroke, while permissive HTN may be beneficial, there are data supporting reducing SBP if it is >200 mmHg or if DBP is >120 mmHg, by 10–15% in 24 h to prevent hemorrhagic conversion or risk of rebleeding.

Recommended Reading

Clinical Trials and Meta-Analyses

ALLHAT Officers and Coordinators for the ALLHAT Collaborative Research Group. Major outcomes in high-risk hypertensive patients randomized to angiotensin-converting enzyme inhibitor or calcium channel blocker vs diuretic: The Antihypertensive and

Lipid-Lowering Treatment to Prevent Heart Attack Trial (ALLHAT). *JAMA* 2002;**288**: 2981–2916.

Dahlof B, Sever PS, Poulter NR et al.; ASCOT Investigators. Prevention of cardiovascular events with an antihypertensive regimen of amlodipine adding perindopril as required versus atenolol adding bendroflumethiazide as required, in the Anglo-Scandinavian Cardiac Outcomes Trial-Blood Pressure Lowering ARM (ASCOT-BPLA): a multicentre randomised controlled trial. *Lancet* 2005;**366**:895–906.

Neal B, MacMahon S, Chapman N; Blood Pressure Lowering Treatment Triallists' Collaboration. Effects of ACE inhibitors, calcium antagonists, and other blood-pressure-lowering drugs: results of prospectively designed overviews of randomized trials. *Lancet* 2000;**356**:1955–1964.

Staessen JA, Gasowski J, Wang JG et al. Risks of untreated and treated isolated systolic hypertension in the elderly: meta-analysis of outcome trials. *Lancet* 2000;**355**:865–872.

Guidelines

Chobanian AV, Bakris GL, Black HR et al. The Seventh Report of the Joint National Committee on Prevention, Evaluation, and Treatment of High Blood Pressure: the JNC 7 report. *JAMA* 2003;**280**:2560–2572.

Rosendorff C, Black HR, Cannon CP et al. Treatment of hypertension in the prevention and management of ischemic heart disease: a scientific statement from the American Heart Association Council for High Blood Pressure Research and the Councils on Clinical Cardiology and Epidemiology and Prevention. *Circulation* 2007;**115**:2761–2788.

Varon J, Marik PE. The diagnosis and management of hypertensive crisis. *Chest* 2000;**118**: 214–227.

II Coronary Artery Disease

4 Stable Angina

Joshua Lehrer and William F. Fearon

Department of Internal Medicine, Division of Cardiology, Stanford University School of Medicine, Stanford, CA, USA

Stable angina is a clinical syndrome characterized by discomfort in the chest, jaw, shoulders, arms, or back, usually elicited by exertion and improved by rest or sublingual nitroglycerin (NTG) administration. It results from hemodynamically obstructive coronary artery disease (CAD). Current treatment strategies focus on medical therapy to improve survival and prevent myocardial infarction (MI), and medical therapy with or without revascularization to treat anginal symptoms.

Etiology

- Regional myocardial ischemia, usually caused by obstructive atheromatous plaque in one or more large epicardial coronary arteries.
- Less often caused by hypertrophic cardiomyopathy, aortic stenosis, vasospasm, inflammatory coronary arteritis, bridging, cocaine abuse, anomalous coronary origin (up to 6.6% incidence in suspected CAD) or other rare conditions.
- Usually provoked by increased myocardial oxygen demand ("demand angina") or by transient decreased oxygen delivery ("supply angina").

Clinical Presentation

This is based on historic features and can be classified as:
- Typical angina:
  - Discomfort of characteristic quality and duration (Box 4.1)
  - Provoked by exertion or emotional stress
  - Relieved by rest or NTG
- Atypical angina:
  - Discomfort not meeting criteria for typical angina

A Practical Approach to Cardiovascular Medicine, First Edition. Edited by Reza Ardehali, Marco Perez, Paul Wang.

Box 4.1 Anginal symptoms

Classic (typical)	Atypical, noncardiac
Discomfort described as squeezing, tightness, burning	Discomfort described as pleuritic, sharp, pricking, knife-like, pulsating, choking
Radiation to shoulder, neck, jaw, inner arm (usually left), or epigastrium (less often); band-like discomfort	Involves chest wall; is positional, tender to palpation; radiation patterns variable
Predictable onset, often with exercise, in the morning, after large carbohydrate-rich meal, cold temperatures	Random onset
Lasts 3–15 min	Lasts seconds, hours, or all day
Abates when stressor is gone or NTG is taken	Variable response to NTG

Box 4.2 Canadian Cardiovascular Society functional classification

I	Ordinary physical activity does not cause angina. Angina with strenuous, rapid, or prolonged exertion
II	Slight limitation of ordinary activity due to angina. Can walk more than two blocks and climb more than one flight of stairs
III	Marked limitation of ordinary activity. Can walk one to two blocks and climb more than one flight of stairs
IV	Inability to carry out any physical activity without discomfort; rest angina may be present

- Noncardiac:
  - Includes esophageal spasm, chest wall and pulmonary pathology.
- Unstable angina (see Chapter 5).

Diagnosis

- **History:**
  - Characteristic symptoms (Boxes 4.1 and 4.2)
  - CAD risk factors (age, tobacco, hypercholesterolemia, diabetes, hypertension, family history of premature CAD, past cerebrovascular accident or peripheral arterial disease)
  - Predictors of multivessel or left main (LM) disease:
    - Typical symptoms
    - Prior MI
    - Diabetes mellitus (DM).

- **Physical exam:**
  - S3, S4, or rub (indicative of failing left ventricle, stiff and hypertrophic left ventricular wall, or pericarditis, respectively)
  - Mitral regurgitation (MR) or apical systolic murmur (MR may be due to papillary muscle ischemia)
  - Paradoxically split S2 [evidence of left bundle branch block (LBBB)]
  - Rales [coronary heart failure (CHF)]
  - Evidence of vascular disease [carotid bruit, abdominal aortic aneurysm (AAA)]
  - Pain with palpation of chest wall (noncardiac chest pain).
- **Laboratory assessment:**
  - CBC, creatinine, fasting glucose, fasting lipid panel
  - Consider CRP, Lp(a), BNP.
- **Rest ECG** (>50% are normal):
  - May be obtained on initial visit and during any episode of angina
  - Ambulatory ECG monitoring if suspected vasospastic angina.
- **Chest X-ray:**
  - Suspected CHF, valvular disease, pericardial disease
  - Suspected significant lung disease.
- **Echocardiogram:**
  - If significant valvular disease or left ventricular (LV) dysfunction is suspected
  - To assess for regional wall motion abnormalities.
- **Noninvasive imaging:**
  - Coronary calcium [by electron beam (EBCT) or noncontrast multi-slice CT]:
    – A negative test may be useful to rule out significant CAD
    – Problematic for following progression of known coronary disease
  - Multislice CT angiography:
    – Excellent for diagnosis of coronary anomalies
    – Negative test rules out CAD
    – Useful for assessing coronary artery bypass graft (CABG) patency
    – Limited by: motion artifacts (requires beta-blocker to slow heart rate); calcium artifacts; no functional information (such as contrast run-off or collaterals); use of contrast.
- **Stress testing:**
  - Exercise ECG:
    – Consider for diagnosis in patients with intermediate pretest probability
    – Less accurate in women due to lower pretest probability
    – Do not use for CAD diagnosis if established CAD; baseline ECG abnormalites (V-paced, LBBB, Wolff–Parkinson–White, significant ST depression, digoxin therapy); asymptomatic patient (hold beta-blocker if possible unless test purpose is to titrate medical therapy)

- Stress imaging (echo, nuclear, magnetic resonance):
  - Exercise stress preferred or pharmacologic
  - Use for diagnosis in patients with intermediate pretest probability; prior CABG or percutaneous coronary intervention (PCI); baseline ECG abnormalities or digoxin (above)
  - Myocardial perfusion imaging (versus stress echo) preferred if LBBB or V-paced
  - Myocardial perfusion imaging (versus stress echo) is less accurate in women.
- **Invasive coronary angiography:**
  - Known or possible CAD in survivors of sudden cardiac death (SCD) or serious ventricular arrhythmia
  - Uncertain diagnosis after noninvasive testing
  - Patients who cannot have noninvasive testing due to illness, disability or obesity
  - Occupational requirement for a definitive diagnosis
  - Suspicion for a nonatherosclerotic etiology:
    - Spasm, Kawasaki's arteritis, radiation-induced vasculopathy
    - High pretest probability of LM or three-vessel CAD
    - Angina with CHF or LV dysfunction
    - High-risk criteria on noninvasive testing (see Box 4.1)
    - Disabling chronic stable angina despite maximal medical therapy.

Risk Stratification

- Exercise ECG testing:
  - Strongest prognostic marker is maximal exercise capacity:
    - Measured by metabolic equivalents (METs), maximum workload, double product
  - Significant exercise-induced ST depression or elevation
  - Can quantify risk with Duke treadmill score (see Chapter 24)
- Stress imaging:
  - Preferred after PCI or CABG.

Treatment

- **Improve prognosis:**
  - Medical therapy:
    - Antiplatelet agent: Aspirin (ASA) first line, clopidogrel if ASA intolerant. Dual antiplatelet therapy may be useful for secondary prevention (avoid selective COX-2 inhibitors; if NSAIDs required, concomitant ASA recommended; dypridamole not recommended)
    - Statin for all CAD patients with goal LDL <70 mg/dL)
    - Beta-blocker if post-MI or CHF
    - ACE-I if CHF or DM

- The following are of no benefit and may be harmful: initiation of hormone replacement therapy (HRT); vitamin C and E; chelation therapy; acupuncture; coenzyme Q10
- Identify and treat risk factors: HTN – risk of CAD doubles for each 20 mmHg rise; elevated LDL or low HDL; tobacco; DM; depression
- Physical activity 30 min 5–7 x/week.
- Revascularization:
  - Significant LM disease
  - Three-vessel disease and one of the following: objective evidence of large ischemic area; LV dysfunction; severe proximal LAD disease
- **Minimize or abolish symptoms:**
  - Medical therapy:
    - Sublingual nitroglycerin (SL NTG)
    - Long-acting nitrates
    - Beta-blocker (not in pure vasospastic angina)
    - Calcium channel antagonist
    - Ranolazine
    - Usually multiple classes of agents are required.
  - Revascularization:
    - PCI: superior to medical management in relief of angina, but can safely be deferred even in patients with multivessel disease and objective ischemia (COURAGE trial); procedural success >90%, <1% periprocedural mortality; no proven reduction in death or MI
    - CABG: greatest benefit for low EF and large ischemic territory; leads to lower rates of revascularization; higher rates of procedural stroke when compared to PCI.

EVIDENCE-BASED PRACTICE

Clinical Outcomes Utilizing Revascularization and Aggressive Drug Evaluation (COURAGE) Trial

Context: Medical therapy versus PCI in the management of stable angina pectoris.

Goal: To evaluate if PCI improves outcomes in CAD with stable angina.

Method: 2287 patients randomized to aggressive medical therapy ± PCI with bare metal stent. All had objective evidence of ischemia. Important exclusions: Class IV angina, LM disease, ejection fraction (EF) <30%, high-risk stress test (hypotensive response or dramatic ST depression).

Results: No difference in all-cause mortality or nonfatal MI; improvement in angina in PCI group at 3 months but no difference in symptoms at 3 years.

Take-home message: Initial strategy in stable angina should be optimizing medical therapy unless LM disease or heart failure.

EVIDENCE-BASED PRACTICE

PCI for nonacute coronary artery disease: a quantitative 20-year synopsis and a network meta-analysis
Context: Medical therapy versus PCI in the management of stable angina pectoris.
Goal: Systematic meta-analysis of all trials comparing medical therapy and PCI.
Method: >25000 patients, 61 RCTs all comparing two or more of percutaneous transluminal coronary angioplasty (PTCA), bare metal stent, drug-eluting stent, and medical therapy.
Results: No reduction in death or MI with PCI. Advances in PCI technology have reduced target vessel revascularization but not death or MI.
Take-home message: Validated COURAGE results in a larger population.

EVIDENCE-BASED PRACTICE

Bypass Angioplasty Revascularization Investigation 2 Diabetes (BARI 2D)
Context: The optimal treatment strategy for patient with diabetes and stable CAD.
Goal: To evaluate if revascularization offers benefit over intensive medical therapy in patients with DM and stable CAD.
Methods: 2368 patients with DM and stable CAD randomly assigned to revascularization (PCI or CABG) with intensive medical therapy or intensive medical therapy alone (medical therapy included either insulin-sensitization or insulin-provisional therapy).
Results: There was no difference in survival rates and freedom from major cardiovascular events among the two groups.
Take-home message: There is no difference in the rates of death and major cardiovascular events between patients undergoing revascularization and those receiving medical therapy.

EVIDENCE-BASED PRACTICE

Synergy between PCI with Taxus and Cardiac Surgery (SYNTAX Trial)
Context: CABG vs PCI in the drug-eluting stent (DES) era.
Goal: To evaluate outcomes in PCI with DES versus CABG in stable three-vessel CAD.
Method: Randomized clinical trial of 1800 patients with three-vesselor LM disease.
Results: Less revascularization in CABG group. Similar rates of death and MI. Lower rates of stroke in PCI group. More complete revascularization in CABG group. Less complex patients (based on SYNTAX score) did equally well with PCI.
Take-home message: If three-vessel disease, complex patients should be referred for CABG, but this also depends on patient preference weighing repeat procedures (PCI group) versus higher stroke risk (CABG).

EVIDENCE-BASED PRACTICE

Intensive lipid lowering with Simvastatin and Ezetimibe in Aortic Stenosis (SEAS Trial)

Context: Benefit of PCI versus CABG for patients in whom both are feasible.

Goal: To compare the effectiveness of PCI and CABG in patients for whom revascularization is clinically indicated.

Methods: 23 RCTs including 5019 patients randomized to PCI and 4944 randomized to CABG.

Results: CABG is more effective in relieving angina and leads to less revascularization, but has a higher risk of procedural stroke. Ten-year survival is similar for both procedures.

Take-home message: Both procedures offer similar long-term survival benefit, but the revascularization rate is higher for PCI.

CLINICAL PEARLS

- The Framingham risk score is a valuable tool, available on the Internet for patient risk stratification during a clinic visit.
- Atypical presentations are more common in women and the elderly.
- The concomitant administration of ibuprofen antagonizes platelet inhibition by ASA.
- PCI improves symptoms but does not decrease MI or mortality.
- CABG improves mortality for LM, three-vessel CAD, and LV dysfunction three-vessel CAD and DM; and two-vessel CAD with severe proximal LAD obstruction.

Recommended Reading

Clinical Trials and Meta-Analyses

Bhatt D, Topol E. Clopidogrel added to aspirin versus aspirin alone in secondary prevention and high-risk primary prevention: Rationale and design of the Clopidogrel for High Atherothrombotic Risk and Ischemic Stabilization, Management, and Avoidance (CHARISMA) trial. *Am Heart J* 2004;**148**:263–268.

Boden B, O'Rourke RA, Teo KK et al.; COURAGE Trial Research Group. Optimal medical therapy with or without PCI for stable coronary disease. *N Engl J Med* 2007;**356**:1503–1516.

Serruys PW. Randomized comparison of coronary artery bypass surgery and stenting for the treatment of multivessel disease. *N Engl J Med* 2001;**344**:1117–1124.

Serruys PW, Morice MC, Keppetein AP et al. Percutaneous coronary intervention versus coronary-artery bypass grafting for severe coronary artery disease. *N Engl JMed* 2009;**360**:961–972.

Trikalinos TA, Alsheikh-Ali AA, Tatsioni A, Nallamothu BK, Kent DM. Percutaneous coronary interventions for non-acute coronary artery disease: a quantitative 20-year synopsis and a network meta-analysis. *Lancet* 2009;**373**:911–918.

Guidelines

Fox K, Garcia MA, Ardissino D et al., ESC Committee for Practice Guidelines (CPG). Guidelines on the management of stable angina pectoris: executive summary. The Task Force on the Management of Stable Angina Pectoris of the European Society of Cardiology. *Eur Heart J* 2006;**27**:1341–1381.

Smith SC Jr, Allen J, Blair SN et al.; AHA/ACC; National Heart, Lung, and Blood Institute. AHA/ACC guidelines for secondary prevention for patients with coronary and other atherosclerotic vascular disease: 2006 update: endorsed by the National Heart, Lung, and Blood Institute. *Circulation* 2006;**113**:2363–2372.

Review Articles

Abrams J. Chronic stable angina. *N Engl J Med* 2005;**352**:2524–2533.

5   Unstable Angina and Non-ST Elevation Myocardial Infarction

Joshua Lehrer and David P. Lee

Department of Internal Medicine, Division of Cardiology, Stanford University School of Medicine, Stanford, CA, USA

Acute coronary syndrome includes all clinical presentations consistent with myocardial ischemia. Unstable angina/non-ST elevation myocardial infarction (UA/NSTEMI) comprises a high-risk subset of this group in which myocardial ischemia occurs.

- **UA**: new or worsening symptoms of ischemia with or without electrocardiographic (ECG) changes but without elevated biomarkers.
- **NSTEMI**: elevated biomarkers for myocardial necrosis (troponin or CK-MB), ischemic symptoms, ECG changes [two of three WHO criteria of myocardial infarction (MI)].

Etiology

- Nonocclusive (or intermittently occlusive) coronary thrombus and/or plaque rupture
- Coronary embolism
- Dynamic coronary obstruction (spasm, increased demand with fixed stenosis)
- Coronary artery dissection [e.g. acute coronary syndromes (ACS) in peripartum women]
- Severe atherosclerotic narrowing without thrombus
- Secondary UA (conditions increasing demand). The "5 H's":
  - Hyperthyroidism
  - Hemoglobin (low)
  - Hypertension
  - High temperature
  - Hypertrophic cardiomyopathy.

A Practical Approach to Cardiovascular Medicine, First Edition. Edited by Reza Ardehali, Marco Perez, Paul Wang.

Box 5.1 Likelihood of obstructive CAD

	High	Intermediate	Low
History	Symptoms same as prior angina History of MI ECG or hemodynamic changes with pain	Absence of high likelihood features and: • Typical chest pain • Atypical chest pain with DM or two other risk factors • Male >70 • Female >60	Absence of high or intermediate features and: • Atypical chest pain • Recent cocaine use • One risk factor but not DM
Exam	Hypotension, transient MR, pulmonary edema	Extracardiac vascular disease	Chest discomfort reproduced with palpation
ECG	ST depression, marked symmetrical TWI precordial leads	Q-waves ST depressions <0.5 mm TWI >1 mm in leads with tall R	T-wave flattening or inversion <1 mm in leads with tall R Normal ECG
Cardiac markers	Elevated	Normal	Normal

DM, diabetes mellitus; TWI, T-wave inversion

Clinical Presentation

- Rest angina
- New-onset (<2 months) severe exertional angina
- Increasing exertional angina (intensity, duration, and/or frequency)

Diagnosis (Box 5.1)

- **History:**
  - Nature of symptoms:
    - Typical: chest discomfort, radiation to jaw, neck, arm, shoulder, back, epigastric; unexplained dyspnea, pain >20 min
    - Atypical for myocardial ischemia – pleuritic, solely abdominal, localizable to a finger tip, reproducible with palpation, brief duration (seconds), radiation to extremities
  - Male gender [higher pretest odds of coronary artery disease (CAD)]
  - Previous MI or known obstructive CAD
  - Presence of other CAD risk factors [tobacco, hypertension (HTN), dyslipidemia, diabetes mellitus (DM), peripheral artery disease (PAD)]

- **ECG:**
  - Transient ST depression ≥0.5 mV during rest pain
  - T-wave inversion, especially >2 mV
  - Transient ST elevation
  - Normal ECG insufficient to confer low risk (4% UA, 1–6% NSTEMI)
  - If nondiagnostic, serial ECGs increase sensitivity (15–30-min intervals):
    - Consider leads V7–V9 in nondiagnostic ECG to identify ST elevation from left circumflex occlusion
- **Physical examination:**
  - Exclude noncardiac causes of chest pain (e.g. pneumothorax, musculoskeletal, GI-related)
  - Signs of heart failure [rales, elevated jugular venous pressure (JVP), S3, edema]
  - New or worsening mitral regurgitation (MR) (may be due to papillary muscle ischemia)
  - If new diastolic murmur, consider alternate diagnosis of aortic dissection with secondary aortic insufficiency and coronary ischemia
- **Biomarkers:**
  - Troponin (Tn) is more sensitive and specific than CK-MB
  - Measure at 6–8 h intervals × 2–3 times
  - Alternatives may include delta CK-MB and Tn at 0 and 2 h or myoglobin + CK-MB/Tn at 0 and 90 min
- **Other studies:**
  - CBC, BMP (renal failure confers worse prognosis), TFTs, BNP
  - CXR if pulmonary edema or hemodynamic instability
  - Lipid panel.

Risk Assessment (Box 5.2)

- **Risk assessment tools:**
  - TIMI risk score: validated for UA/NSTEMI patients to predict 30-day and 1-year mortality. 1 point for age ≥65 years, ≥3 CAD risk factors (FHx, HTN, chol, DM, active smoker), known CAD stenosis >50%, Aspirin (ASA) use in past 7 days, recent <24 h severe angina, cardiac markers, ST deviation ≥0.5 mm; risk score 0/1, 2, 3, 4, 5, 6/7 risk of death, MI, or urgent revascularization 5, 8, 13, 20, 26, 41%, respectively (www.timi.org)
  - GRACE: models based on GRACE clinical database have been validated for inhospital and 6-month mortality (www.outcomes-umassmed.org/grace)
- **Patient triage:**
  - Telemetry:
    - Positive biomarkers
    - ECG changes consistent with myocardial ischemia

Box 5.2 Risk assessment

	High-risk (at least one of following)	Intermediate-risk (no high-risk features and one of following)	Low-risk (no high- or intermediate-risk features and one of following)
History	Accelerating symptoms past 2 days	Prior MI, extracardiac vascular disease, CABG, prior ASA use	
Pain	Rest pain >20 min, ongoing	Rest pain >20 min, resolved	New-onset or progressive angina without prolonged rest pain
Clinical findings	Pulmonary edema, new or worse MR, S3, rales, hypotension, tachy- or brady-cardia Age >75	Age >70 years	
ECG	Rest angina with transient ST changes >0.05 mV New BBB New VT	TWI >0.2 mV Pathologic Qs	Normal or unchanged ECG during chest discomfort
Cardiac markers	Elevated	Slightly elevated	Normal

BBB, bundle branch block; CABG, coronary artery bypass graft; TWI, T-wave inversion; VT, ventricular tachycardia.

- CCU/ICU admission:
  - Evidence of ongoing ischemia
  - Hemodynamic or electrical instability (VT).

Treatment

- Anti-ischemic and analgesic therapy:
  - Oxygen
  - SL or IV nitroglycerin (NTG):
    - Not if sildenafil used in past 24 h or tadalafil in past 48 h, hypotension, bradycardia, right ventricular (RV) infarct
    - Caution in hypertrophic cardiomyopathy (HCM) and severe valvular aortic stenosis
    - Works by preload reduction
  - Oral or IV beta-blocker:
    - Avoid in patients at high risk for cardiogenic shock (age >70, hypotension, bradycardia or tachycardia, >6 h since symptom onset), and in patients with atrioventricular (AV) block
    - If contraindication to beta-blocker, can use non-dihydropyridine calcium channel blocker (CCB) such as diltiazem
  - Oral (not IV) angiotensin-converting enzyme inhibitor (ACE-I) or angiotensin receptor II blocker (ARB) in first 24 h if no contraindications [especially if congestive heart failure (CHF) or ejection fraction (EF) <40%]
  - Discontinue NSAIDs
  - Consider intra-aortic balloon pump (IABP) for recurrent ischemia on maximum medical therapy or for hemodynamic instability before or after percutaneous coronary intervention (PCI)
- Antiplatelet therapy (reduces risk of MI by 33%):
- ASA 325 mg:
  - Clopidogrel acceptable if ASA intolerant
- If patient is a candidate for early invasive management (see below):
  - Upstream clopidogrel load of 300 mg (usually delayed until time of diagnostic angiography in case of planned CABG); plasugrel 60 mg load per TRITON
  - Upstream glycoprotein (GP) IIb/IIIa inhibitor (do not use abciximab unless PCI is imminent)
- Anticoagulant therapy (reduces ischemic events by 33%):
- Unfractionated heparin (UFH), low-molecular-weight heparin (LMWH), bivalirudin (not FDA approved for ACS), fondaparinux all acceptable
- If early conservative management:
  - May be of benefit for LMWH or fondaparinux over UFH
- Early invasive (angiography within 48 h) versus early conservative management:
- Invasive (intermediate-to-high-risk patients):
  - Refractory angina on maximal medical therapy

- – Prior CABG or PCI within 6 months
- – CHF
- – Hemodynamic or electrical instability
- – Initially stabilized patient at high risk of adverse clinical events (especially NSTEMI patients)
- – Benefit from GP IIb/IIIa inhibition + clopidogrel
- Conservative:
  - – Extensive comorbidities
  - – Low likelihood of ACS (Box 5.3)
  - – Lack of consent for PCI
  - – GP IIb/IIIa reserved for patients with ongoing ischemia
- Hemodynamic support:
- IABP or percutaneous ventricular support:
  - – Ischemia refractory to medical management
  - – Cardiogenic shock
  - – High-risk angiogram [significant left main (LM) disease]
- Percutaneous ventricular support.

Box 5.3 Need for angiography in ACS

Immediate	Urgent	Deferred
Hypotension	Recent PCI or CABG (<6 months)	TIMI score 0–2
New CHF	New ST depressions	No high-risk
Persistent rest angina	Increased troponin I (TnI)	features
Sustained VT	Recurrent angina with minimal activity	Should have stress
New MR	EF <40%	test instead within
New VSD	TIMI score >2	48h of discharge

CABG, coronary artery bypass graft; CHF, chronic heart failure; EF, ejection fraction; MR, mitral regurgitation; PCI, percutaneous coronary intervention; TIMI, thrombolysis in myocardial infarction; VSD, ventricular septal defect; VT, ventricular tachycardia

---

EVIDENCE-BASED PRACTICE

Routine versus selective invasive strategies in patients with acute coronary syndromes: a collaborative meta-analysis of randomized trials
Context: Benefit of early angiography and PCI in USA/NSTEMI.
Goal: To evaluate outcomes in early versus selective invasive strategies in USA/NSTEMI.
Methods: 9212 patients from seven major RCTs (including TIMI/TACTICS 18, FRISC II, RITA 3).
Results: Early invasive strategy: during hospitalization, increase in mortality; remainder of follow-up, decrease in mortality and in nonfatal MI; overall decrease in nonfatal MI. No decrease in death or MI in patients with negative TnI.

> **Take-home message:** Routine invasive strategy was more beneficial in reducing MI, severe angina, and hospitalization when compared to selective invasive strategy. But note that the negative ICTUS study (no benefit for early invasive strategy in all patients with positive TnI) was performed after this meta-analysis.

Predischarge Risk Stratification

Low- or intermediate-risk patients free of ischemia for 12–24 h:
- Stress test with imaging for patients with:
  - Resting ST depression
  - Left ventricular hypertrophy (LVH)
  - Bundle branch block (BBB) or intraventricular conduction defect (IVCD)
  - Digoxin therapy:
- If stress test is not low risk, proceed to elective angiography
- If low-risk stress test, then consider:
  - Indefinite ASA
  - Clopidogrel 1 month to 1 year
  - Anticoagulation 48 h to 8 days
- Evaluate LVEF in definite ACS in patients without planned angiography.

Revascularization

- PCI:
  - High-risk features and amenable lesion
  - One or two-vessel CAD with moderate- or high-risk noninvasive test
  - Saphenous vein graft (SVG) lesions in poor candidate for reoperation
  - LM >50% in poor operative candidates
  - If PCI planned:
    - Load clopidogrel 600 mg
    - Prasugrel 60 mg is more potent than clopidogrel but at a cost of higher bleeding complications [Note: prasugrel use is discouraged in patients >75 years, patients with a history of cerebrovascular accident (CVA), weight <60 kg]
    - GP IIb/IIIa in TnI + or other high risk patients (reasonable to omit if using bivalirudin)
    - Discontinue anticoagulation downstream of PCI in uncomplicated intervention
- CABG preferable to PCI in selected patients if:
  - LM obstruction >50%
  - Three-vessel CAD (especially if EF <50%)
  - Two-vessel CAD + prox LAD *and* EF <50%
  - In diabetic patients with prior CABG and multiple SVG stenosis, reoperation may be preferable to PCI if left internal mammary artery (LIMA) graft to LAD is possible

- If CABG is planned:
  - Discontinue clopidogrel 5–7 days or plasugrel 7 days before elective CABG
  - Discontinue tirofiban/eptifibatide 4h before
  - Continue UFH
  - If LMWH, change to UFH 12–24h before
  - If fondaparinux, change to UFH 24h before
  - If bivalirudin, change to UFH 3h before.

Discharge Care

- Cardiac rehabilitation program
- Continue anti-ischemic therapy required inhospital if not revascularized
- SL NTG
- Antiplatelet therapy:
  - ASA 75–162mg indefinitely
  - If bare metal stent (BMS): ASA 162–325 for ≥1 month, then 75–162mg *and* clopidogrel 1 month to 1 year (minimum 2 weeks)
  - If drug-eluting stent (DES): ASA 162–325 for ≥3 months; if sirolimus-eluting stent (SES), ≥6 months; if paclitaxel-eluting stent (PES) *and* clopidogrel ≥12 months. All DES at least 12 months dual antiplatelet; plasugrel should also be considered in this list
  - Prasugrel may be substituted for clopidogrel and has a lower risk of stent thrombosis, but higher rate of bleeding complications

---

EVIDENCE-BASED PRACTICE

Trial to assess Improvement in Therapeutic Outcomes by optimizing platelet Inhibition with prasugrel Thrombolyis In Myocardial Infarction 38 (TRITON-TIMI 38)

Context: Does prasugrel reduce stent thrombosis compared to clopidogrel?

Goal: To valuate prasugrel versus clopidogrel in moderate-to-high-risk ACS patients.

Method: RCT 13608 patients with moderate-to-high-risk ACS, including NSTEMI and STEMI, scheduled to undergo PCI were randomized to prasugrel or clopidogrel for 6–15 months.

Results: Prasugrel reduced the composite endpoint of death, nonfatal MI or stroke from 12.1% to 9.9% (driven by reduction in nonfatal MI). Increase in major and life-threatening bleeding, however, was higher in those receiving prasugrel (2.4% vs 1.8%).

Take-home message: Prasugrel reduces nonfatal MI after PCI in ACS at the expense of higher bleeding complications.

- Beta-blocker:
  - Indefinitely in all patients without contraindications
- Long-term ACE-I or ARB:
  - HTN
  - DM
  - EF <40%
  - Consider ACE + ARB if persistent symptomatic CHF symptoms
- CCB:
  - For ischemic symptoms if beta-blockers are contraindicated or ineffective
- Lipids:
  - Begin statin therapy regardless of baseline level
  - Goal of therapy <70 mg/dL LDL
  - Consider adding fibrate or niacin if HDL<40 or TG >200 mg/dL
- Other considerations:
  - Omega-3-fatty acid
  - Discontinue hormone replacement therapy in women after UA/NSTEMI
  - Discourage use of antioxidant supplements (vitamin C, E, folate).

CLINICAL PEARLS

- UA and NSTEMI are indistinguishable on presentation (only defined retrospectively by biomarkers).
- Relief of chest pain with SL NTG does not predict CAD in the acute setting and should not be used as a triage tool.
- Performance of >5 METs without ischemia on exercise treadmill test (ETT) confers a good prognosis.
- Low-risk stress test <1% annual cardiac mortality, high risk >4% mortality.
- A normal ECG does not rule out ACS.
- ST segment elevation in aVR = higher prevalence of LM or three-vessel disease.
- TWIs alone are not predictors of ischemic events, but deep symmetrical TWI across the precordium is often due to LAD ischemia.
- >50% of patients older than 65 present with dyspnea and no chest pain.
- GP IIb/IIIa inhibitor is of greatest benefit in patients undergoing PCI; also useful for higher-risk medically treated patients (no PCI).
- Benzodiazepine and CCBs are indicated for cocaine/methamphetamine chest pain or vasospasm.
- Patients with angina symptoms post CABG should have low threshold for angiography.
- Prinzmetal's angina (coronary vasospasm) – angiography for transient ST elevations; nitrate/CCB therapy is indicated in patients with normal angiograms.
- In syndrome X (normal epicardial coronaries with presumed microvascular disease), nitrates, beta-blockers, CCBs alone or in combination may be beneficial.

Recommended Reading

Clinical Trials and Meta-Analyses

de Winter RJ, Windhausen F, Cornel JH et al. Early invasive versus selectively invasive management for acute coronary syndrome. *N Engl J Med* 2005; **353**:1095–1104.

Mehta SR, Cannon CP, Fox KA et al. Routine vs. selective invasive strategies in patients with acute coronary syndromes: a collaborative meta-analysis of randomized trials. *JAMA* 2005;**293**:2908–2917.

Wiviott SD, Braunwald E, McCabe CH et al. Prasugrel versus clopidogrel in patients with acute coronary syndromes. *N Engl J Med* 2007; **357**:2001–2005.

Guidelines

ACC/AHA 2007 Guidelines for the management of patients with unstable angina/non-ST-elevation myocardial infarction – Executive summary. *J Am Coll Cardiol* 2007;**50**:652–726.

Cannon CP, Weintraub WS, Demopoulos LA; TACTICS (Treat Angina with Aggrastat and Determine Cost of Therapy with an Invasive or Conservative Strategy) – Thrombolysis in Myocardial Infarction 18 Investigators. Comparison of early invasive and conservative strategies in patients with unstable coronary syndromes treated with the glycoprotein IIb/IIIa inhibitor tirofiban. *N Engl J Med* 2001;**344**:1879–1887.

Cohen M, Demers C, Gurfinkel EP et al. A comparison of low-molecular-weight heparin with unfractionated heparin for unstable coronary artery disease. Efficacy and Safety of Subcutaneous Enoxaparin in Non–Q-Wave Coronary Events Study Group. *N Engl J Med* 1997;**337**:447–452.

Fox KAA, Mehta SR, Peters R et al.; Clopidogrel in Unstable angina to prevent Recurrent ischemic Events Trial. Benefits and Risks of the combination of clopidogrel and Aspirin in patients undergoing surgical revascularization for non-ST-elevation acute coronary syndrome. *Circulation* 2004;**110**:1202–1208.

Review Articles

Bavry AA, Kumbhani DJ, Rassi AN, Bhatt DL, Askari AT. Benefit of early invasive therapy in acute coronary syndromes, *J Am Coll Cardiol* 2006;**48**:1319–1325.

6 ST-Elevation Myocardial Infarction

Yen Tibayan

Department of Internal Medicine, Division of Cardiology, Stanford University School of Medicine, Stanford, CA, USA

Etiology

ST-elevation myocardial infarction (STEMI) results usually from thrombotic occlusion of an epicardial coronary artery:

- Rupture or erosion of the fibrous cap of a vulnerable atherosclerotic plaque can result in platelet activation, thrombin formation, and thrombus generation, leading to vessel occlusion and myocardial ischemia/infarction. In >90% of patients with STEMI, angiographic evidence of coronary thrombus is present.
- Given the abrupt and occlusive nature of the coronary thrombosis in STEMI, myocardial necrosis is generally not limited to the subendocardium but extends transmurally to the outer half of the ventricular wall.

Clinical Presentation

- Typical: patients with STEMI commonly present with angina pectoris usually at rest
- Atypical: shortness of breath, weakness, diaphoresis, nausea, and light-headedness can occur in the absence of chest pain, especially in woman, diabetics, and the elderly
- Low output: infarction of a substantial portion of the left ventricle can result in evidence of low cardiac output (hypotension, sinus tachycardia, diaphoresis, cool skin, impaired cognition) and elevated filling pressures [elevated jugular venous pressure (JVP), pulmonary rales]

A Practical Approach to Cardiovascular Medicine, First Edition. Edited by Reza Ardehali, Marco Perez, Paul Wang.

© 2011 Blackwell Publishing Ltd. Published 2011 by Blackwell Publishing Ltd.

- Arrhythmias: ventricular tachycardia and fibrillation
- Right ventricular (RV) infarct [right coronary artery (RCA) occlusion]:
  - Arrhythmias: sinus bradycardia and/or atrioventricualar (AV) block
  - RV failure: right ventricular infarction involving occlusion of the proximal RCA can manifest as hypotension and jugular venous distension without pulmonary edema.

Diagnosis

Electrocardiography (ECG)
- ST elevations >1 mm (0.1 mV) in at least two anatomically contiguous leads
- New left bundle branch block (LBBB) in the presence of high clinical suspicion
- Localization by ECG:
  - Anterior: V1–V6
  - Anteroseptal: V1–V3
  - Lateral: V4–V6, I, aVL
  - Inferior: II, III, aVF
  - Posterior: V7–V9, prominent R-waves and ST depressions V1–V2
  - Right ventricle: V4R, V5R, V6R
- Differential diagnosis of ST elevation on ECG:
  - Acute pericarditis
  - Early repolarization
  - Left ventricular hypertrophy (LVH) with strain
  - Hypertrophic cardiomyopathy
  - Wolff–Parkinson–White syndrome
  - Brugada syndrome
  - Tako–Tsubo syndrome (stress-induced cardiomyopathy).
  - Coronary vasospasm can also result in ST elevations, though ECG changes are often transient
  - Aortic dissection with coronary compromise can lead to ST elevations.

Treatment

Timing is Essential
- A fundamental principle in the management of STEMI is prompt recognition and reperfusion therapy. Expeditious revascularization correlates with improved short- and long-term outcomes.
- Goal total ischemic time from symptom onset: 120 min or less. AHA guidelines emphasize patient education regarding symptoms of myocardial ischemia and early prehospital and hospital triage:
  - Goal door-to-fibrinolysis time: 30 min or less
  - Goal door-to-balloon time: 90 min or less.

Box 6.1 Choice of reperfusion strategy during STEMI

Fibrinolysis preferred if	*Primary PCI preferred if*
Early presentation (≤3h from symptom onset) and delay to invasive strategy (see below)	Skilled PCI laboratory available with surgical back-up: • Medical contact-to-balloon <90 min • (Door-to-balloon)–(door-to-needle) time <1 h
Invasive strategy is not an option: • Catheterization laboratory not available • Vascular access difficulties • Lack of access to a skilled PCI laboratory	High-risk STEMI: • Cardiogenic shock • Killip class ≥3
Delay to invasive strategy: • Prolonged transport • (Door-to-balloon) – (door-to-needle) time ≥1 h • Medical contact-to-balloon ≥90 min	Contraindications to fibrinolysis, including high risk for intracranial and other major hemorrhage Late presentation: • Symptom onset ≥3 h ago

---

Reperfusion Therapy (Box 6.1)

- Mainstay of treatment for STEMI remains rapid restoration of blood flow to the compromised myocardium.
- Reperfusion can be accomplished either pharmacologically or mechanically. In a meta-analysis of 23 RCTs, primary percutaneous coronary intervention (PCI) was superior to fibrinolytic therapy in reducing death, reinfarction, and stroke after STEMI.
- Mortality benefit of primary PCI over fibrinolysis is time dependent. Therefore, primary PCI is recommended if a timely intervention (door-to-balloon time <90 min or PCI-related delay <60 min) at a skilled PCI laboratory is available.

Fibrinolysis

- Pharmacologic fibrinolysis (Table 6.1) is indicated for patients presenting within 12h of symptom onset with ST elevations, new LBBB, or ST depressions V1–V3 consistent with posterior infarct.
- Fibrinolysis is the preferred reperfusion strategy in hemodynamically stable patients presenting within 3h of symptom onset when there is a delay to primary PCI (such that door-to-balloon time – door-to-needle time exceeds 1h).

Table 6.1 Comparison of fibrinolytic agents

	Streptokinase	Alteplase	Reteplase	Tenecteplase-tPA
Dose	1.5 MU over 30–60 min	Up to 100 mg in 90 min (based on weight)	10 U x 2 (30 min apart)	30–50 mg based on weight
Bolus administration	No	No	Yes	Yes
Half-life (min)	20	5	15	18
Antigenic	Yes	No	No	No
Allergic reaction	Yes	No	No	No
Systemic fibrinogen depletion	Marked	Mild	Moderate	Moderate
90-min patency rate (approximate %)	50	75	60–70	75
TIMI 3 flow (%)	32	54	60	63

- Fibrinolysis improves survival in STEMI, with a significant 18% relative reduction in 35-day mortality (9.6% fibrinolysis versus 11.5% placebo).
- ACC/AHA guidelines mandate door-to-needle time ≤30 min.
- Major complication of fibrinolysis is bleeding, with intracranial hemorrhage occurring at a rate of 0.3–1.3%.
- **Absolute contraindications:**
  - Prior hemorrhagic stroke
  - Ischemic stroke within 3 months
  - Intracranial neoplasm or vascular lesion
  - Active bleeding or bleeding diathesis (excluding menses), suspected aortic dissectionSignificant head or facial trauma within 3 months.
- **Relative contraindications** include:
  - BP >180/110 mmHg
  - Ischemic stroke in the past 3 months
  - Cardiopulmonary resuscitation (CPR) >10 min
  - Major surgery within 3 weeks
  - Recent internal bleeding within 2–4 weeks
  - Active peptic ulcer
  - Noncompressible vascular punctures
  - Pregnancy
  - Chronic anticoagulation with warfarin
  - For streptokinase – prior exposure.
- Adjuvant anticoagulant therapy (weight-based unfractionated heparin, enoxaparin, or fondaparinux) should be given for a minimum of 48 h with fibrinolysis.

Rescue PCI
- Current fibrinolytic regimens have 75% 90-min patency rates, a significant number of vessels fail to open or to achieve normal TIMI 3 flow, and >10% of opened vessels reocclude or have high-grade stenosis leading to recurrent angina during hospitalization.
- In meta-analysis of randomized trials of therapy after failed fibrinolysis, "rescue" PCI was associated with significant reductions in heart failure and reinfarction and a nonsignificant trend toward reduced mortality compared with conservative management, at the cost of increased risk of stroke and minor bleeding.
- Recommended in:
  - Cardiogenic shock (Class I recommendation for age <75, Class II for age ≥75)
  - Severe congestive heart failure (Class I)
  - Hemodynamically compromising ventricular arrhythmias (Class I)
  - Persistent ischemic symptoms (Class IIa)
  - Failure to resolve ST-segment elevation >50% at 90 min after fibrinolytic therapy in patients with moderate or large area of myocardium at risk (Class IIa).

EVIDENCE-BASED PRACTICE

Danish Trial in Acute Myocardial Infarction-2 (DANAMI-2 Trial)
Context: Comparison of PCI with fibrinolytic therapy in acute MI.
Goal: To evaluate outcomes in patients with primary PCI with bare metal stent (BMS) versus fibrinolysis with alteplase.
Method: RCT, 1572 patients with STEMI were randomized to angioplasty or accelerated treatment with intravenous alteplase.
Results: Study was discontinued prematurely due to reduction in the primary end-point of mortality, reinfarction, or stroke at 30 days with primary PCI (8.0 versus 13.7%). Mortality benefit was noted only in high-risk patients (TIMI risk score ≥5).
Take-home message: Reperfusion therapy involving transfer of patients to a treatment for primary angioplasty is superior to on-site fibrinolysis, providing transfer takes <2h.

Primary PCI
- **Indications:**
  - STEMI presenting within 12h of symptom onset, if PCI can be performed in a timely fashion (door-to-balloon time ≤90min) by skilled operators (≥75PCIs/year) at experienced facilities (≥36 primary PCI procedures/year)
  - Primary PCI reasonable in older patients (≥75 years old) with good functional capacity, or
  - Patients with onset of symptoms within the previous 12–24h who present with congestive heart failure (CHF), hemodynamic or electrical instability, or persistent ischemic symptoms.
- **Benefit:**
  - Primary PCI improved survival in STEMI compared with fibrinolytic therapy in a meta-analysis of 23 randomized trials (21 lives saved per 1000 patients treated)
  - Benefit is time-dependent, such that the two strategies become equivalent in mortality benefit at "PCI-related delay" (door-to-balloon time – door-to-needle time) of 110min.
- **Stents:**
  - **Bare-metal stent (BMS)** placement during primary PCI reduced restenosis, reocclusion, and need for target vessel revascularization (TVR) compared to balloon angioplasty alone in the Stent PAMI and CADILLAC trials
  - Role of **drug-eluting stents (DES)** in primary PCI is less clear. DES appears safe to use in STEMI, with low incidence of stent thrombosis. However, as the incidence of target vessel revascularization (TVR) is

relatively low after BMS placement in STEMI, the benefits of DES may not be as pronounced and should be weighed against the need for long-term clopidogrel use.
- **Adjuvant medications**:
  - Unfractionated heparin (70–100 U/kg without GP IIb/IIIa inhibitor; 50–70 U/kg with GP IIb/IIIa inhibitor) or enoxaparin (1 mg/kg SQ bid)
  - Clopidogrel: administer loading dose, then 75 mg PO qd (minimum of 1 month for BMS and 1 year for DES)
  - GP IIb/IIIa inhibitors: administer abciximab, tirofiban, or eptifibatide before primary PCI and continue for 12–18 h (abciximab) or 18–24 h (tirofiban or eptifibatide). Cessation of infusion should occur with significant bleeding or thrombocytopenia
- **"No reflow:"**
  - No reflow (TIMI 0–1 flow) may occur after primary PCI, reflective of microvascular dysfunction secondary to vasospasm or distal embolization of plaque or thrombus
  - Associated with increased mortality
  - Intracoronary verapamil, adenosine, or nitroprusside are routinely employed as treatment
  - Aspiration thrombectomy prior to balloon dilatation of culprit vessel may decrease incidence of no reflow.

Facilitated PCI
- A planned reperfusion strategy using full-dose fibrinolytic therapy followed by immediate PCI may be harmful.
- Attempts at improving outcomes with reduced-dose fibrinolysis prior to "facilitated" PCI have resulted in higher coronary patency rates prior to PCI, but with no improvement in mortality or infarct size and at the cost of higher rates of bleeding.

Acute Surgical Reperfusion
- Primary PCI and fibrinolysis are mainstays of the early reperfusion strategy for STEMI. However, in the subsets of patients who are not candidates for PCI or fibrinolysis or in patients who fail PCI with persistent chest pain and significant myocardial territory at risk or hemodynamic instability, emergency surgical revascularization can be considered, with understanding of the higher risk of emergency coronary artery bypass graft (CABG) compared with elective operation.
- Patients with significant LM or severe multivessel disease, especially if complicated by cardiogenic shock within 36 h of STEMI or by life-threatening ventricular arrhythmias, may be offered early surgical revascularization.
- Revascularization after STEMI:
  - Patients treated with fibrinolysis and who have no high-risk features (heart failure, systemic hypoperfusion, recurrent chest pain) can undergo functional noninvasive study to dictate further management

- Patients with depressed EF or ongoing ischemia have increased long-term morbidity and mortality and may benefit from further revascularization.

Ancillary Therapy to Reperfusion in STEMI

Ancillary therapy focuses on maintaining vessel perfusion, preventing reocclusion, limiting myocardial injury, and aiding positive remodeling:

Aspirin (ASA)

- In the ISIS-2 trial, ASA use in STEMI resulted in a significant 23% reduction in 5-week cardiovascular mortality.
- ASA (initial dose 162–325 mg) should be given to patients with suspected STEMI as early as possible and continued daily indefinitely.

EVIDENCE-BASED PRACTICE

Second International Study of Infarct Survival (ISIS-2)
Context: The benefits of antiplatelet therapy in acute MI.
Goal: To compare intravenous streptokinase, oral ASA, or both in acute MI.
Method: RCT, 17 187 patients with acute MI randomized to 1 h of streptokinase infusion or 1 month of ASA; or neither or both treatments
Results: ASA reduced 5-week vascular mortality (23% reduction), equivalent to that seen with streptokinase (25% reduction) and additive when streptokinase and ASA were administered together (42% reduction). No increase in major bleeding or hemorrhagic stroke
Take-home message: Routine use of ASA in all suspected acute MI patients is required.

Clopidogrel

- Addition of clopidogrel to ASA reduces risk of ischemic events in patients undergoing PCI.
- Should be started for patients for whom PCI is planned and continued for at least 1 month after BMS implantation and for at least 1 year after DES implantation.
- Can be administered as initial loading dose of 300 or 600 mg, with the higher load associated with a steady state of platelet inhibition after 2 h.
- 75 mg PO qd for at least 14 days should be given to patients with STEMI, regardless of whether they undergo reperfusion with fibronolytic therapy or do not receive reperfusion therapy.
- Should be withheld for at least 5 days and preferably 7 days prior to CABG, unless bleeding risk is outweighed by urgency for surgery.

EVIDENCE-BASED PRACTICE

Abciximab as adjunctive therapy to reperfusion in STEMI: a meta-analysis
Context: GP IIb/IIIa use as an additional antiplatelet agent in patients with STEMI.
Goal: To evaluate utility of adjunctive GP IIb/IIIa use in STEMI patients undergoing reperfusion by PCI.
Method: 11 RCTs of abciximab use in STEMI: 27 115 patients in the abciximab group compared with 14 513 patients in the control group.
Results: Significant reductions in mortality at 30 days (2.4 versus 3.4% with placebo) and 6–12 months (4.4 versus 6.2%) and in reinfarction at 30 days (1.0 versus 1.9%); without increase in bleeding.
Take-home message: Adjunctive abciximab therapy improves survival in STEMI patients undergoing PCI (but not those receiving fibrinolyis).

EVIDENCE-BASED PRACTICE

Clopidogrel and Metoprolol in Myocardial Infarction Trial (COMMIT CCS-2)
Context: Clopidogrel use in acute MI
Goal: To evaluate utility of adjunctive clopidogrel use in acute MI in reperfusion by PCI or fibrinolysis.
Method: RCT 45 582 patients with acute MI, 93% with STEMI or new LBBB. Half the patients were randomized to clopidogrel 75 mg daily or placebo in addition to ASA 162 mg/day until discharge or up to 4 weeks in hospital.
Results: At 16 days the primary end-points of death and the composite of death, repeat MI, or stroke were significantly lower in the patients who received clopidogrel (7.5% versus 8.1% and 9.3% versus 10.1%, respectively).
Take-home message: Adjunctive clopidogrel therapy reduces mortality and major vascular events in acute MI patients.

Glycoprotein IIb/IIIa Inhibitors
- Not recommended with fibrinolysis.
- Significant mortality benefit with PCI.
- Administer abciximab, tirofiban, or eptifibatide before primary PCI and continue for 12–18 h (abciximab) or 18–24 h (tirofiban or eptifibatide). Cessation of infusion should occur with significant bleeding or thrombocytopenia.

Anticoagulant Therapy
- Aims to prevent intraprocedural thrombosis in primary PCI and to prevent reocclusion after fibrinolysis.

- Patients undergoing primary PCI should receive unfractionated heparin. Heparin is usually discontinued following successful PCI.
- Patients undergoing fibrinolysis should receive anticoagulant therapy (unfractionated heparin, enoxaparin, or fondaparinux) for a minimum of 48 h and preferably for the duration of the index hospitalization, up to 8 days.

Beta-blockers
- Benefits of beta-blockage after STEMI must be weighed against possible worsening of heart failure and cardiac output.
- Oral beta-blocker therapy should be initiated in the first 24 h for patients who do not have any of the following:
  - Signs of heart failure
  - Evidence of low cardiac output state
  - Increase risk for cardiogenic shock
  - Other relative contraindications to beta blockade (PR >0.24 s, second- or third-degree heart block, active asthma).
- Long-term use of oral beta-blockers for secondary prevention in patients with moderate or severe LV failure should be initiated after hemodynamic stabilization with gradual titration scheme.

Renin–Angiotensin–Aldosterone Axis Inhibitors
- Angiotensin-converting enzyme inhibitor (ACE-I; captopril). The ISIS-4 trial (oral captopril) and GISSI-3 trial (lisinopril) both demonstrated improved mortality with ACE-I use initiated within the first 24 h of STEMI. ACE inhibition was most beneficial in patients with depressed ejection fraction (EF) and heart failure.
- An ACE-I should be administered orally within the first 24 h of STEMI to patients with anterior infarction, pulmonary congestion, or LVEF <40%, in the absence of hypotension or known contraindication. ACE inhibitor can also be considered for other STEMI patients. Initiation of ACE inhibitor after STEMI should start with low dose and close monitoring for hypotension.
- For patients with MI complicated by left ventricular systolic dysfunction or heart failure and who are intolerant of ACE-I, angiotensin receptor blockers (ARBs) (valsartan, candesartan) may be an alternative.
- Aldosterone blockers can be considered in patients with STEMI with heart failure or low EF, with close monitoring of renal function and potassium.

HMG-CoA Reductase Inhibitors
Statin therapy should be initiated during hospitalization for STEMI and continued upon discharge with a goal LDL <70 mg/dL

Nitroglycerin (NTG)
Given its marginal treatment benefit, NTG may be administered for persistent angina, CHF, or hypertension in STEMI patients. However, it should be

avoided in patients who cannot tolerate NTG in combination with beta-blockers or ACE-Is.

Morphine Sulfate
May be given for chest pain associated with STEMI.

Secondary Prevention after STEMI

- Cardiac rehabilitation
- Smoking cessation
- Dietary modification
- Physical activity
- Lipid management
- Hypertension control
- Diabetic management
- Medications (ASA, clopidogrel, ACE-I, beta-blocker, statin)

Complications of STEMI

- STEMI can result in a low cardiac output (CO) state and pulmonary edema. The differential diagnosis of hypotension in STEMI includes:
  - Low CO
  - Arrhythmias (tachy- or brady-arrhythmias)
  - Hypovolemia (i.e. secondary to retroperitoneal bleeding)
  - Contrast reaction
  - Adverse reaction to adjuvant medications (beta-blocker, ACE-I)
  - RV infarct: hypotension may respond to aggressive volume repletion and in severe cases dobutamine or inhaled nitric oxide.
- **Mechanical complications of STEMI** [acute mitral regurgitation (MR), VSD, and free wall rupture have a bimodal time distribution: 24h and 3–5 days]:
  - Acute MR secondary to papillary muscle dysfunction or rupture
  - Ventricular septal rupture
  - Free wall rupture
  - Ventricular aneurysm
- **Recurrent ischemia/infarction after STEMI:**
  - Ischemic chest pain should be differentiated from nonischemic pain, including pericarditis
  - Ischemic chest pain should prompt optimization of medical therapy and anticoagulation if not already given
  - If new or recurrent ST elevations are present on ECG, patient should undergo emergency cardiac catheterization and revascularization with PCI or CABG as dictated by anatomy
  - If cardiac catheterization is not an option, repeat fibrinolysis may be appropriate

- If ST elevations are not present on ECG, timing of cardiac catheterization can be dictated by symptoms, hemodynamic stability, and response to medical management.
- **Management of STEMI with hemodynamic instability:**
  - Echocardiography and Swan-Ganz catheterization may help guide management
  - Intra-aortic balloon pump for afterload reduction and augmentation of cardiac output and coronary blood flow may be considered in cardiogenic shock, acute MR, ventricular septal rupture, or ongoing ischemia with large area of myocardium at risk.

CLINICAL PEARLS

- Time is muscle – time to reperfusion is more important than method of reperfusion.
- At presentation, a patient with acute coronary symptoms (ACS) should be asked about use of cocaine and sildenafil.
- To diagnose RV infarction, perform right-sided pericordial ECG and look for ST elevation in V4R.
- Delayed fibrinolysis (>12 h after onset of event) should be avoided since it has been shown to increase mortality.
- Risk factors for free wall rupture post-MI include absence of previous MI (previous MI could be "protective") and late thrombolysis.
- Spontaneous coronary dissection is a life-threatening entity, usually diagnosed with angiography. PCI of the affected vessel is indicated in symptomatic patients with refractory ischemia. There is a risk of entering the false lumen with the wire and propagating the dissection with the stent.
- In posterior MI, look for: R/S >1 in V1 and V2, R-wave >0.04 in V1 and V2, significant ST depression in V1 and V2, and upright T-waves in same leads with dominant R-waves.
- Acute MR is usually associated with inferior infarct involving posterior papillary muscle rupture. This is due to single blood supply to posterior papillary muscle from the dominant coronary artery.
- Pericarditis can produce ST elevation mimicking MI but will *not* produce reciprocal ST depression (look for PR depression, except in aVR).
- Inferior MI could lead to: first-degree block (intranodal) or second-degree Mobitz type I. Both are transient and both can lead to transient third-degree complete heart block. Anterior MI could lead to second-degree Mobitz type II which could progress to complete heart block, justifying implantation of a pacemaker.
- Accelerated idioventricular rhythm (AIVR) (slow VT) is common after successful reperfusion.
- Discontinue NSAIDs in all MI patients.
- Beware beta-blockers and nitrates in inferior MI with RV involvement.
- 7.5% of STEMIs have "normal" coronaries.

Recommended Reading

Clinical Trials and Meta-Analyses

Andersen HR, Nielsen TT, Rasmussen K et al. A comparison of coronary angioplasty with fibrinolytic therapy in acute myocardial infarction. *N Engl J Med* 2003;**349**:733–742.

Chen ZM, Jiang LX, Chen YP et al.; COMMIT (ClOpidogrel and Metoprolol in Myocardial Infarction Trial) Collaborative Group. Addition of clopidogrel to aspirin in 45 852 patients with acute myocardial infarction: randomized placebo-controlled trial. *Lancet* 2005;**366**: 1607–1621.

De Luca G, Suryapranata H, Stone GW et al. Abciximab as adjunctive therapy to reperfusion in acute ST-segment elevation myocardial infarction: a meta-analysis of randomized trials. *JAMA* 2005;**293**:1759–1765.

Fibrinolytic Therapy Trialist' (FTT) Collaborative Group. Indications for fibrinolytic therapy in suspected acute myocardial infarction: collaborative overview of early mortality and major morbidity results from all randomized trials of more than 1000 patients. *Lancet* 1994;**343**:311–322.

Gruppo Italiano per lo Studio della Sopravvivenza nell'infarto Miocardico (GISSI). GISSI-3: effects of lisinopril and trandermal glyceryl trinitrate singly and together on 6-week mortality and ventricular function after acute myocardial infarction. *Lancet* 1994;**343**: 1115–1122.

ISIS-2 (Second International Study of Infarct Survival) Collaborative Group. Randomised trial of intravenous streptokinase, oral asprin, both, or neither among 17 187 cases of suspected acute myocardial infarction: ISIS-2. *Lancet* 1988;**2**:349–360.

ISIS-4 (Fourth International study of Infarct Survival) Collaborative Group. ISIS-4: a randomized factorial trial assessing early oral captopril, oral mononitrate, and intravenous magnesium sulphate in 58,050 patients with suspected acute myocardial infarction. *Lancet* 1995;**345**:669–685.

Stone GW, Grines CL, Cox DA; Controlled Abciximab and Device Investigation to Lower Late Angioplaty Complications (CADILLAC) Investigators. Comparison of angioplasty with stenting, with or without abciximab, in acute myocardial infarction. *N Engl J Med* 2002;**346**:957–966.

Guidelines

Antman EM, Hand M, Armstrong PW et al. 2007 focused update of the ACC/AHA 2004 guidelines for the management of patients with ST-elevation myocardial infarction: a report of the American College of Cardiology/American Heart Association task force on practice guidelines (writing group to review new evidence and update the ACC/AHA 2004 guidelines for the management of patients with St-elevation myocardial infarction). *J Am Coll Cardiol* 2008;**51**:210–247.

Review Articles

Gelfand EV, Cannon CP. Myocardial infarction: contemporary management strategies. *J Intern Med* 2007;**262**:59–77.

Heart Failure

7 Care of the Cardiomyopathic Patient

Nicholas J. Leeper, Reza Ardehali, and Michael Fowler

Department of Internal Medicine, Division of Cardiology, Stanford University School of Medicine, Stanford, CA, USA

Cardiomyopathy

Cardiomyopathy is broadly defined as "a disease of the myocardium associated with cardiac dysfunction," and may manifest with systolic pump failure or with an abnormality of diastolic relaxation. As a primary myocardial disease or a consequence of myocardial injury or infiltration, symptomatic heart failure develops as a result of the cardiovascular system's inability to meet the metabolic needs of the tissues or to respond to elevation in cardiac filling pressures. The most common discharge diagnosis for patients over age 65, congestive heart failure (CHF), is responsible for over $33 billion of healthcare expenditures per year in the United States, with mortality rates in excess of 50% at 5 years for patients with advanced disease.

Etiology and Classification

Systolic Dysfunction [depressed left ventricular ejection fraction (LVEF)]
Figure 7.1 shows an overview of the common causes of dilated cardiomyopathy and systolic pump failure.

Diastolic Dysfunction (preserved LVEF)
- "Hypertensive heart disease" is a frequent cause of CHF with preserved contractility.
- Often associated with left ventricular hypertrophy (LVH) and echocardiographic parameters of impaired relaxation.

A Practical Approach to Cardiovascular Medicine, First Edition. Edited by Reza Ardehali, Marco Perez, Paul Wang.

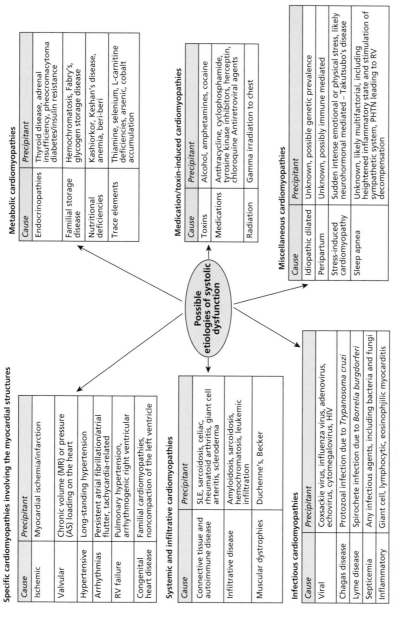

Figure 7.1 Common causes of dilated cardiomyopathy and systolic pump failure. MR, mitral regurgitation; AS, aortic stenosis; SLE, systemic lupus erythematosus; PHTN, pulmonary hypertension; RV, right ventricle

Specific cardiomyopathies involving the myocardial structures

Cause	Precipitant
Ischemic	Myocardial ischemia/infarction
Valvular	Chronic volume (MR) or pressure (AS) loading on the heart
Hypertensive	Long-standing hypertension
Arrhythmias	Persistent atrial fibrillation/atrial flutter, tachycardia-related
RV failure	Pulmonary hypertension, arrhythmogenic right ventricular
Congenital heart disease	Familial cardiomyopathies, noncompaction of the left ventricle

Systemic and infiltrative cardiomyopathies

Cause	Precipitant
Connective tissue and autoimmune disease	SLE, sarcoidosis, celiac, rheumatoid arthritis, giant cell arteritis, scleroderma
Infiltrative disease	Amyloidosis, sarcoidosis, hemochromatosis, leukemic infiltration
Muscular dystrophies	Duchenne's, Becker

Infectious cardiomyopathies

Cause	Precipitant
Viral	Coxsackie virus, influenza virus, adenovirus, echovirus, cytomegalovirus, HIV
Chagas disease	Protozoal infection due to *Trypanosoma cruzi*
Lyme disease	Spirochete infection due to *Borrelia burgdorferi*
Septicemia	Any infectious agents, including bacteria and fungi
Inflammatory	Giant cell, lymphocytic, eosinophjlic myocarditis

Metabolic cardiomyopathies

Cause	Precipitant
Endocrinopathies	Thyroid disease, adrenal insufficiency, pheocromacytoma diabetes/insulin resistance
Familial storage disease	Hemochromatosis, Fabry's, glycogen storage disease
Nutritional deficiencies	Kashiorkor, Keshan's disease, anemia, beri-beri
Trace elements	Thiamine, selenium, L-carnitine deficiencies, arsenic, cobalt accumulation

Medication/toxin-induced cardiomyopathies

Cause	Precipitant
Toxins	Alcohol, amphetamines, cocaine
Medications	Anthracycline, cyclophosphamide, tyrosine kinase inhibitors, herceptin, chloroquine Antiretroviral agents
Radiation	Gamma irradiation to chest

Miscellaneous cardiomyopathies

Cause	Precipitant
Idiopathic dilated	Unknown, possible genetic prevalence
Peripartum	Unknown, possibly immune mediated
Stress-induced cardiomyopathy	Sudden intense emotional or physical stress, likely neurohormonal mediated – Takutsubo's disease
Sleep apnea	Unknown, likely multifactorial, including heightened inflammatory state and stimulation of sympathetic system, PHTN leading to RV decompensation

Possible etiologies of systolic dysfunction

- Note that outcomes for patients with heart failure due to diastolic dysfunction are as poor as for those with depressed systolic function.
- Tailored therapy for the patient with diastolic dysfunction is not available due to a lack of clinical data, yet BP management appears to be paramount, in addition to standard heart failure therapy.

Restrictive Cardiomyopathy (Box 7.1)

Box 7.1 Comparison between constrictive and restrictive cardiomyopathy		
Feature	*Constrictive pericarditis*	*Restrictive cardiomyopathy*
History	Previous pericarditis, cardiac surgery, trauma, radiotherapy, connective tissue disease, tuberculosis, malignancy	Myeloma, sacrcoidosis, chronic inflammation, multisystem involvement
Physical exam Auscultation	Kussmaul's sign, paradoxical pulse	Later S3, low pitched, "triple rhythm"
JVP	Early S3, high-pitched "pericardial knock" X and Y dips brief and "flicking," not conspicuous positive waves	Mitral (MR) and tricuspid regurgitation (TR) usually present X and Y dips less brief, may have conspicuous A- or V-wave
ECG	P-waves reflect intra-atrial conduction delay	P-waves reflect right or left atrial hypertrophy or overload.
Plain chest radiograph	Pericardial calcification in 20–30%	Pericardial calcification rare
Echocardiogram	Pericardial thickening Abrupt septal movement ("notch") in early diastole Respiratory variation in mitral and tricuspid flow velocity in >25% of cases	Increased wall thickness MR and TR Pronounced left atrial enlargement
Hemodynamics	Equilibration of diastolic pressures in all cardiac chambers (RVEDP ≈ LVEDP) (usually RVEDP >1/3 RVSP)	LVEDP often 5 mmHg >RVEDP
MRI/CT	Thick pericardium	Normal pericardium
Endomyocardial biopsy	Normal, or nonspecific abnormalities	May reveal infiltrative disease (i.e. amyloid)

JVP, jugular venous pressure; RVEDP, right ventricular end-diastolic pressure; LVEDP, left ventricular end-diastolic pressure; RVSP, right ventricular systolic pressure

- A cardiomyopathy characterized by an abnormality of relaxation and filling due to infiltration or stiffening of the heart, though systolic function may be impaired in advanced cases.
- Causes include:
  - Amyloidosis (primary AL plasma cell dyscrasia, secondary AA inflammatory proteins, or "senile" age-associated somatic mutations of prealbumin with deposition)
  - Sarcoidosis
  - Radiation-induced scarring
  - Glycogen storage disease
  - Idiopathic etiologies.
- Because of their impaired diastolic function, patients with restrictive disease develop marked atrial enlargement and atrial arrhythmias, which are poorly tolerated and predispose to stroke risk.
- Marked LVH with relatively low ECG voltages are hallmarks of the disease.
- Pericardial constriction is the most common differential diagnosis to entertain in these patients.

Hypertrophic Obstructive Cardiomyopathy (HOCM) (Box 7.1)

- Autosomal dominant sarcomeric gene mutation resulting in myocyte hypertrophy and disarray (affects ~1:500 individuals, over 400 mutations now identified).
- Commonly associated with asymmetric thickening of the interventricular septum, which results in an obstruction to outflow of blood across the aortic valve.
- Mitral valve dysfunction and ventricular arrhythmias also frequently accompany the diagnosis.
- Important cause of sudden cardiac death in young adults.
- Specific therapy includes beta-blockade to improve LV filling, lessen obstruction, and prevent arrhythmia.
- Implantable cardioverter defibrillator (ICD) therapy has an important role in many cases.

CLINICAL PEARLS

- Patients with diastolic pathology are particularly intolerant of atrial fibrillation, as loss of atrial contraction can dramatically reduce left atrial emptying, LV filling, and LV stroke volume in the setting of a stiff ventricular wall.
- Doppler echocardiography is normally used to establish the presence of diastolic dysfunction. In patients with impaired relaxation, assessment of mitral valve inflow velocity may demonstrate diminished early diastolic filling velocity, manifested by an abnormally low E-wave, and increased late diastolic filling, manifested by an increased A-wave; as a result, the E/A ratio is <1.

- Amyloid fibrils may bind digoxin, angiotensin-converting enzyme inhibitors (ACE-Is), and calcium channel blockers (CCBs) with high affinity, making their use in this cohort dangerous.
- Pericardial disease and constrictive cardiomyopathy may present with similar symptoms, preserved LVEF on echo, with a history of trauma, chronic infection, rheumatic disease, malignancy, pericardectomy, etc. Evaluation for pericardial effusion, pericardial thickening on CT, and pulsus paradoxus may be useful.
- Classes of medications that should be avoided or used with caution in HOCM patients include: vasodilators (fall in peripheral resistance in setting of outflow obstruction leading to hypotension), aggressive use of diuretics (reduce preload and less LV filling), digoxin (adverse hemodynamic effect of positive inotrope).
- First-degree family members of HOCM patients should have genetic screening due to high penetrance of the disease.
- Surgical myomectomy or septal alcohol ablation is normally considered in HOCM patients with severe LV outflow obstruction and recurrent syncope and/or heart failure symptoms despite persistent pharmacotherapy.

Diagnosis and Work-up of New-Onset CHF

Signs and Symptoms at Presentation
- Exercise intolerance, dyspnea at rest and/or on exertion, cough, fatigue
- Peripheral edema
- Abdominal distension and discomfort
- Orthopnea, paroxysmal nocturnal dyspnea
- Palpitations [especially if concurrent atrial fibrillation or nonsustained ventricular tachycardia (NSVT)]
- Chest pain [atypical or if related to coronary artery disease (CAD)]
- Anorexia (thought to be due to poor splenchnic circulation, bowel edema, and nausea/vomiting as a result of hepatic congestion)

Misleading Symptoms
- Cough attributed to pulmonary disease, yet due to pulmonary edema
- Cultural differences in description of symptoms
- Sedentary lifestyle leading to underreporting of dyspnea or angina, nausea, anorexia, bloating attributed to hepatobiliary disease, yet due to right ventricular (RV) pressure overload

Physical Exam
- Cardiac: S3, PMI, S4, regularity (new-onset atrial fibrillation), JVP/hepatojugular reflex (HJR)
- Pulmonary: crackles, wheezes
- Abdominal: hepatic distension, HJR, ascites
- Peripheral: edema, diminished pulses, coolness of skin

Diagnostic Tests
- Transthoracic echocardiography (TTE):
  - Assess for regional wall motion abnormalities
  - Measure LVEF (<30% severe dysfunction, >55% normal)
  - Measure diastolic indices for restrictive/diastolic dysfunction
  - Measure right atrial and pulmonary artery pressures, determined by peak velocity across tricuspid valve
  - Assess valvular function
  - Note pericardial thickening, pericardial effusion
- Serum tests:
  - BNP: useful if very low (<100) or markedly abnormal for diagnosis
  - Troponin (rules out ischemia)
  - TFTs
  - Serum (SPEP) and urine protein electrophoretic pattern (UPEP) if amyloid suspected
  - Iron studies if hemochromatosis suspected
- Radiology:
  - Chest X-ray: may see pulmonary edema, cardiomegaly
  - Coronary angiogram and right heart catheterization.

Management

Lifestyle Modification
- Low-salt diet:
  - Importance of diet *cannot be overemphasized*. Diuretics can nearly always be reduced or discontinued with adherence to a low-salt diet
  - A *"fresh food" or "no-added salt" diet* is recommended for compliance (2 g sodium diet is another quotable diet, but is often confusing to patients). Examples should focus on avoidance of processed food, as salt is added to these foods, i.e. pork (not ham or bacon), milk (not cheese), cucumber (not pickles), etc.
  - Obviously, all preserved/packaged foods are troublesome (canned soups, lunch meats, bottled salad dressings, etc.) as are restaurant foods
  - Educational focus on salt avoidance (not cholesterol, fat, or fluid intake) is paramount, and a significant part of patient visit time may be dedicated to dietary education when dealing with the cardiomyopathic patient.
- Smoking cessation and graded exercise programs are indicated as well.

Identification of Reversible Factors
Screen for:
- Anemia
- Thyroid disease (hyper or hypo)
- Occult arrythmias/tachycardia
- Uncontrolled hypertension
- Sleep apnea

Box 7.2 Medical interventions with proven benefit

Therapy	Mechanism of action	Landmark clinical trials
ACE-I/ARB	Vasodilators, afterload reducers, renal-protective Prevent negative remodeling	CONSENSUS, SOLVD, SAVE, CHARM-Alternative, Val-HeFT, Elite-2
Beta-blockers	Limit myocardial oxygen utilization, block catecholamine-induced injury, sensitize beta-receptors, induce positive remodeling	MERIT-HF, COPERNICUS, US-Cardvedilol Trials, COMET, MDC, etc.
Hydralazine + nitrates	Function as balanced vasodilators, improve symptoms, exercise capacity, and survival	V-HeFT I, V-HeFT II, A-HeFT
Aldosterone antagonists	Mild K+-sparing diuretic with aldosterone-blocking properties via the mineralocorticoid receptor Reduces CHF admissions, sudden cardiac death, and total mortality	RALES, EPHESUS
Implantable cardioverter defibrillator (ICD)	Delivers electrical antiarrhythmic therapy to rescue both ischemic and nonischemic patients from malignant tachycardias Note most CRT devices include ICD technology	SCD-HeFT, MADIT-II, DINAMITE, CABG-Patch, DEFINITE
Cardiac resynchronization therapy (CRT)	Resynchronize the heart to improve contractile efficiency, timing, and ejection fraction Results in beneficial remodeling, improved symptoms, and lower mortality	CARE-HF, COMPANION

Medical Therapies

Medical interventions with proven survival benefit in patients with heart failure due to systolic dysfunction are summarized in Box 7.2.

Diuretics

- Indicated for relief of congestion (elevated neck veins, peripheral edema, crackles, etc.) but do not improve survival.
- Loop diuretics commonly prescribed first (e.g. lasix).
- Diuresis can be augmented by giving thiazide agent (HCTZ) ~30 min prior to loop diuretic.

- Caution needed for electrolyte derangement and laboratory work-up is usually indicated 1 week after initiation or escalation of a diuretic medication. Remember that dose can typically be weaned down with aggressive salt education!
- Typical starting dose: furosemide 40 mg PO bid. Titrate as needed.

Digoxin

- Improves symptoms and reduces hospitalizations but does not reduce mortality.
- Therapeutic window is narrow and toxicity is commonly seen in patients with renal insufficiency (ST changes on ECG, bradycardia, nausea, anorexia, etc.).
- Used for rate control if concurrent tachyarrythmia in heart failure patient, or as palliative therapy if still symptomatic after the addition of the agents described below.
- Follow renal function and levels closely (therapeutic window 0.5–0.9 ng/ml).
- Typical starting dose (normal creatinine clearance): digoxin 0.125 mg PO qid.

ACE Inhibitors

- ACE-Is (equivalent efficacy to ARBs) are mandatory for all heart failure patients without an obvious contraindication or significant renal failure.
- Associated with dramatic survival improvement in all heart failure patients with any severity of symptoms and at all levels of EF.
- Also reduce MI and heart failure admissions, with benefits independent of beta-blockers.
- Function to vasodilate, afterload-reduce the heart, and block harmful neurohormones.
- Typical starting dose: lisinopril 5 mg PO qid [may uptitrate in the first several weeks after making sure that electrolytes and glomerullar filtration rate (GFR) are stable].
- Aim for doses in the range of 20–40 mg/day as tolerated by SBP >90 mmHg).

Other Vasodilators

- Other vasodilators, such as hydralazine and nitrates, are effective at improving survival and symptoms in heart failure, but are less effective than ACE-Is from a mortality point of view, and thus should be used as second-line agents *after* maximal beta-blocker and ACE-I therapy has been titrated.
- Black patients, on the other hand, may derive particular benefit from these vasodilators compared to whites, due in part to differing levels of sympathetic nervous system and renin–angiotensin axis activity.
- Hydralazine–nitrate combinations should also be added if intolerant of ACE-Is, or if vasodilation is particularly desired, as in the patient with significant MR.

- Typical starting dose: hydralazine 10 mg PO tid and nitroglycerin (NTG) 60 mg PO qid, started simultaneously. Aim for doses in the range of hydralazine 25 mg tid to qid with NTG 90 mg PO qid.
- Alpha-blockers and CCBs do not have therapeutic roles as vasodilators in heart failure (though they are not dangerous if needed for other reasons).

Beta-blockers
- Along with ACE inhibitors, beta-blockers represent perhaps the most important medical breakthrough in medical heart failure therapy in the last 30 years.
- With profound survival benefits in NYHA Class II–IV patients, and improved outcomes at all EFs, these drugs are indicated for nearly every patient with cardiomyopathy (caution needed in decompensated heart failure).
- Although there is impressive survival data for the beta1 selective drugs (such as metoprolol succinate), many believe that carvedilol is the most effective drug in this class (and likely induces the least insulin resistance).
- Typical starting dose: carvedilol 3.125 mg PO bid – uptitrate by doubling dose *every 1–2 weeks* (not sooner) to goal of 25 mg PO bid.
- It is important to aim for a target dose of 25 mg PO bid of carvedilol to achieve maximal benefit, and to coach patient about maneuvers to limit orthostasis when rising from bed, etc.
- Common reasons for intolerance include fluid overload when initiating drug, so patient must be euvolemic.
- *Severe* reactive airway disease is another contraindication, but beware the history of "COPD" in the heart failure patient as this may reflect "cardiac asthma" – pulmonary function tests (PFTs) can be a useful guide.

Aldosterone Antagonists/K+-Sparing Diuretics
- Though only weak diuretic agents, the K+-sparing diuretics/aldosterone inhibitors spironolactone and eplerenone have important roles in symptomatic heart failure and provide survival benefits of up to 30% in Class III patients, as well as in post-infarct patients with reduced EFs.
- Also may help prevent sudden cardiac death (SCD) by reducing hypokalemia-related arrythmias, but conversely can cause significant and life-threatening hyperkalemia, particularly in patients with renal insufficiency.
- Initiation of spironolactone requires K+/Cr checks at time of prescription and at 1 and 3 weeks post initiation of therapy. Use spironolactone in Class III patients, with low EF (<40% post MI) and Cr <2.5.
- Starting dose: spironolactone 25 mg PO qid, no titration.
- Eplerenone has similar effects without hormonal side effect of gynecomastia. Should be added after beta-blocker and ACE-I.

> **CLINICAL PEARLS**
>
> - Be sure to inquire about stimulant use, OTC weight loss drugs containing amphetamines, and to limit alcohol consumption (particularly in toxin-related cardiomyopathy). NSAIDs induce fluid retention and tramadol should be only analgesic used by the cardiomyopathic patient. Beware of fluid retention from glitazone class of drugs in diabetic patients.
> - Exercise intolerance in heart failure may be exacerbated by inadequate rate control of fast arrhythmias, such as atrial fibrillation in the heart failure patient. Evaluate by checking heart rate during ambulation in hallway or on exercise test. Better rate control with exercise (despite adequate resting beta-blockade) may improve symptoms dramatically.
> - When adding amiodarone therapy to a patient on digoxin, an empiric reduction in the digoxin dose by one-half is indicated to prevent drug interaction and toxicity.

Diastolic Dysfunction-Specific Therapy
- With the increasing prevalence of hypertensive heart disease and CHF with preserved EF (who have similar mortality rates to patients with depressed contractility), it is important to treat these patients aggressively.
- Although there are no data regarding specific therapies for diastolic dysfunction, *blood pressure control is key* (often requiring combinations of ACE-Is and dihydropiridene CCBs, such as amlodipine).
- Beta-blockers are somewhat less well tolerated (delayed relaxation) and long-term benefit with this class of drugs is less clear.
- Teaching patients on salt restriction is of paramount importance.

Device Therapies

ICDs
- While the medical advances listed above have dramatically improved survival over the last several decades, devices such as the ICD have accounted for an *additional* ~30% mortality benefit in the cardiomyopathic patient.
- The ability to prevent death from malignant arrythmias (ventricular tachycardia) in both the ischemic *and* nonischemic heart failure patient has made these devices mandatory in selected patients, *even in the absence of prior dyssrythmia.*
- Refer for ICD placement as primary prophylaxis in any patient with an EF <35%, class II–III symptoms, and who is on a rationale medical regimen (i.e. carvedilol and ACE-Is have been titrated with no medication-related recovery of contractile function).
- Trials suggest waiting 6 months post-infarct prior to implantation, and defibrillators should not be placed at the time of bypass surgery.
- Secondary prevention for those who have sustained SCD or syncope related to VT should have defibrillators implanted with EFs <40%.

Resynchronization Therapy

- Dyssynchrony, typically due to left bundle branch block (LBBB) and the resultant uncoordinated contraction of the LV, portends increased mortality and is associated with progressive symptoms and mitral regurgitation.
- By placing pacemaker leads in both ventricles and activating them simultaneously, the heart can essentially be "retimed" to contract in a synchronous manner with improved efficiency and hemodynamic parameters.
- Additionally, this resynchronization therapy causes beneficial remodeling, lessens MR, reduces hospital admissions, and has been associated with significant survival benefit.
- Although selection criteria will likely be refined in the coming years due to high rates of nonresponders, biventricular ICDs are currently indicated for patients with Class III–IV CHF, EFs <35%, a wide QRS (>120 ms), who are in sinus rhythm.
- They are indicated for patients with ischemic as well as nonischemic cardiomyopathy with concomitant conduction disease.

Left Ventricular Assist Device (LVAD)

- A mechanical circulatory device used to partially support the failing left ventricle.
- Continuous flow LVADs use either centrifugal pumps or axial flow pumps. In centrifugal pumps, rotors accelerate the blood circumferentially hence forcing blood to the outer rim of the pump, whereas in the axial flow pumps the rotors are cylindrical with helical blades, causing the blood to accelerate in the direction of the rotor's axis.
- A recent study from the HeartMate II clinical trial concluded that continuous flow LVADs provide effective hemodynamic support for at least 18 months in patients awaiting heart transplant, with improvement of both functional status and quality of life.
- As of January 2010, HeartMate II was approved by the FDA in the US for destination therapy.

CLINICAL PEARLS

- Sinus tachycardia and peripheral vasoconstriction is typically seen in advanced heart failure patients who have low cardiac output. This is directly correlated with the severity of cardiac dysfunction.
- All patients with an established diagnosis of heart failure should receive an annual flu shot.
- Patients with newly diagnosed heart failure must undergo coronary angiogram if there is any suggestion of CAD as a cause for ischemic cardiomyopathy.
- ACE-Is may be particularly useful for the prevention of chemotherapy-related cardiomyopathy. Early use of enalapril in high-risk, troponin-positive subjects

(Continued)

post-chemotherapy has been shown to result in dramatic protection against systolic dysfunction.

- Always minimize RV pacing. Setting high back-up rates (lower rate limits) that cause the RV to be paced induces an iatrogenic LBBB and is associated with significantly worse incidences of heart failure symptoms and mortality. Thus, set lower rate limits of ~40 bpm to minimize RV pacing and allow use of the native conduction system.

Recommended Reading

Clinical Trials and Meta-Analyses

Bangalore S, Wild D, Parkar S, Kukin M, Messerli FH. Beta-blockers for primary prevention of heart failure in patients with hypertension insights from a meta-analysis. *J Am Coll Cardiol* 2008;**52**(13):1062–1072.

Flather MD, Yusuf S, Køber L et al.; ACE-Inhibitor Myocardial Infarction Collaborative Group. Long-term ACE-inhibitor therapy in patients with heart failure or left-ventricular dysfunction: a systematic overview of data from individual patients. *Lancet* 2000;**355**: 1575–1581.

Muthumala A, Drenos F, Elliott PM, Humphries SE. Role of beta adrenergic receptor polymorphisms in heart failure: systematic review and meta-analysis. *Eur J Heart Fail* 2008; **10**(1):3–13.

Taylor AL, Ziesche S, Yancy C et al.; African-American Heart Failure Trial Investigators. Combination of isosorbide dinitrate and hydralazine in blacks with heart failure. *N Engl J Med* 2004;**351**(20):2049–2057.

Guidelines

Hunt SA, Abraham WT, Chin WT et al. 2009 focused update incorporated into the ACC/ AHA 2005 Guidelines for the Diagnosis and Management of Heart Failure in Adults: a report of the American College of Cardiology Foundation/American Heart Association Task Force on Practice Guidelines: developed in collaboration with the International Society for Heart and Lung Transplantation. *Circulation* 2009;**119**(14):e391–479.

Review Articles

Ezekowitz JA, McAlister FA. Aldosterone blockade and left ventricular dysfunction: a systematic review of randomized clinical trials. *Eur Heart J* 2009;**30**(4):469–477.

Maeder MT, Kaye DM. Heart failure with normal left ventricular ejection fraction. *J Am Coll Cardiol* 2009;**53**(11):905–918.

McAlister FA, Ezekowitz JA, Wiebe N et al. Systematic review: cardiac resynchronization in patients with symptomatic heart failure. *Ann Intern Med* 2004;**141**(5):381–390.

8 Pulmonary Hypertension and Right Heart Failure

Matthew T. Wheeler[1] and Roham T. Zamanian[2]

[1]Department of Internal Medicine, Division of Cardiology, and
[2]Department of Internal Medicine, Division of Pulmonary and Critical Care, Stanford University School of Medicine, Stanford, CA, USA

Pulmonary hypertension (PHTN) is characterized by elevated pulmonary arterial and/or venous pressures. It is a rare, female-predominant disorder. Once correctly diagnosed (usually as late as 1–2 years after initiation of symptoms) there is a >50% mortality rate at 5 years.

Right heart failure (RHF) is a clinical syndrome of impaired function of the right ventricle. The most common cause is left heart failure (LHF). RHF (systolic and diastolic) is the cause of death in patients with PHTN. The natural history of RHF and its severity is not well understood in patients with PHTN.

Pulmonary Hypertension

Etiology and Classification
PHTN is classified into five categories:
- **Group 1: Pulmonary artery hypertension (PAH):**
  - Familial (FPAH) (may be caused by mutations in *BMPR2,* and possibly serotonin or endoglin genes)
  - Idiopathic (iPAH) defined as those in whom all other risk factors have been excluded; prevalence of 1 case in 1 million
  - Associated (APAH) with collagen vascular disease (scleroderma, CREST), congenital systemic-to-pulmonary shunts, portal hypertension, HIV infection, drugs/toxins, and several other conditions
  - PAH with venous or capillary involvement; pulmonary veno-occlusive disease (PVOD), pulmonary capillary hemangiomatosis (PCH)
  - Hematologic disorders: sickle cell anemia, splenectomy, hereditary hemorrhagic telangictasia.
- **Group 2: PHTN with left heart disease:**
  - Atrial, ventricular, or valvular left heart disease.

A Practical Approach to Cardiovascular Medicine, First Edition. Edited by Reza Ardehali, Marco Perez, Paul Wang.
© 2011 Blackwell Publishing Ltd. Published 2011 by Blackwell Publishing Ltd.

- **Group 3: PHTN with lung disease and/or hypoxemia:**
  - Chronic obstructive pulmonary disease (COPD)
  - Interstitial lung disease
  - Obstructive sleep apnea or sleep-disordered breathing
  - Alveolar hypoventilation, high altitude, developmental lung disease.
- **Group 4: PHTN due to chronic thromboembolic disease:**
  - Thromboembolic obstruction, nonthrombotic embolism (tumor, fat, parasites).
- Group 5: PHTN due to other causes:
  - Sarcoid, histiocytosis X, lymphangiomatosis, external compression of pulmonary vessels, pulmonary stenosis.

Risk Factors for PAH
See Box 8.1.

Presentation of PAH
- Symptoms:
  - Dyspnea, exercise intolerance, fatigue, chest pain, syncope
  - Hemoptysis, hoarseness due to recurrent laryngeal nerve stretching.
- Signs:
  - Fixed or paradoxically split P2; loud/palpable P2
  - Pulmonic regurgitation (Graham Steel) murmur
  - Lung exam typically unrevealing in PAH
  - Elevated jugular venous pressure (JVP), right ventricular (RV) heave, hepatomegaly, and/or edema with RHF.

Box 8.1 Risk factors for PAH

Risk factor	Definite	Likely	Possible
Drugs/toxins	(dex)Fenfluramine	Amphetamines	Cocaine
	Aminorex	L-tryptophan	Amphetamine
	Diethylpropion		
Disease	Congenital heart disease	Rheumatoid arthritis	Thyroid diagnosis
	Intracardiac shunts		
	HIV		
	Schistosomiasis		
	Scleroderma		
	Lupus		
	Portal HTN		
Demographic	Female		Pregnancy
			Obesity
			Insulin resistance

Box 8.2 Specific tests for determining PHTN etiology

Etiology	Preferred test	Additional tests
Chronic thromboembolism	VQ scan	Pulmonary angiogram; CT angiography (pulmonary embolism)
COPD, interstitial lung disease	PFTs	High-resolution chest CT
Sleep apnea	Polysomnography	

- Occult disease is occasionally discovered on routine exam or incidental testing.
- Prospective screening for PHTN:
  - Screening by echocardiography for presence of disease in patients with connective tissue disease, HIV, and possibly in known familial primary PHTN
  - Screening is currently not recommended for patients exposed to appetite suppressants in absence of symptoms.

Diagnostic Evaluation (Box 8.2)

- Once diagnosis is suspected, initial evaluation focuses on determination of the degree of PHTN and the evaluation of possible coexistent conditions (as seen in the classification system).
- If high clinical suspicion for a coexisting condition, i.e. connective tissue disease in patient with dermatologic findings supportive of scleroderma, it is mandatory to tailor testing toward the suspected etiology.
- **Routine tests**:
  - Echo (transthoracic, TTE) tricuspid regurgitant velocity to estimate right ventricular systolic pressure (RVSP):
    - RV size and RVEF; LV size and LVEF
    - Tricuspid, pulmonary, mitral valve function and morphology
    - Congenital heart disease, ASD, VSD; consider bubble study
  - ECG:
    - Right axis deviation, right ventricular hypertrophy (RVH) (R in V1 > 7 mm, R V1 plus S V5/6 > 10 mm)
    - RV strain with ST, T changes; ischemia, infarction, arrhythmia
  - CXR:
    - Signs of chronic pulmonary disease, fibrosis, interstitial lung disease, prominent PA shadows, peripheral pruning of pulmonary vasculature, enlarged right atrium (RA):
    - Loss of retrosternal airspace on lateral (RVH).

- **Laboratory tests:**
  - Routine: LFT, CBC, ESR, uric acid, lipid panel
  - BNP: distinct difference in mortality in patients who have >150 pg/mL NT-pro-BNP at presentation. This finding may also be applicable in the setting of active therapy
  - Infectious: HIV, hepatitis screen, schistosomiasis Ab
  - Thyroid function
  - Autoimmune: ANA, DS-DNA, Scl-70, anticentromere Ab, RF
  - Hypercoagulable work-up: protein C&S, Factor V Leiden, antithrombin III, anticardiolipin, antiphospholipid Abs.
- **Functional tests:**
  - 6-min walk test: used to follow response to therapy and progression of disease in conjunction with New York Heart Association (NYHA) classification. Traditionally the primary end-point in clinical trials. However, its limitations (especially in NYHA I and II patients) keep it from being an ideal surrogate of disease. A distance of <380 m indicates "high risk" with a poor prognosis
  - Cardiopulmonary exercise testing: peak VO_2 and heart rate (HR) response have been used in clinical trials and appear useful. Limited by the lack of expertise and standardization across centers.
- **Right heart catheterization:**
  - Remains the gold standard for diagnosis of PAH
  - Includes:
    – Saturations: inferior vena cava (IVC), high superior vena cava (HSVC), low superior vena cava (LSVC), mid RA, RV, right, left, and main pulmonary artery (RPA, LPA, MPA). If possible, LA, PVs, and AO
    – Pressures: RA, RV, PA, pulmonary capillary wedge pressure (PCWP); left ventricular end-diastolic pressure (LVEDP) may be needed (Figure 8.1)
    – Hemodynamics: cardiac output. Fick versus Td are debated. Fick most useful if VO_2 is measured (metabolic cart); Td most valid in patients with least TR
    – Vasodilator testing (see below).
- **Vasodilator testing** (Table 8.1):
  - Standard of care for patients with iPAH and mean pulmonary artery pressure (PAP) > 40 mmHg. Also useful in other APAH
  - Contraindicated in WHO Group 2 (pulmonary venous hypertension; Box 8.3) as it may precipitate pulmonary edema

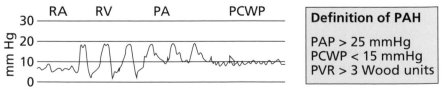

Figure 8.1 Pressures in right heart catheterization

Table 8.1 Vasodilator testing

Agent	Dose	Increment	Side effects
Epoprostenol	2–10 ng/kg/min IV	1–2 ng/kg/min q5–15 min	Headache, flushing, shortness of breath (SOB)
Adenosine	50–250 µg/kg/min IV	50 µg/kg/min q2 min	Chest pressure, SOB
NO	10–80 ppm inhaled	Single dose for 5 min	

Box 8.3 WHO functional classification of PHTN

I	Patients with PHTN in whom there is no limitation of usual physical activity; ordinary physical activity does not cause increased dyspnea, fatigue, chest pain, or presyncope
II	Patients with PHTN who have mild limitation of physical activity. There is no discomfort at rest, but normal physical activity causes increased dyspnea, fatigue, chest pain, or presyncope
III	Patients with PHTN who have a marked limitation of physical activity. There is no discomfort at rest, but less than ordinary activity causes increased dyspnea, fatigue, chest pain, or presyncope
IV	Patients with PHTN who are unable to perform any physical activity at rest and who may have signs of right ventricular failure. Dyspnea and/or fatigue may be present at rest, and symptoms are increased by almost any physical activity

PHTN, portal hypertension

- Test is considered positive if mean PAP decreases ≥ 10 mmHg to a mean of <40 mmHg with *no* decrement in cardiac output
- If test is positive, trial of calcium channel blocker (CCB) is appropriate in iPAH. Less than 5% of patients with PAH are vasoreactive and only ~7% of those who qualify for testing will be long-term responders to CCBs.

Treatment

General Principles
- Treat underlying/contributing disease (Figure 8.2).
- Treat symptomatic patients with advanced therapy.
- Advanced therapy initiation by experienced clinical PHTN center.
- Interventions to be considered in all patients with PHTN include:
  - **Oxygen:**
    - All patients with hypoxemia, 1–4 l NC to keep O_2 saturation >90% at rest, and with exercise and sleep if possible
    - Survival in COPD better with continuous versus nocturnal (may cause hypercapnia in endstage COPD)

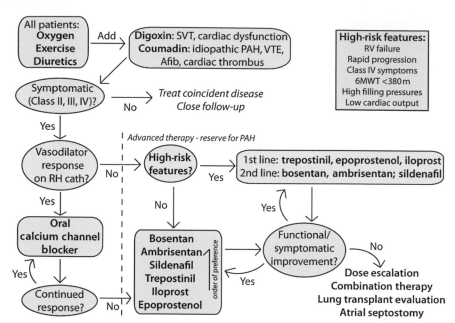

Figure 8.2 Treatment algorithm for pulmonary hypertension. PAH patients with WHO functional Class II–IV should be evaluated for advanced therapy. SVT, supraventricular tachycardia; VTE, venous thromboembolic disease; Afib, atrial fibrillation; 6MWT, 6-min walk test

- – Generally lower O_2 saturations (at rest and peak exercise) in patients with congenital heart disease and Eisenmenger physiology (R to L shunt)
- **Exercise:** graded, moderate exercise improves exercise tolerance, does not change hemodynamics, may improve outcomes
- **Diuresis:** indicated for volume overload, no mortality benefit; beware alkalosis, K^+.

Routine Therapy
- **Coumadin:**
  - Anticoagulation recommended for all patients with idiopathic PAH, thromboembolic PHTH, atrial fibrillation, intracardiac thrombus
  - Goal INR 2–3 (though some recommend 1.5–2.0 or 2.0–2.5)
  - Beware higher risk of bleeding with PHTN, connective tissue diagnosis.
- **Digoxin:**
  - Controls HR in SVT with RV dysfunction
  - Improves LVEF in PHTN due to COPD
  - Unclear if beneficial without cardiac dysfunction
  - Beware increased risk of toxicity, interactions with other meds.
- **Calcium channel blockers:**
  - Initiate only if meet vasoreactivity criteria on RH catheterization

- Nifedipine, diltiazem, amlodipine
- Follow-up to assess for functional improvement; if none, consider alternate treatment
- Generally considered alternative to advanced therapy.
- **Monitoring response to routine therapy:**
  - Repeat TEE including RVSP
  - Repeat 6-min walk test and NYHA evaluation
  - Close clinical follow-up for assessment of symptom progression.

Advanced Therapy

Current guidelines recommend advanced therapy to be started for patients with NYHA Class II, III, or IV symptoms. Initiation should be done by a specialist in the treatment of PHTN, generally at a clinical PHTN center. Although exceptions exist, current literature supports the use of advanced therapies for patients with PAH (WHO Group 1) *only*!

Frequent clinical reassessment is warranted in all patients on advanced therapy.

Prostacyclins

Act as pulmonary and systemic arterial vasodilators, also platelet inhibitors.
- **Epoprostenol (Flolan®):**
  - IV formulation only, requires continuous infusion; half-life <6 min
  - Initiation as inpatient, starting at 1–2 ng/kg/min via central venous catheter
  - Indicated for Class III and Class IV PAH patients
  - Usual chronic dosing 25–40 ng/kg/min
  - Heat and light sensitive; requires extensive patient/caregiver training
  - Common side effects: headache, nausea, diarrhea, flushing
  - *Dangers:* abrupt discontinuation may lead to rebound PHTN, shock, and catheter-based infection.
- **Trepostinil (Remodulin®):**
  - IV and SC formulation, half-life 3–4 h, requires continuous infusion
  - Initiate at 2–4 ng/kg/min, uptitrate weekly; maintenance dose 60–120 ng/kg/min
  - Indicated for Class II, III, IV PAH patients
  - SC formulation adverse effect of severe site pain/erythema
  - IV infusion associated with higher incidence of Gram-negative bacteremia
  - Recent addition of inhaled formulation (Tyvaso®).
- **Iloprost (Ventavis®)**
  - Aerosolized prostacyclin analog, inhaled to minimize systemic effects
  - Immediate acting with half-life of 30 min. Effects lost by 1.5–2 h
  - Initiate at 2.5 µg; if tolerated 5 µg/dose 6–9 times daily
  - Approved for Class III, IV PAH patients.

Endothelin Antagonists
Antagonize endothelin A and/or B receptors, inhibiting pulmonary artery vasoconstriction and smooth muscle proliferation.
- **Bosentan (Tracleer®):**
  - Oral, nonselective endothelin receptor antagonist
  - Initiate at 62.5 mg bid, then stable dose at 125 mg bid after 1 month
  - Functional benefit; survival benefit based on long-term follow-up
  - Risk of hepatotoxicity, teratogenic, increased peripheral edema (requires monthly LFT, CBC, and pregnancy test)
  - Recommended first-line therapy for Class II, alternative for Class III, IV
  - Only specially licensed pharmacies and prescribers may dispense
  - Consider potential drug–drug interactions
  - May decrease efficacy of sildenafil when combined.

EVIDENCE-BASED PRACTICE

Bosentan Randomized Trial of Endothelin Antagonist Therapy (BREATHE-1))
Context: Oral therapy for PAH addressing novel mechanism.
Goal: To compare bosentan (endothelin receptor antagonist) at two doses to placebo.
Method: Multicenter, double-blind RCT. 213 Class III or IV PAH patients, treated for 16 weeks.
Results: Bosentan treatment improved functional class in 38%, 6MWD improved by 44 m, decreased clinical worsening.
Take-home message: Oral bosentan improves function and delays clinical worsening in PAH.

- **Ambrisentan (Letairis®):**
  - Oral, once daily, selective endothelin receptor A antagonist
  - Initial dose 2.5 mg/day, increase to max 10 mg/day
  - Improved hemodynamics and function in trials
  - Less risk of elevated LFTs as compared with bosentan; teratogenic
  - May result in diuretic-resistant edema
  - Only specially licensed pharmacies and prescribers may dispense.

Phosphodiesterase Inhibitors
- **Sildenafil (Revatio®):**
  - Oral phosphodiesterase-5 inhibitor (Viagra)
  - Dose at 20 mg three times daily (PHTN centers have experience with use of up to 80 mg tid)
  - Functional improvements maintained at 1 year of treatment, longer data not currently published
  - Studied in combination with epoprostenol, iloprost, or bosentan

- Side effects include headache, flushing, dyspepsia, epistaxis
- Must avoid nitrates (risk of severe hypotension) and alpha agonists.
- **Tadalafil (Adcirca®):**
  - Oral phosphodiesterase inhibitor
  - Dose at 20 or 40 mg once daily
  - Similar cautions as for sildenafil apply.

Lung Transplantation

Reserved for patients failing medical therapy, with advanced disease, and expected 1-year survival less than that for transplantation.

Atrial Septostomy

- Reserved for refractory syncope, severe RHF to increase systemic blood flow, bypass high pressure pulmonary circuit
- Will decrease arterial saturation but may improve systemic oxygen delivery
- Procedure-related mortality 15–20% in the first 24 h
- Contraindications include anemia and significant hypoxemia.

Right Heart Failure

Etiology

RHF may be due to pressure and/or volume overload of the right ventricle (Box 8.4).

Presentation

- **Acute:** hepatic congestion; elevated JVP; if severe – hypotension, shock, arrhythmia:
  - With RVMI: chest pain, nausea, vomiting, syncope, bradycardia (nodal involvement)
  - With pulmonary embolism (PE)/PHTN: cough, dyspnea, chest pain, tachycardia, hemoptysis
  - With sepsis: fever, tachycardia, hypotension, also endocarditis signs.
- **Chronic:** hepatic congestion, congestive cirrhosis, elevated JVP, peripheral edema/fluid overload, dyspnea on exertion, exercise intolerance, palpitations, RV heave, cardiac cachexia, ascites.

Diagnostic Evaluation

- **Echo:**
  - RV function, size, and shape
  - RA size
  - Tricuspid regurgitation
  - Estimated RVSP and right atrial pressure (IVC diameter and distensibility).

Box 8.4 Common causes for RV dysfunction

Mechanism of RV dysfunction	Etiologies
Pressure overload	**Left-sided HF (most common)**
	Pulmonary embolism (common)
	PHTN
	Systemic RV; double-chambered RV
	Right ventricular outflow tract (RVOT) obstruction, pulmonary stenosis
Volume overload	Tricuspid regurgitation, pulmonary regurgitation
	ASD/VSD
	Anomalous pulmonary, coronary return
	Carcinoid
Ischemia/infarction	**RVMI (common)**
Myocardial pathology	Cardiomyopathy
	Arrhythmogenic right ventricular dysplasia (ARVD)
	Septic cardiomyopathy
Other	Constrictive pericarditis
	Tricuspid stenosis, superior vena cava (SVC) stenosis
	Complex congenital defects (tetralogy of Fallot, Ebstein's, transposition of the great arteries, double outlet RV)

ASD/VSD, atrial septal defect/ventricular septal defect; HF, heart failure; PHTN, portal hypertension; RV, right ventricle; RVMI, right ventricular myocardial infarction

---

- **ECG:**
  - RVMI – ST elevation > 1 mm in V3R to V5R
  - RVH, right atrial enlargement (RAE), right axis deviation (RAD), repolarization abnormalities
  - Tachy-, brady-arrhythmias
- **MRI:**
  - Improved windows, 3D evaluation of RV size and shape
  - Fibrosis, dysplasia
- **Catheterization:**
  - R ± L heart with coronaries (consider coronary compression from large PA)
  - Evaluation for PHTN
  - Acutely for PCI in RVMI
- **Laboratory tests:**
  - Metabolic panel, LFTs
  - Cardiac enzymes, BNP
  - Coags, PHTN labs as described above

- **Functional tests:**
  - Cardiopulmonary
  - Exercise test, 6MWT.

Treatment

Acute Right Heart Failure
- **Treat underlying etiology:**
  - RVMI:
    - Involvement of RV increases mortality significantly in acute MI
    - Reperfusion of RV branches of right coronary artery (RCA) improves RV function, reduces heart block, improves outcomes
    - RV function recovers significantly with time
  - PE:
    - Anticoagulation
    - Thrombolysis if hemodynamically unstable
    - Consider thrombectomy in selected patients
  - PHTN:
    - Inhaled NO (do not withdraw abruptly as it can cause rebound PHTN)
    - IV epoprostenol/inhaled iloprost
    - Inotropic support.
- **Optimize volume status:**
  - If volume overload – gentle diuresis (500–1000 mL/day) if unresponsive to diuretics, continuous venovenous hemoflitration (CVVH) or ultrafiltration
  - In acute MI, acute PE, and absolute hypovolemia, may need 300 continuous venovenous hemofiltration 600 mL NS challenge, even with normal or mildly elevated RA pressures
  - Volume challenge in patients with PHTN is not recommended, unless central venous pressure (CVP) is monitored and fluid is absolutely necessary.
- **Treat hypotension/low cardiac output:**
  - Avoid high inspiratory pressures, autoPEEP
  - Inotropic/vasopressor support:
    - Dobutamine preferred (2–5 µg/kg/min)
    - Dopamine for augmentation
    - Milrinone if tachyarrhythmia
    - Inhaled NO if PAH component (may need to avoid in PVH)
  - Mechanical unloading if refractory:
    - Atrial septostomy
    - Limited data with right ventricular assist device (RVAD) and extracorporeal membrane oxygenation (ECMO) in adults
  - Consideration for transplantation if persistent RV failure.
- Maintain sinus rhythm:
  - Cardioversion if unstable

- Antiarrhythmics
- Sequential AV pacing/resynchronization as appropriate
- Electrolyte maintenance.

EVIDENCE-BASED PRACTICE

Effect of reperfusion in acute RV infarction

Context: RVMI leads to RHF and high mortality. Does RV reperfusion improve outcome?

Goal: To reperfuse patients with RVMI and evaluate them for functional and survival improvements.

Method: Single-center, prospective case series. 53 patients with acute RVMI underwent attempted reperfusion of RV infarct-related artery.

Results: 7/12 who were not reperfused died versus 1/41 who were reperfused. RV function and arrhythmic events were reduced in the reperfusion group.

Take-home message: Reperfusion of RV branches in RVMI reduces mortality.

Chronic Right Heart Failure

Management and treatment of RHF in many ways mirrors treatment of LHF. Significantly fewer data are available to guide treatment. Staging is similar to revised AHA Stages A–D for LHF:
- **Stage A:** at risk for RHF:
  - Routine echo to follow-up
  - Lifestyle modifications.
- **Stage B:** evidence of RV dysfunction:
  - Monitor closely
  - Consider corrective surgery of congenital or valvular lesions
  - Consider warfarin
  - Implantable cardioverter defibrillator (ICD) if indicated.
- **Stage C:** RHF with symptoms:
  - Diuretics for volume management
  - Diet, sodium restriction; daily weights
  - Graded exercise program
  - Digoxin for improvement CO (best studied in PH)
  - Aggressive treatment of arrhythmias, valvular dysfunction
  - Consider resynchronization therapy.
- **Stage D:** Refractory RHF:
  - Decision on level, goals of care
  - Evaluation for heart or heart/lung transplantation
  - Atrial septostomy (PHTN with persistent RV failure)
  - Chronic inotropic support
  - RVAD
  - Arrhythmia management.

CLINICAL PEARLS

- Abrupt interruption of epoprostenol infusion can be life-threatening.
- PHTN oral agents can improve function and outcomes.
- Advanced PHTN therapies are most appropriate for patients with proven PAH, and potentially dangerous for those with "secondary" PHTN.
- Patients with acute MI with RV involvement should undergo immediate revascularization.
- There are no clear data supporting use of beta-blockers, ACE-Is, or aldosterone antagonists in isolated RHF.
- Consider ICD implantation in patients with RHF given high risk of sudden arrhythmic death (similar to LHF).

Recommended Reading

Clinical Trials and Meta-Analyses

Bowers TR, O'Neill WW, Grines C, Pica MC, Safian RD, Goldstein JA. Effect of reperfusion on biventricular function and survival after right ventricular infarction. *N Engl J Med* 1998;**338**:933–940.

Galiè N, Ghofrani HA, Torbicki A et al.; Sildenafil Use in Pulmonary Arterial Hypertension (SUPER) Study Group. Sildenafil Citrate Therapy for Pulmonary Arterial Hypertension. *NEJM* 2005;**353**:2148–2157.

Rubin LJ, Badesch DB, Barst RJ et al. Bosentan therapy for pulmonary arterial hypertension. *N Engl J Med* 2002;**346**:896–903.

Guidelines

McLaughlin VV, Archer SL, Badesch DB et al.; American College of Cardiology Foundation Task Force on Expert Consensus Documents; American Heart Association; American College of Chest Physicians; American Thoracic Society, Inc; Pulmonary Hypertension Association. ACCF/AHA 2009 expert consensus document on pulmonary hypertension a report of the American College of Cardiology Foundation Task Force on Expert Consensus Documents and the American Heart Association developed in collaboration with the American College of Chest Physicians; American Thoracic Society, Inc.; and the Pulmonary Hypertension Association. *J Am Coll Cardiol* 2009;**53**:1573–1619.

Review Articles

Haddad F, Doyle R, Murphy DJ, Hunt SA. Right Ventricular Function in Cardiovascular Disease. Part II: pathophysiology, clinical importance, and management of right ventricular failure. *Circulation* 2008;**117**:1717–1731.

McLaughlin VV, McGoon MD. Pulmonary artery hypertension. *Circulation* 2006;**114**: 1417–1431.

Zamanian RT, Haddad F, Doyle RL, Weinacker AB. Management Strategies for Patients with Pulmonary Hypertension in the Intensive Care Unit. *Crit Care Med* 2007;**35**:2037–2050.

9 Heart Transplantation

Jesus Almendral, Robert Maranda, and Sharon Hunt

Department of Internal Medicine, Division of Cardiology, Stanford University School of Medicine, Stanford, CA, USA

History

- First human-to-human heart transplant performed by Christian Barnard on December 3, 1967 in Cape Town, South Africa.
- On January 6, 1968, Norman Shumway from Stanford performed the first adult heart transplant in the United States.
- Over 100 heart transplant procedures were performed in 1968, with poor outcomes and survival measured in weeks and months (15% survival at 1 year).
- Enthusiasm for the procedure rapidly waned until only two centers remained with active programs (Stanford and Medical College of Virginia).
- Introduction of cyclosporine in the early 1980s and the development of newer immunosuppressive agents shortly after led to a dramatic improvement in outcomes and a resurgence of interest.
- In 2006, over 3200 cardiac transplant procedures were performed worldwide.
- Survival is now much better with approximately 85% of patients alive at 1 year, 5-year survival of 66%, and median survival of 10 years.

Indications

- Systolic heart failure with severe functional limitation (NYHA Class III–IV heart failure) despite maximum medical therapy, especially if maximum oxygen uptake (VO_2 max) $< 12–14\,mL/kg/min$ on exercise testing. Underlying causes may include ischemic, idiopathic, congenital, or acquired valvular heart disease.
- Refractory angina not amenable to surgical or percutaneous revascularization.

A Practical Approach to Cardiovascular Medicine, First Edition. Edited by Reza Ardehali, Marco Perez, Paul Wang.

- Refractory life-threatening arrhythmia despite antiarrhythmic medications, implantable cardioverter defibrillator (ICD) therapy, ablation.
- Severe symptomatic hypertrophic or restrictive cardiomyopathy refractory to treatment.
- Cardiac tumors with low likelihood of metastasis.

Contraindications

- Older age; patients over age 65 may be considered if they do not have significant comorbidities.
- Severe pulmonary hypertension despite vasodilator challenge [transplanted heart with normal right ventricle (RV) may develop acute RV failure if subjected abruptly to high pulmonary pressures]:
  - PA systolic pressure > 60 mmHg (or >50% of systemic pressure)
  - Pulmonary vascular resistance >4–5 Wood units
  - Mean transpulmonary gradient > 15 mmHg.
- Active systemic infection:
  - Immunosuppression likely would exacerbate infectious process
  - May be listed after infection adequately treated.
- Active malignancy or recent malignancy with high risk of recurrence (<5 years):
  - Exceptions include nonmelanoma skin cancers, primary cardiac tumors limited to the heart, and low-grade prostate cancers
  - Oncology consultation is recommended.
- Diabetes mellitus with poor control and/or end-organ damage:
  - Usual HbA1c >7.5
  - Neuropathy, nephropathy, proliferative retinopathy.
- Marked obesity with BMI > 30 kg/m^2 or >140% of ideal body weight.
- Severe peripheral or cerebrovascular disease not amenable to revascularization.
- Irreversible, severe renal, hepatic or pulmonary disease (combined heart/kidney, heart/liver, and heart/lung transplants are done in select centers):
  - Creatinine clearance < 40–50 mL/min
  - Bilirubin > 2.5 mg/dL (not due to hepatic congestion), transaminases >2 x normal (may need liver biopsy to exclude cirrhosis or other intrinsic liver disease)
  - FVC and FEV1 <40% of predicted.
- Active peptic ulcer disease.
- Recent or unresolved pulmonary infarction (due to high probability of progressing to pulmonary abscess after initiating immunosuppression).
- Psychosocial factors:
  - History of poor compliance with medications or follow-up appointments
  - Uncontrolled psychiatric illness severe enough to jeopardize adherence to medical regimen

- Lack of adequate family or social support
- Active or recent substance abuse (alcohol, tobacco, illicit drugs) – typically should be abstinent for >6 months
- Cognitive impairment severe enough to limit comprehension of medical regimen
- Failure to establish stable address or telephone number.

Transplant Evaluation

- **Medical history:**
  - Meets indication for transplantation?
  - Have adequate medical, device, or surgical interventions been attempted?
  - No significant contraindications?
- **Psychosocial evaluation:**
  - Assess understanding and willingness to undergo transplant and chronic immunosuppression
  - Assess adequacy of family and social support
  - Formal screening for psychiatric illness and substance abuse.
- **Diagnostic testing:**
  - Unless critically ill, all patients should have the tests shown in Box 9.1 as part of the transplant evaluation.

Box 9.1 Tests needed prior to heart transplant evaluation

- Routine blood tests: CBC, metabolic profile, LFTs, TFTs, cholesterol profile, iron studies, PT/PTT, RPR, HbA1c (if diabetic), panel reactive antibody, HLA phenotype, hepatitis, HIV and syphilis serologies
- Purified protein derivative (PPD) testing with controls
- Echocardiogram and/or multigated acquisition (MUGA)
- Electrocardiogram
- Chest X-ray
- Pulmonary function test
- Cardiopulmonary stress testing with maximum VO_2 measurement
- Right heart catheterization with measurement of pulmonary vascular resistance (may use intravenous nitroprusside or inhaled nitric oxide to document reversibility if pulmonary hypertension is present)
- 24-h urine collection for creatinine clearance and total protein
  For patients ≥50 years old and all diabetic patients:
- Carotid/transcranial Dopplers
- Noninvasive lower extremity arterial studies (ABI)
- Age- and sex-appropriate cancer screening (PSA, pap smear, mammogram, colonoscopy)

Decisions on candidate acceptability are typically made by a multidisciplinary committee consisting of transplant surgeons, transplant cardiologists, social workers, psychologist, and nurses.

Cardiac Donor Selection Criteria

Optimal donors should meet the following criteria:
- Age <55 years
- No history of chest trauma or cardiac disease
- No prolonged hypotension or hypoxemia
- Meets hemodynamic criteria:
  - Mean arterial pressure (MAP) > 60 mmHg
  - CVP 8–12 mmHg
  - Inotropic support < 10 µg/kg/min (dopamine or dobutamine) and cardiac index > 2.4 L/min
- Normal ECG
- Normal echocardiogram
- Normal coronary angiography if coronary artery disease (CAD) is suspected
- Negative HBsAg, HCV, HIV serologies

Some centers have an "alternate list" of potential recipients (older, less ideal candidates), who are considered for suboptimal donor hearts.

Donor Management

- Aggressive hemodynamic and metabolic management of donors has been shown to result in higher organ retrieval rates.
- Typical management should include correction of:
  - Volume deficits: keep CVP 5–10, Hct ~30%
  - Metabolic derangements: avoid acidosis, hypoxemia, hypercarbia
  - Hormonal abnormalities: replacement with arginine vasopressin, triiodothyronine, methylprednisolone, and/or insulin may be necessary [of particular importance if initial donor ejection fraction (EF) is <45%].

Donor and Recipient Matching

- Parameters typically include only ABO compatibility and body size matching.
- Body size is of particular importance if pulmonary hypertension is present.
- Given limits of ischemic time and small numbers of donors, HLA matching is not practical.
- If recipient panel reactive (PRA) antibody titer is high (indicative of recipient presensitization from previous transfusions, pregnancy, infections, etc.), a prospective cross-match with donor lymphocytes is done (currently many/most use "virtual cross-match" with avoidance of prespecified donor HLA antigens).

Organ Allocation and Prioritization

- In the United States, recipient waiting list is maintained by the United Network of Organ Sharing (UNOS), a private organization under contract to the federal government.
- Recipients and donors are matched according to priority status (Box 9.2) and time accrued on the waiting list, distance from donor site, blood type, and body size.
- Distribution is first done locally (within 500 miles of donor site), then regionally.

Surgical Technique

- **Biatrial technique:**
  - Original technique of orthotopic cardiac transplantation (donor heart placed in same position as the explanted heart), first developed by Richard Lower and Norman Shumway while working at Stanford in the 1960s
  - Involves resection of the native recipient heart at the midatrial level, leaving a cuff of left and right atrium, and transection of the great vessels just above the semilunar valves
  - Donor heart is explanted in the same fashion and anastomosed at the level of the atria with the donor right atrium connected to the recipient right atrial cuff with the same technique performed on the left side. The pulmonary veins remain in place in the recipient left atrium
  - Donor and recipient aorta and pulmonary artery are anastomosed with continuous sutures
  - Although largely successful, this technique often results in postoperative tricuspid and mitral insufficiency, largely related to the abnormal geometry and increased size of the newly reconstructed atria
  - Sinus node dysfunction and heart block requiring pacemaker implantation also occur occasionally after transplantation, related to damage to the sinoatrial (SA) node during harvesting and implantation.
- **Bicaval technique:**
  - In the early 1990s, the surgical technique was modified to address the issues of valve insufficiency and sinus node dysfunction
  - First described by Dreyfus and colleagues in 1991, the bicaval technique involves making the right atrial anastomoses at the level of the inferior (IVC) and superior vena cava (SVC) rather than at the mid-right atrium. The left atrial anastomosis is the same
  - This technique preserves right atrial architecture and results in less tricuspid valve regurgitation and decreased incidence of sinus node dysfunction and heart block
  - Currently the method of choice in most transplant centers.

Box 9.2 UNOS Status Code for Medical Urgency (priority status)

Status 1A

Patient is admitted to the listing transplant hospital ICU and has at least one of the following:
- Mechanical circulatory support that includes at least one of the following:
  - Left and/or right ventricular assist device (VAD) – may be listed for 30 days at any point after implant once felt to be clinically stable
  - Total artificial heart
  - Intra-aortic balloon pump (IABP)
  - Extracorporeal membrane oxygenation (ECMO)
- Mechanical circulatory support for >30 days with evidence of device-related complications:
  - Thromboembolism
  - Device infection
  - Mechanical failure
  - Life-threatening arrhythmias
- Mechanical ventilation
- Continuous infusion of a single high-dose inotrope (dobutamine $\geq$ 7.5 µg/kg/min or milrinone $\geq$ 0.5 µg/kg/min) or multiple intravenous inotropes with continuous hemodynamic monitoring of left ventricular filling pressures (usually via a pulmonary artery catheter)[1]
- Does not meet any of the above criteria but felt to have an urgency and potential for benefit comparable to other candidates of same status[2]

Status 1B

- Left and/or right VAD after >30 days as status 1A
- Continuous infusion of an intravenous inotrope
- May be admitted to hospital (not necessarily in a transplant center) or may be an outpatient

Status 2

- Any patient who does not meet the criteria for status 1A or 1B
- Usually an outpatient

Status 7

- Temporarily unsuitable to receive an organ transplant (active infection, acute renal failure, awaiting insurance clearance, etc.)

[1]Status 1A under this criterion is valid for 7 days with a one-time 7-day renewal
[2]Status 1A under this criterion is valid for 14 days and must be recertified by an attending physician, subject to review by the applicable UNOS Regional Review Board and the UNOS Thoracic Organ Transplantation Committee

Immunosuppression

General Principles

- Purpose of immunosuppression is to reduce the intensity of the immune response to the cardiac allograft (transplanted heart) to a sufficient degree that allows the body's acceptance of the foreign tissue while minimizing short- and long-term toxicity.
- High-dose immunosuppression is typically started immediately postop to minimize the risk of early rejection and to facilitate graft acceptance.
- A three-drug regimen consisting of corticosteroids, a calcineurin-inhibitor (cyclosporine or tacrolimus), and an antiproliferative agent [mycophenolate mofetil (MMF)] is commonly employed.
- Corticosteroids are gradually tapered and often discontinued within the first 6–12 months, and the remaining drugs are continued indefinitely, although with lower target blood levels over time.
- Sirolimus [mammalian target of rapamycin (mTOR) inhibitor], which has been shown to retard smooth muscle cell proliferation, is sometimes substituted for MMF if transplant vasculopathy develops, since sirolimus can retard progression of the disease.
- In patients who develop renal dysfunction, a calcineurin inhibitor (CNI)-free regimen consisting of sirolimus and MMF is sometimes used.
- Typical starting dose and target trough levels of commonly used immunosuppressive agents are shown in Table 9.1.

Induction Therapy

- Usually started in the immediate post-transplant period to provide intense immunosuppression at time of most intense alloimmune response.
- Allows delayed initiation of CNIs in patients with renal failure post-transplant.
- Typical agents include:
  - Polyclonal antibody rabbit antithymocyte globulin (RATG)
  - Monoclonal antibody OKT3 (muromonab), which binds to the CD3 cell surface molecule on T cells, causing cell death
  - IL-2 receptor blocker (daclizumab, basiliximab) which binds to the TAC subunit of the IL-2 receptor of activated T cells.
- In 2007, 51% of post-transplant patients received some form of induction therapy, although routine use remains controversial as some studies suggest no change in 1-year survival and benefits are limited to delay in onset of first rejection.

Maintenance Therapy

Corticosteroids

- **Clinical use:**
  - Typically combined with a CNI and an antiproliferative agent during the first 6–12 months post-transplant as part of a three-drug regimen

Table 9.1 Immunosuppressive drugs commonly used in cardiac transplantation

Drug	Typical dose	Target level in conjunction with mycophenolate mofetil (MMF)	Target level in conjunction with sirolimus
Corticosteroids			
Methylprednisolone Prednisone	500 mg IV prior to coming off cardiopulmonary bypass (CBP), then 125 mg IV q8h x 3 doses POD #1 0.6–1.0 mg/kg/day x first 1–3 weeks, then tapered to 0.1 mg/kg/day by third month, then decreased gradually with each negative or low-grade biopsy until discontinued in the first 6–12 months	None – levels not followed	None – levels not followed
Calcineurin inhibitors			
Cyclosporine	IV: 0.5–1 mg/h continuously postop to achieve target levels Oral: start 3–8 mg/kg/day divided into two doses and increase over 3–4 days to achieve target 12-h trough level	*0–1 month*: 300–350 ng/mL *1–6 months*: 250–350 ng/mL *6–12 months*: 150–250 ng/mL *>12 months*: 100–150 ng/mL	*0–6 months*: 100–150 ng/mL *6–12 months*: 75–125 ng/mL *>12 months*: 50–100 ng/mL
Tacrolimus	IV: 0.01–0.05 mg/kg/day as continuous infusion to achieve target level Oral: start 1–2 mg bid and progressively increase to achieve target 12-h trough level	*0–1 month*: 15–20 ng/mL *1–6 months*: 12–15 ng/mL *6–12 months*: 8–12 ng/mL *>12 months*: 5–10 ng/mL	*0–6 months*: 5–10 ng/mL *6–12 months*: 5–7 ng/mL *> 12 months*: 3–5 ng/mL
Antiproliferative agents			
Mycophenolate mofetil	IV dosing equivalent to oral dose: 1000–1500 mg bid fixed dose – titrated to side effects Some centers titrate dose to achieve 12-h trough levels in first year, although controversial	Mycophenolic acid (MPA) level 2.5–5 µg/mL	MMF discontinued and sirolimus substituted in setting of cardiac allograft vasculopathy (CAV)
Azathioprine	1–2 mg/kg/day – dose titrated to keep WBC >3, platelet count >100 000 or Hct >27	None – levels not typically followed	None – levels not typically followed
mTOR inhibitor			
Sirolimus	1–5 mg once daily	24-h trough level of 5–10 ng/mL	None

- High doses are used in the early postoperative period and then are gradually tapered over several months
- Also used as pulse therapy for acute rejection.
- **Mechanism of action:**
  - Anti-inflammatory effects by inhibiting leukotrienes and prostaglandins
  - Retards nuclear gene transcription, leading to decreased expression of IL-2, TNF-α, and interferon-γ
  - Also reduces MHC expression, suppresses macrophage function, and induces leukocyte apoptosis.
- **Dosing:**
  - Solumedrol 500 mg IV given prior to coming off CPB
  - Solumedrol 125 mg IV q8h x 3 doses given on first postoperative day
  - Prednisone 0.6–1.0 mg/kg/day for first 1–3 weeks, then tapered gradually with each negative or low-grade biopsy until discontinued in the first 6–12 months
  - Protocols are highly variable depending on the transplant program.
- **Side effects:**
  - New-onset diabetes mellitus: 5–10% will require medications
  - Obesity: dose-related, due to increased appetite
  - Cushingoid facies
  - Myopathy: typically proximal muscle weakness
  - Psychiatric: insomnia, euphoria, confusion, psychosis (rare)
  - Hypertension: usually due to fluid and salt retention, especially when combined with CNIs
  - Cataracts: occurs in 5–10%
  - Peptic ulcer disease
  - Bone disorders: osteoporosis, avascular necrosis especially with prolonged exposure.

Calcineurin Inhibitors
- **Clinical use:**
  - Cyclosporine and tacrolimus
  - Form the cornerstone of chronic maintenance protocols
  - Introduced about 10 years after cyclosporine, tacrolimus is now used by more than half of transplant programs due to a slightly more favorable side effect profile
  - CNIs are metabolized in the liver via cytochrome P-450 and have significant interaction with many commonly used drugs; hence levels must be frequently monitored (Box 9.3).

Cyclosporine
- Initially introduced in the early 1980s, its use has dramatically reduced episodes of acute rejection and improved survival rates.

Box 9.3 Common drug interactions with calcineurin inhibitors

Increases levels	*Decreases levels*
Calcium channel blockers:	**Anticonvulsants:**
Diltiazem	Phenobarbital
Verapamil	Phenytoin
Nicardipine	Carbamazepine
Antifungal agents:	**Antibiotics:**
Fluconazole	Rifampin
Itraconazole	Rifabutin
Ketoconazole	
Voriconazole	
Posaconazole	
Macrolide antibiotics:	**Miscellaneous:**
Azithromycin	St John's wort
Clarithromycin	Octreotide
Erythromycin	
Miscellaneous:	
Allopurinol	
Amiodarone	
Bromocriptine	
Colchicine	
Danazol	
Metoclopramide	
Oral contraceptives	
Grapefruit juice	

- Currently available in three formulations: Sandimmune, Neoral, Gengraf.
- Sandimmune is the oldest formulation and has a 30% bioavailabilty.
- Neoral microemulsion and its generic equivalent, Gengraf, have better bio-availability with absorption less dependent on bile flow.
- **Mechanism of action:**
  - Blocks calcineurin-dependent cell signal transduction leading to inhibition of IL-2 and IFN-γ production, which are critical for T-cell proliferation and differentiation
  - Blocks T-cell cycle at G0–G1 phase and limits activation of cytotoxic T cells
  - Also inhibits T-cell dependent B-cell proliferation.

- **Dosing:**
  - IV: 0.5–1 mg/h continuous infusion post-op if unable to tolerate oral intake to achieve target level
  - Oral: 3–8 mg/kg/day divided into two doses and increased over 3–4 days to achieve target trough level.
- **Side effects/toxicity:**
  - Nephrotoxicity: due partly to renal arteriolar vasoconstriction from local prostaglandin inhibition
  - Hypertension: occurs in >80% of patients due to intrarenal vasoconstriction
  - Hepatotoxicity: uncommon, level related, reversible
  - Hyperkalemia due to inhibition of Na^+/K^+ ATPase activity in distal tubule
  - Metabolic acidosis
  - Hypomagnesemia
  - Hyperuricemia
  - Neurologic: hand tremors, seizures (rare), white matter degeneration
  - Hypertrichosis/hirsutism
  - Gingival hyperplasia
  - Hyperlipidemia
  - Post-transplant lymphoproliferative disorder (PTLD).

Tacrolimus
- Initially called FK-506; brand name Prograf.
- First used in 1989 as replacement for cyclosporine in liver transplant patients with intractable rejection.
- **Mechanism of action:**
  - Chemically unrelated to cyclosporine but has similar action
  - Prodrug that combines with FK-binding protein forming a complex that binds and inactivates calcineurin.
- **Dosing:**
  - IV: 0.01–0.05 mg/kg/day as continuous infusion
  - Oral: initial dose 1–2 mg bid, progressively increased to achieve target trough level.
- **Side effects/toxicity:**
  - Nephrotoxicity: dose related
  - Neurologic: tremor, headache, insomnia; rarely, confusion, seizure, psychosis
  - Diabetes mellitus: incidence slightly higher than with cyclosporine
  - Hyperkalemia: common and usually responds to dose reduction
  - Hypertension and hyperlipidemia: less common than with cyclosporine
  - PTLD: incidence similar to cyclosporine (2%).

Compared to cyclosporine emulsion, tacrolimus has a lower discontinuance rate and a 39% reduction in acute rejections at 6 month and a 31% reduction at 1 year. There is less post-transplantation hypertension but more new-onset diabetes mellitus with tacrolimus than with cyclosporine. One-year survival and the incidence of renal failure and malignancy are similar in both groups.

Antiproliferative Agents
- **Clinical use:**
  - MMF and azathioprine
  - Typically combined with a CNI as part of maintenance immunosuppression regimen
  - MMF more commonly used due to better side effect profile and evidence of lower incidence of transplant vasculopathy.

Mycophenolate Mofetil
- Cellcept (MMF) or Myfortic (mycophenolic acid – enteric coated formulation).
- Some suggestion that Myfortic may be better tolerated with less GI side effects.
- Unlike CNIs, has no renal toxicity but can cause mild bone marrow suppression.
- **Mechanism of action:**
  - Prodrug that is metabolized to mycophenolic acid (MPA) by gastric and hepatic hydrolysis
  - Blocks de novo purine synthesis pathway used by lymphocytes
  - Selectively inhibits T- and B-cell lymphocyte proliferation
  - Rapidly absorbed in GI tract and has 90% bioavailability
  - Typically given on an empty stomach – food delays absorption.
- **Dosing:**
  - Target dose: 1000–1500 mg of MMF twice a day
  - IV dosing equivalent to oral dose
  - Usually given in a fixed dose with adjustments made based on side effects
  - Limited data on the relationship between drug levels and efficacy and side effects
  - Trough levels usually not monitored, although some programs aim for trough level between 2.5 and 5 μg/ml, especially in the early post-transplant period (first 3–6 months)
  - 250 mg of Cellcept is equivalent to 180 mg Myfortic.
- **Side effects/toxicity:**
  - GI: nausea and vomiting, diarrhea, less commonly gastritis and cholestasis
  - Leukopenia
  - Side effects usually respond to dose reduction.

Azathioprine (Imuran)
- Older agent largely supplanted by MMF as use is limited due to side effect profile, particularly myelosuppression.

- **Mechanism of action:**
  - Purine analog which impairs DNA synthesis and blocks de novo purine synthesis pathway
  - Inhibits T- and B-cell proliferation
  - Hepatically metabolized.
- **Dosing:**
  - 1–2 mg/kg/day with dose titrated to keep WBC > 3, platelet count > 100 000 or Hct > 27
  - Blood levels not typically followed
  - Caution with allopurinol (xanthine oxidase inhibitor) as combined use increases azathioprine levels four-fold and increases toxicity.
- **Side effects/toxicity:**
  - Myelosuppression: major side effect; dose related and reversible, responds to dose reduction or drug discontinuance
  - Malignancies: increased incidence primarily of skin cancers due to chromosomal breakage
  - Alopecia: reversible
  - Hepatotoxicity: rare
  - Pancreatitis
  - Megaloblastic anemia
  - Metabolism blocked by concomitant use of allopurinol and can lead to severe bone marrow hypoplasia if interaction is not recognized.

Proliferation Signal Inhibitors/mTOR Inhibitors

- **Clinical use:**
  - Sirolimus (Rapamune) and everolimus (Certican)
  - Everolimus is currently used in Europe and is undergoing Phase III trials in the United States
  - Newer class of agents which block proliferation of T and B cells, as well as vascular smooth muscle cells
  - Typically used in patients with CAV, as sirolimus has been shown to retard disease progression due to its antiproliferative effects on vascular smooth muscle cells
  - Also occasionally substituted for CNIs in patients with renal insufficiency (CNI-free regimen) due to lack of nephrotoxic effects
  - Sirolimus potentiates action and side effects of CNIs
  - Lower levels of cyclosporine or tacrolimus should be maintained when used in combination with sirolimus.
- **Mechanism of action:**
  - Prodrug which blocks mTOR, a cytoplasmic serine/threonine kinase critical in cell signaling, causing cell cycle arrest in mid-to-late G1 phase
  - Inhibits cell proliferation by impairing their response to growth-promoting lymphokines
  - Also retards mTOR-mediated endothelial and smooth muscle cell proliferation in blood vessels and airways.

- **Dosing:**
  - 1–5 mg/day to achieve 24-h trough level of 5–10 ng/mL.
- **Side effects/toxicities:**
  - Elevated cholesterol and triglycerides
  - Stomatitis
  - Poor wound healing
  - Lower extremity edema due to capillary "leak," unrelated to volume overload
  - Pneumonitis/interstitial lung disease
  - Occasional thrombocytopenia and leucopenia.

Infection prevention

- Strategies include vaccination, universal precautions, and pre-emptive therapy.
- Vaccination status should be considered pretransplant as vaccination is less effective in immunosuppressed patients.
- All live vaccines are contraindicated in immunosuppressed patients.
- **Pretransplant:**
  - Determine need for vaccination for tetanus, measles, mumps, rubella, pertusis, diphtheria, polio, pneumococcal pneumonia, influenza
  - Verify cytomegalovirus (CMV), human immunodeficiency virus (HIV), varicella, toxoplasmosis status
  - Verify hepatitis B and hepatitis C status and provide hepatitis B vaccination as appropriate and as time allows
  - Verify TB status either by skin testing or serology (Quantiferon) and provide isoniazid prophylaxis as appropriate
  - All patients should receive yearly influenza vaccine as well as pneumococcal vaccine very 3–5 years.
- **Post-transplant universal precautions:**
  - Use of a Hepa-filter mask advised for the first 3 months after transplant when outdoors
  - Routine hand-washing after contact with raw foods, secretions, feces, or soil
  - Avoid close contact with persons with respiratory illness
  - Avoid well and lake water, raw foods, undercooked meats, unpasteurized dairy products, or unwashed fruits or vegetables
  - Avoid environments with known pathogens (e.g. construction sites).
- **Pre-emptive therapy:**
  - Targeted against pathogens which typically cause infections in immunocompromised host
  - Specific agent and duration of use varies among transplant centers and local experience
  - Cytomegalovirus (CMV):
    – Dependent on CMV status of donor and recipient

    – CMV-positive donor to negative recipient poses highest risk
    – CMV-negative donor to negative recipient poses lowest risk
    – Oral valganciclovir used for 6–12 months with dose adjusted for renal function and WBC count
- *Candida albicans*:
    – Nystatin swish and swallow or clotrimazole troches given for the first 3 months
- *Pneumocystis jiroveci*:
    – Trimethoprim/sulfamethoxazole (TMP/SMX) 80/400 mg once daily or 160/800 mg three times a week for 1 year (some programs continue it indefinitely)
    – TMP/SMX also effective for *Toxoplasma gondii*, *Isospora belli*, *Cyclospora cayetanensis*, and Nocardia and Listeria species
    – For sulfa-allergic patients, alternatives include atovaquone, pentamidine and dapsone, all of which have narrower coverage compared to TMP/SMX.

Post-Transplant Mortality

Causes of Death Post-transplant (according to the ISHLT 2008 Report)

- **Early mortality:**
  - First 30 days post-transplant:
    – Graft failure: 42%
    – Non-CMV infection: 13%
    – Multiorgan failure: 12%
    – Technical factors: 8%
  - 1–12 months post-transplant:
    – Non-CMV infection: 33%
    – Graft failure: 18%
    – Acute rejection: 12%
- **Late mortality:**
  - 1–3 years post-transplant:
    – Graft failure: 23%
    – CAV: 14%
    – Non-CMV infection: 13%
    – Malignancy: 10%
  - 5 years post-transplant:
    – CAV and late graft failure (likely due to CAV): 33%
    – Malignancies: 23%
    – Non-CMV infections: 11%.

Post-transplant Morbidities/Complications

Acute rejection
- Despite modern immunosuppression, up to 40% of patients develop acute rejection in the first post-transplant year.

Box 9.4 Stanford Medical Center Biopsy and Clinic Follow-up Schedule

Biopsy schedule

4 weekly biopsies starting at week 2 post-transplant
Every 2 weeks until month 3
Monthly until month 6
Every 2 months until 12 months
Every 3–4 months until year 3
Every 6 months until year 5
Biopsies typically discontinued after year 5

Clinic follow-up

Twice a week for first month
Weekly–biweekly for first 3 months
Monthly until 6 months
Every 2 months until 12 months
Every 4 months until year 3
Every 6 months until year 5
Annually >5 years

- Death from rejection is 6.4% in the first 30 days and 12.4% from 1 to 12 months.
- Mortality progressively declines down to 2% at >5 years.
- 5% develop severe hemodynamic compromise (decreased left ventricular systolic function, CI < 2.0, PA saturation < 50%, elevated PCWP, profound dyspnea or fatigue).
- Most, however, are asymptomatic and detected through routine echocardiogram and surveillance biopsy.
- As the incidence is highest in the early post-transplant period, frequent surveillance biopsies and clinic follow-up are performed in the first 3 months and then gradually decreased (Box 9.4).
- Noninvasive monitoring for acute cellular rejection (ACR) by gene expression profiling of peripheral lymphocytes (Allomap®) for patients 6–12 months post-transplant is being performed in some centers, although still not widely accepted.
- An Allomap® score of <34 has a 99.2% negative predictive value for moderate to severe cellular rejection, but positive predictive value is poor.

Types of Rejection
- **Hyperacute rejection:**
- Usually occurs within minutes to hours and triggered by high levels of preformed antibodies either against epitopes of the HLA or ABO systems

(in rare cases of transplantation across a major blood group) of the donor heart
- Causes rapid activation of the complement cascade leading to endothelial damage and microvascular thrombosis causing graft loss
- Rarely seen now due to rigorous ABO cross-matching and avoidance of donors with HLA antigens that the recipient has high antibody levels against.
- **Acute cellular rejection (ACR):**
  - Most common type of rejection, with incidence commonly peaking at 1 month post-transplant, then declining rapidly over next 5 months and reaching a low steady level at 1 year
  - Predominantly a T-cell-mediated response against the cardiac allograft, leading to mononuclear inflammatory infiltrates causing myocardial damage
  - Diagnosed by biopsy with severity dependent on degree of lymphocytic infiltration and myocardial damage and graded according to the standardized ISHLT classification (Box 9.5)
  - Treatment depends on severity of rejection and typically consists of pulse steroids, and augmentation of immunosuppression ± cytolytic therapy (rATG, OKT3)
  - Recurrent or recalcitrant rejection sometimes treated with total lymphoid irradiation (TLI).
- **Acute antibody-mediated rejection (AMR or humoral rejection):**
  - Mediated by B cells and involves antibodies directed against donor antigens on the endothelial surface of the allograft coronary vasculature
  - Resulting immunoglobulin deposition and complement activation leads to neutrophil and macrophage infiltration of the vessel wall, causing increased vascular permeability and microvascular thrombosis, and eventual graft dysfunction
  - More likely to lead to hemodynamic compromise and has a worse prognosis
  - Suspect AMR when hemodynamic instability occurs in setting of a low-grade cellular endomyocardial biopsy result
  - Diagnosis based on a combination of:
    - Clinical evidence of graft dysfunction
    - Presence of circulating antibodies against known donor HLA antigens
    - Endomyocardial biopsy showing: histologic findings of capillary endothelial swelling, macrophage, and/or neutrophil capillary infiltration, and interstitial edema and/or hemorrhage and fibrin in the vessels; positive immunofluorescence staining for immunoglobulin (IgG, IgM) and complement deposition (C3d, C4d, C1q); positive staining of macrophages within capillaries for CD68 and C4d staining of capillaries by paraffin immunohistochemistry

Box 9.5 1990 and 2004 ISHLT Grading System for Acute Cellular Rejection and Typical Treatment

ISHLT Grade 2004 (Revised)	ISHLT Description 2004 (Revised)	ISHLT Grade 1990	ISHLT Description 1990	Treatment
0 R	No rejection	0	No rejection	None
1R (mild)	Interstitial and/or perivascular infiltrate with up to one focus of myocyte damage	1 (mild) 1A focal	Focal perivascular and/or interstitial infiltrate without myocyte damage	None – treatment not shown to alter outcomes
		1B diffuse	Diffuse infiltrate without myocyte damage	
		2 (moderate – focal)	One focus of infiltrate with associated myocyte damage	
2 R (moderate)	Two or more foci of infiltrate with associated myocyte damage	3 (moderate) 3A focal	Multifocal infiltrate with myocyte damage	Pulse steroids (methylprednisolone 500–1000 mg/day IV × 3 days) with or without cytolytic antibody therapy (rATG, OKT3) depending on hemodynamic stability
3 R (severe)	Diffuse infiltrate with multifocal myocyte damage ± edema, ±hemorrhage, ±vasculitis	3B diffuse	Diffuse infiltrate with myocyte damage	Pulse steroids (methylprednisolone 500–1000 mg IV daily x 3 days) with or without cytolytic antibody therapy (rATG, OKT3) depending on hemodynamic stability
		4 (severe)	Diffuse, polymorphous infiltrate with extensive myocyte damage ± edema, ±hemorrhage, ±vasculitis	

Box 9.6 1990 and 2004 ISHLT Grading System for Acute Antibody-mediated Rejection and Typical Treatment

ISHLT Grade 2004 (Revised)	ISHLT Description 2004 (Revised)	ISHLT Description 1990	Treatment
AMR 0	Negative for acute AMR No histologic or immunopathologic features of AMR	Humoral rejection (positive immunofluorescence, vasculitis or severe edema in absence of cellular infiltrate) recorded as additional information required	None
AMR 1	Positive for AMR Histologic features of AMR Positive immunofluorescence or immunoperoxidase staining for AMR (+ CD68, C4d)		Pulse steroids (methylprednisolone 500–1000 mg/day IV × 3 days followed by plasmapheresis and IVIg with or without rituximab and/or cyclophosphamide (depending on hemodynamic stability)

- Treatment consists of pulse steroids, plasmapheresis, IVIg, ± rituximab or cyclophosphamide (Box 9.6).

Post-transplant Infections

- Early diagnosis and determination of specific microbiologic etiology is essential and often requires invasive diagnostic procedures.
- It is a significant cause of death within the first year post-transplant but remains a threat throughout the patient's lifetime due to chronic immunosuppression.
- Infections usually occur in a predicable pattern according to time post-transplant:
  - <1 month:
    - Typically due to technical or nosocomial factors
    - Bacterial infections from aspiration, catheter or wound infections
    - Hospital-acquired infections with MRSA or VRE
    - Opportunistic infections uncommon as full effects of immunosuppression not yet reached
  - 1–6 months:

- Viral: polyomavirus BK, adenovirus, influenza, hepatitis (HCV)
- Fungal infections: cryptococcus neoformans,
- Mycobacterium tuberculosis
- Pneumocystis, CMV, herpes virus infections, nocardia, listeria, toxoplasma uncommon due to routine use of prophylaxis with TMP-SMZ and valganciclovir
- \>6 months:
  - Community-acquired bacterial pneumonia and urinary tract infection
  - Fungal pathogens: aspergillus, atypical molds, candida, mucor species
  - Late viral infections: CMV, hepatitis (HBV, HCV), herpes simplex virus (HSV)
  - Atypical pathogens: nocardia, rhodococcus.

Malignancy

- Transplant patients have higher risk of developing malignancies compared to the general population due to chronic immunosuppression.
- Malignancies account for 23% of deaths in long-term survivors >5 years post-transplant.
- By 10 years post-transplant, 33% of patients develop a type of malignancy, with the great majority being skin cancers (20% of recipients by 10 years), often quite aggressive.
- PTLD often related to latent Epstein-Barr virus (EBV) infection occurs in 2–5%.
- Regular use of sun screen, avoidance of excessive sun exposure, and annual dermatologic evaluation should be emphasized.
- Age- and gender-specific cancer-screening guidelines should be rigorously followed.

Cardiac Allograft Vasculopathy

- Often diffuse and rapidly progressive.
- Major issue limiting long-term survival.
- Exact mechanism incompletely understood but likely has immunologic and nonimmunologic components:
  - Traditional risk factors: hypertension, dyslipidemia, diabetes mellitus
  - Immunologic (HLA mismatch, recurrent AMR)
  - Infectious (CMV).
- Incidence ~10% at 1 year, and 30–50% by 5 years.
- Early CAV typically silent but late manifestations include heart failure, syncope, MI, ventricular tachycardia, bradyarrhythmias, sudden death.
- Most transplant programs do annual coronary angiography to monitor for CAV.
- Coronary intravascular ultraouns (IVUS): gold standard for diagnosing CAV defined as mean intimal thickness >0.5 mm.
- Baseline angiogram and IVUS soon after transplant useful in differentiating donor atherosclerosis from CAV on later studies.

- Survival as low as 18–20% at 1 year after an initial ischemic event.
- Proliferation signal inhibitors/mTOR inhibitors (sirolimus and everolimus) have been shown to delay progression of CAV.
- PCI useful in small minority of patients with focal disease but does not significantly alter prognosis due to progressive and diffuse nature of allograft vasculopathy.
- Only definitive treatment is retransplantation.

CLINICAL PEARLS

- Chronic HIV infection that is well-treated with HAART with low viral loads is not considered an absolute contraindication, but most transplant centers still consider HIV a contraindication.
- Immunosuppression is associated with a higher incidence of new malignancy (particularly skin and lymphatic), as well as a higher risk of recurrence or more aggressive behavior of a previous malignancy.
- Adequate family and social support pre- and post-heart transplant must be carefully evaluated.
- In patients with biatrial heart transplant, it is not unusual to see distinct "extra" P-waves on ECG, one from patient's own remnant atrium and one from the transplanted atrium, which precedes each QRS complex.
- In bicaval technique for heart transplant, there is an increased risk of SVC and/or IVC stenosis.
- Since the risk of rejection is highest during the first 3 months, immunosuppression levels are kept highest during this time. Target levels are gradually reduced until after the first year when they are maintained at lower levels for chronic acceptance.
- Corticosteroids used as pulse therapy are the main agents for acute rejection.
- Tacrolimus is now the most commonly used CNI in heart transplant recipients (57% versus 37% cyclosporine).
- Suspect acute AMR when hemodynamic instability occurs in setting of a low-grade cellular endomyocardial biopsy result.
- Statins have been shown to decrease the incidence of CAV.

Recommended Reading

Clinical Trials and Meta-Analyses

Mancini D, Pinney S, Burkhoff D et al. Use of rapamycin slows progression of cardiac transplantation vasculopathy. *Circulation* 2003;**108**:48–53.

Ye F, Ying-Bin X, Yu-Guo W, Hetzer R. Tacrolimus versus cyclosporine microemulsion for heart transplant recipients: A meta-analysis. *J Heart Lung Transplant* 2009;**28**:58–66.

Guidelines

Stewart S, Winters GL, Fishbein MC et al. Revision of the 1990 Working Formulation for the Standardization of Nomenclature in the Diagnosis of Heart Rejection. *J Heart Lung Transplant* 2005;**24**:1710–1720.

Review Articles

Baran DA. Induction therapy in cardiac transplantation: When and why? *Heart Failure Clin* 2007;**3**:31–41.

Fishman JA. Infection in Solid-Organ Transplant Recipients. *N Engl J Med* 2007; **357**(25):2601–2614.

Hunt SA. Taking heart – cardiac transplantation past, present and future. *N Engl J Med* 2006;**355**(3):231–235.

Mehra MR. The emergence of genomic and proteomic biomarkers in heart transplantation. *J Heart Lung Transplant* 2005;**24**:S213–218.

Sipahi I, Starling R. Cardiac allograft vasculopathy: An update. *Heart Failure Clin* 2007; **3**:87–95.

Tan CD, Baldwin III WM, Rodriguez ER. Update on cardiac transplant pathology. *Arch Pathol Lab Med* 2007;**131**:1169–1191.

Taylor DO, Edwards LB, Aurora P et al. Registry of the International Society for Heart and Lung Transplantation: Twenty-fifth Official Adult Heart Transplant Report – 2008. *J Heart Lung Transplant* 2008;**27**:943–956.

IV Valvular and Vascular Disease

10 Valvular Heart Disease

Reza Ardehali and Ingela Schnittger

Department of Internal Medicine, Division of Cardiology, Stanford
University School of Medicine, Stanford, CA, USA

Cardiac auscultation is the most widely used method to screen for valvular
heart disease. Heart murmurs are produced by:
- High blood flow through orifices
- Forward flow through an irregular/narrow orifice
- Backward flow through an incompetent valve.

All patients with a heart murmur who are symptomatic or have other signs
of cardiac disease should have a complete work-up, including a transthoracic
echocardiogram (TTE). Other murmurs that warrant further evaluation by
TTE include:
- All diastolic murmurs
- Continuous murmurs, excluding venous hum
- Holosystolic murmurs
- Early and late systolic murmurs
- Midsystolic Grade 3 or more.

Certain maneuvers can change the intensity of heart murmurs and help
with correct diagnosis (Box 10.1).

When treating patients with valvular heart disease, three major issues must
be addressed:
- What is the underlying cause contributing to its development?
- Is the structural failure leading to valvular disease severe enough to require
  medical therapy and/or surgical intervention of the diseased valve?
- If surgical intervention is warranted, then what type of procedure is most
  appropriate based on the underlying valvular disease and individual's
  comorbidities?

With this information, appropriate medical management and either serial
follow-up examinations or surgical correction can be achieved.

A Practical Approach to Cardiovascular Medicine, First Edition. Edited by Reza Ardehali,
Marco Perez, Paul Wang.
© 2011 Blackwell Publishing Ltd. Published 2011 by Blackwell Publishing Ltd.

> **Box 10.1 Maneuvers that change murmur intensity**
>
> | Maneuver | Alteration in murmur intensity |
> | --- | --- |
> | Respiration | Inspiration increases venous flow to the right heart, augmenting right-sided murmurs |
> | | Expiration makes left-sided murmurs louder |
> | Isometric handgrip | Increases afterload and peripheral resistance. This reduces murmurs of aortic stenosis (AS) and hypertrophic obstructive cardiophyopathy (HOCM), while increasing murmurs of mitral regurgitation (MR), mitral stenosis (MS), and aortic insufficiency (AI) |
> | Positional changes | Standing leads to a decrease in left ventricular (LV) volume. Most murmurs diminish, except HOCM (becomes louder) and mitral valve prolapse (MVP) (lengthen and intensify) |
> | | Squatting simultaneously increases venous return while augmenting afterload and peripheral resistance. Most murmurs intensify, except HOCM and MVP (usually soften) |
> | Valsalva maneuver | Decreases venous return to right and subsequently left heart, hence reducing LV size. Most murmurs decrease in intensity and length, except HOCM (become louder) and MVP (become longer and louder) |
> | | After release of Valsalva, LV size increases leading to return of right-sided murmurs to baseline earlier |
> | Ventricular premature beats (VPB) | Murmurs due to stenotic semilunar valves increase in intensity in the cycle after a VPB |
> | | By contrast, MR or tricuspid regurgitation (TR) normally do not change (may diminish slightly) |
> | Amyl nitrite | Venodilation, leading to reduced venous return to right heart. Augments HOCM and MVP murmur, while reducing AS murmur |

Aortic Stenosis

Etiology

The etiologies of aortic stenosis (AS) can be divided as follows:

- **Subvalvular:** thought to be caused by an underlying abnormality in the architecture of the LV outflow tract (LVOT), with turbulence leading to progressive LVOT fibrosis. Symptoms may appear during childhood, requiring surgical correction.
- **Supravalvular:** a fixed form of congenital (LVOT) obstruction that occurs as a localized or a diffuse narrowing of the ascending aorta beyond the superior margin of the sinuses of Valsalva.
- **Valvular:**
  - Rheumatic: more frequent in developing countries; pathologically AV commisures are fused

- Bicuspid: affects 1–2% of population. Normally leads to calcification in the fifth or sixth decade of life
- Calcific: the most common cause of AS in the United States.

Clinical Assessment

AS leads to:
- Narrowing of the valve orifice area
- Pressure gradient between the LV and aorta
- Increased afterload, leading to concentric hypertrophy, elevated LV end-diastolic pressure (LVEDP), and impaired relaxation.

Symptoms

- **Angina** develops because of both reduced coronary flow reserve and increased myocardial demand caused by high afterload.
- **Syncope** is typically related to exertion and may be caused by arrhythmias, hypotension, or decreased cerebral perfusion resulting from increased blood flow to exercising muscles without compensatory increase in cardiac output.
- **Congestive heart failure** is due to both diastolic and systolic dysfunction, as a result of an increase in left ventricular filling pressures and impaired myocardial contraction.

Diagnostic Tests

- ECG: LV hypertrophy, left atrial (LA) enlargement.
- TTE: used to evaluate atrioventricular (AV) morphology, transvalvular gradient, AV area, secondary LV remodeling, serial changes over time.

Treatment

Asymptomatic patients with moderate-to-severe AS must be followed closely. There is no effective long-term medical therapy. In the presence of severe AS accompanied by symptoms or with LV dysfunction, surgical replacement of the valve is warranted (Box 10.2 and Figure 10.1).

EVIDENCE-BASED PRACTICE

Intensive lipid lowering with Simvastatin and Ezetimibe in Aortic Stenosis (SEAS Trial)

Context: Benefit of lipid reduction in patients with mild-to-moderate, asymptomatic AS.

Goal: To evaluate if simvastatin and ezetimibe reduce major cardiovascular events.

Method: Double-blind RCT: 1873 patients with mild-to-moderate asymptomatic AS received either 40 mg of simvastatin + 10 mg of ezetimibe or placebo daily.

Results: Combination therapy no better than placebo in reducing aortic valve and cardiovascular events, although therapy reduced the incidence of ischemic cardiovascular events.

Take-home message: Lipid-lowering therapy in asymptomatic patients with mild-to-moderate AS does not reduce major cardiovascular events.

Box 10.2 Summary of cardiac valve disease

Signs/symptoms	Diagnostics	Management
Aortic stenosis		
Angina, syncope, heart failure	TTE is used to assess severity of AS:	Surgical replacement in all patients with symptoms or
Systolic ejection murmur radiating	*Mild* – area 1.5 cm2, mean	asymptomatic patients with LV dysfunction (Figure 10.1)
to neck, delayed carotid upstroke,	gradient < 25 mmHg, jet velocity < 3 m/s	Asymptomatic patients with normal LV function should
S4, soft or paradoxical S2	*Moderate* – area 1.0–1.5 cm2, mean	be followed with serial TTEs to assess AVA, mean
	gradient 25–40 mmHg, jet velocity 3–4 m/s	gradient, LV function, and LVH:
	Severe – area < 1 cm2, mean	*Mild:* 3–5 years, *moderate:* 1–2 years, *severe:* every 6
	gradient > 40 mmHg, jet velocity > 4 m/s	months
Aortic regurgitation		
Dyspnea, orthopnea, PND, angina,	TTE is used to assess severity of AR:	Acute severe AR requires urgent surgical intervention
syncope	*Mild* – PHT > 400 m/s, AI jet/LVOT area	AVR is indicated in patients with severe AR who have
Chronic: diastolic blowing murmur,	<4%, RF <30%	symptoms or are asymptomatic but have LV
hyperdynamic circulation, displaced	*Moderate* – PHT 300–400 m/s, AI jet/LVOT	dysfunction
PMI, Quincke's pulse, Musset sign	area 4–59%, RF 30–49%	Clinical follow-up with serial TTE is indicated in
Acute: short diastolic blowing	*Severe* – PHT <300, AI jet/LVOT area	asymptomatic patients (Figure 10.2)
murmur, soft S1	>60%, RF ≥ 50%.	
Mitral stenosis		
Dyspnea, orthopnea, PND,	TTE is used to assess severity of MS:	PMBV in symptomatic patients (NYHA ≥ II) with
hemoptysis, hoarseness, edema,	*Mild* – area > 1.5 cm2, mean	moderate-to-severe MS, favorable valve morphology,
ascites	gradient < 5 mmHg, PASP < 30 mmHg	absence of LA thrombus or moderate to severe MR
Diastolic rumble following an	*Moderate* – area 1.0–1.5 cm2, mean	MV repair/replacement in symptomatic patients (NYHA
opening snap, loud S1, RV lift, loud	gradient 5–10 mmHg, PASP 30–50 mmHg	III–IV) with moderate-to-severe MS, and not a candidate
P2	*Severe* – area < 1.0 cm2, mean	for PMBV, i.e. unfavorable valve morphology, LA
	gradient > 10 mmHg, PASP > 50 mmHg	thrombus despite anticoagulation, or moderate to
		severe MR (Figure 10.3).

Mitral regurgitation

Dyspnea, orthopnea, PND

Holosystolic apical murmur radiating to axilla, S3, displaced PMI

TTE is used to assess severity of MR:

Mild – VC width < 0.3 cm, RF <30%, regurgitant orifice area < 0.2 cm2

Moderate – VC width 0.3–0.69 cm, RF 30–49%, regurgitant orifice area 0.2–0.39 cm2

Severe – VC width ≥ 0.7, RF ≥ 50%, regurgitant orifice area ≥ 0.4 cm2

MV surgery is generally indicated in all surgically eligible patients with symptomatic acute or chronic severe MR, and in those asymptomatic patients with severe MR and mild-to-moderate LV dysfunction and/or ESD ≥ 40 mm

Tricuspid regurgitation

Signs of RV failure, i.e. dyspnea, ascites, edema

Systolic murmur along the left lower sternal border that may increase on inspiration. Jugular venous distention, with a prominent merged c–v wave and a steep y descent.

Systolic hepatic pulsation

Mild – VC width not defined, jet area < 5 cm2, systolic dominance in hepatic veins

Moderate – VC width < 0.7 cm, jet area 5–10 cm2, systolic blunting in hepatic veins

Severe – VC width > 0.7 cm, jet area > 10 cm2, systolic flow reversal in hepatic veins

TV repair is indicated for severe TR in patients with MV disease requiring MV surgery

TV replacement or annuloplasty is also reasonable in symptomatic patients with severe TR

PND, paroxysmal nocturnal dyspnea; PMI, point of maximal impact; RV, right ventricle; PHT, pressure half-time; LVOT, left ventricular outflow tract; RF, regurgitant fraction; AI, aortic insufficiency; PASP; pulmonary artery systolic pressure; VC, vena contracta; LVH, left ventricular hypertrophy; AVR, atrial valve replacement; PMBV, percutaneous mitral balloon valvotomy; MV, mitral valve; TV, tricuspid valve; ESD, end-systolic diameter

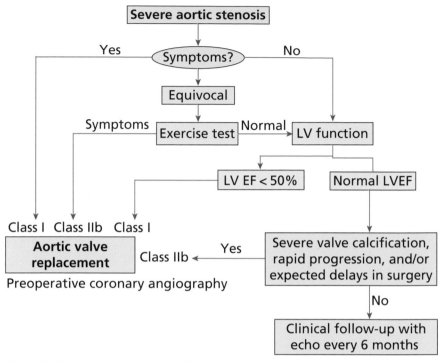

Figure 10.1 Management of patients with severe AS

Aortic Regurgitation

Etiology
The most common causes of acute AR are:
- Infective endocarditis
- Aortic dissection
- Trauma.

   The most common causes of chronic AR are:
- Calcific AV
- Congenital abnormalities
- Endocarditis
- Annuloaortic ectasia
- Collagen-vascular disease
- Hypertension
- Marfan's syndrome.

Clinical Assessment
The clinical presentation of atrial regurgitation (AR) generally is determined by the time course over which regurgitation develops.

Symptoms

- **Acute AR:** a sudden increase in LV filling pressure due to large regurgitant volume, leading to pulmonary congestion, impaired cardiac output, and finally cardiogenic shock.
- **Chronic AR:** a volume overload of LV, leading to an increase in wall thickness and size:
  - There is an initial augmentation in ejection fraction (EF) (a portion of stroke volume regurgitates back into the LV), with a fall in diastolic pressure and a wide pulse pressure
  - Individuals with chronic AR and normal LV function may remain asymptomatic for years.
  - In chronic decompensated AR, further ventricular dilation results in an increase in end-systolic dimension and LVEDP
  - There is impaired LV function which leads to an increase in end-systolic volume and a fall in EF.

The most important markers for poor prognosis are: age, end-systolic dimension, and LV function.

Diagnostic Tests

- ECG: LV hypertrophy, left atrial enlargement.
- TTE: used to evaluate aortic valve and annulus morphology, LV systolic function, and end-systolic dimension. Doppler techniques can be used to evaluate severity of regurgitation, although mild AR is not uncommon and should not be over-interpreted.

Treatment

Immediate surgical treatment is the mainstay of therapy for patients with acute AR. Patients with chronic AR may remain asymptomatic for many years. Surgical intervention is warranted when symptoms occur or there is evidence of LV systolic dysfunction (Box 10.2 and Figure 10.2). In asymptomatic patients with severe chronic AR who have preserved systolic function, the LV dimension can help mandate the need for surgery.

CLINICAL PEARLS

- A common echo finding in bicuspid aortic valve is aortic root dilation. A small subset of bicuspid AV is associated with coarctation of the aorta.
- Acquired von Willebrand syndrome is a common feature in patients with AS that can lead to bleeding, particularly in the GI tract. The abnormality and bleeding is normally improved after AV replacement.
- Avoid aggressive diuresis or vasodilation in patients with congestive heart failure (CHF) and AS, as they are exquisitely preload dependent. Nitrates are contraindicated in severe AS, as it causes profound hypotension.

(Continued)

- Patients with severe AS and low cardiac output may present with low mean gradient in the setting of critically small valve area, due to contractile dysfunction. In these patients, it is useful to determine transvalvular gradient and valve area at rest and during exercise or low-dose dobutamine stress. Patients with severe AS will have a fixed valve area with an increase in gradient.
- Address five basic issues when doing a TTE to evaluate an AS patient: AV morphology, transvalvular gradient, AV area, secondary LV changes, serial changes.
- When doing a TTE for AS study, use continuity equation to calculate AV area.
- Angina experienced in decompensated chronic AR is due to an increase in myocardial O_2 consumption (high myocardial mass), fall in coronary perfusion pressure (low diastolic pressure), and concomitant coronary artery disease (CAD).
- The rapid development of LV failure in acute AR, manifested primarily as pulmonary edema, may warrant urgent surgical intervention.

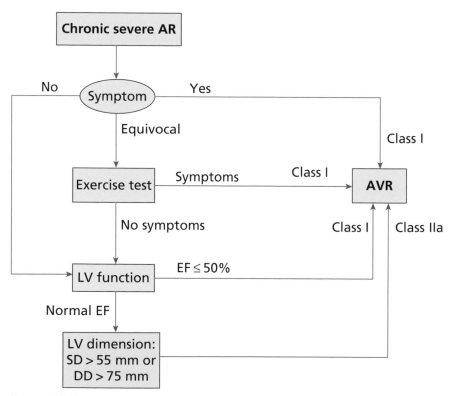

Figure 10.2 Management of patients with severe AR. SD, systolic dimension; DD, diastolic dimension.

Mitral Stenosis

Etiology and Clinical Assessment

The most common cause of mitral stenosis (MS) worldwide is a history of rheumatic carditis. MS is relatively rare in developed countries due to a decline in the incidence of rheumatic heart disease. The majority of rheumatic MS cases encountered in the United States are found in immigrant communities.

The chronic inflammatory reaction leads to:

- Fibrous thickening and calcification of the valve leaflets
- Fusion of the commissures
- Contracture and shortening of the chordae tendinae.

Patients with MS may remain asymptomatic for years, before symptoms typical of left-sided heart failure are observed (elevated left atrial pressure and reduced cardiac output). These include dyspnea on exertion, orthopnea, and paroxysmal nocturnal dyspnea.

Diagnostic Tests

- ECG: evidence of left atrial enlargement demonstrated by a prominent terminal portion of a biphasic P-wave in lead V1, RV enlargement, and rhythm abnormalities, such as atrial fibrillation.
- TTE: used to evaluate the gradient across the mitral valve, presence of MR, LV size and function, and pulmonary artery pressure. Four components are graded in severity for an overall score (4–16) that can help determine whether percutaneous mitral balloon valvotomy (PMVB) can be effective:
  - Leaflet mobility
  - Subvalvular thickening
  - Leaflet calcification
  - Leaflet thickening.

Treatment

In general, surgical intervention is required for individuals with moderate-to-severe MS who have significant functional limitation and/or severe pulmonary hypertension.

- Symptomatic patients (NYHA ≥ II) with moderate or severe MS due to rheumatic disease and valve morphology favorable for PMVB in the absence of left atrial thrombus or moderate-to-severe MR can be effectively treated with PMVB.
- Mitral valve replacement (MVR) (or repair if possible) is indicated in symptomatic patients (NYHA III–IV) with moderate or severe MS when PMVB is contraindicated, i.e. valve morphology not favorable for PMVB, presence of LA thrombus despite anticoagulation, or presence of moderate-to-severe MR (Box 10.2 and Figure 10.3).
- Asymptomatic patients (at rest) with moderate-to-severe MS with valve morphology favorable for PMVB, absence of LA thrombus, and absence of moderate-to-severe MR, should be considered for PMVB if:

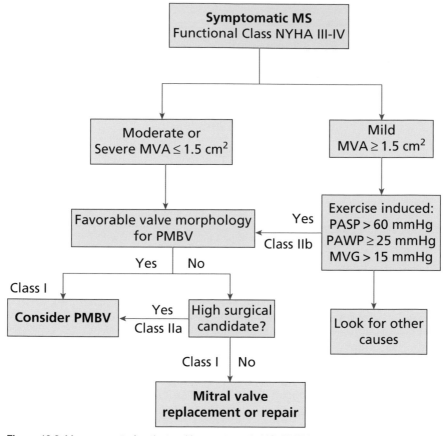

Figure 10.3 Management of patients with symptomatic MS. PMBV, percutaneous mitral balloon valvotomy; PAWP, pulmonary artery wedge pressure; PASP, pulmonary artery systolic pressure; MVA, mitral valve area

- Resting pulmonary artery systolic pressure (PASP) >50 mmHg
- Poor exercise tolerance
- Exercise-induced PASP > 60 mmHg or pulmonary artery wedge pressure (PAWP) ≥ 25 mmHg.

Mitral Regurgitation

Etiology

The most common causes of acute mitral regurgitation (MR) are:

- Ruptured chordae tendinae
- Ruptured papillary muscles
- Infective endocarditis.

The common causes of chronic MR are:

- Mitral valve prolapse (MVP)
- Rheumatic heart disease
- Infective endocarditis
- Drugs such as phentermine–fenfluramine and ergots
- Collagen vascular disorders
- Papillary muscle dysfunction secondary to ischemic heart disease
- MV annular dilation induced by LV enlargement.

Clinical Assessment

The clinical presentation of MR generally is determined by the time course over which valvular incompetence develops.

The hallmark of MR is low cardiac output and LV diastolic volume overload.

- **Acute MR**: an abrupt elevation of LA pressure due to volume overload is transmitted to the pulmonary circulation, resulting in pulmonary congestion, manifested as dyspnea. Patients develop acute heart failure in the presence of normal or high EF.
- **Chronic MR**: the LA enlarges progressively, leading to hypertrophy and LV dilatation:
  - Increased preload, normal afterload, and normal contractile function of the LV in the early stages leads to an elevated stroke volume, which compensates for the regurgitant flow
  - In the late stages, an increase in LV systolic volume, LVEDP, and left atrial pressure (LAP) lead to pulmonary congestion and CHF. As a result, exertional dyspnea and fatigue progress gradually over many years.

Diagnostic Tests

- ECG: LA enlargement, left ventricular hypertrophy (LVH).
- TTE: used to evaluate the severity of MR, valve morphology, LA and LV size, LV function.

Treatment

- **Medical**:
  - **Acute MR:**
    - Medical therapy has a limited role and is aimed at stabilizing hemodynamics in preparation for surgery
    - In normotensive patients with acute MR, consider nitroprusside to decrease the amount of MR, increase forward output, and reduce pulmonary congestion
    - In hypotensive patients with acute MR, combination therapy with dobutamine and nitroprusside and/or intra-aortic balloon pump (IABP) may be of benefit in preparation for surgery
  - **Chronic MR:**
    - In the asymptomatic patients with chronic MR, there is no accepted medical therapy, while those with functional or ischemic MR, may benefit from preload reduction with vasodilators.

- **Surgical:** MV surgery is indicated in:
  - All symptomatic patients with acute severe MR
  - Chronic severe MR and NYHA Class II–IV in the absence of severe LV dysfunction and/or end-systolic dimension ≤ 55 mm
  - Asymptomatic patients with chronic severe MR and mild-to-moderate LV dysfunction, EF 30–60%, and/or end-systolic dimension ≥ 40 mm (Box 10.2 and Figure 10.4).

CLINICAL PEARLS

- A typical TTE finding of rheumatic MS is the "hockey stick" appearance of the anterior valve with restrictive movement of the tip of the leaflet.
- Papillary muscle rupture can occur in 1–2% of post-myocardial infarction (MI) patients (especially in patients with posterior MI), normally days 5–7 post MI. It can lead rapidly to pulmonary congestion. Obtain a stat TTE in anticipation of possible surgical intervention. If hypotensive, may require dobutamine and nitroprusside. IABP may increase forward output and mean atrial pressure, while decreasing LV filling pressure.
- Use the diaphragm of the stethoscope for MVP. Examine the patient in the supine, left decubitus, and sitting position, and listen for a nonejection systolic click shortly after S1, often followed by a mid-to-late crescendo systolic murmur that continues through A2.
- Patient with MVP should have a TTE to assess for MR, valve morphology, and LV function.
- Avoid inotropic drugs in patients who have systolic anterior motion (SAM) and are in hemodynamic compromise. Instead, by increasing afterload, left ventricular end-diastolic volume (LVEDV) will increase and pressure will be improved. The agent of preference is phenylepherine.

Tricuspid Regurgitation

Etiology

In the majority of patients, TR is "secondary," caused by dilatation of the annulus as a result of increased pulmonary and right ventricular pressure. The primary causes of TR include:

- Rheumatic disease
- Infective endocarditis
- Connective tissue disease
- Ebstein's anomaly
- Carcinoid
- Right-sided MI causing papillary muscle dysfunction.

Clinical Assessment

Mild tricuspid regurgitation (TR) is generally clinically insignificant and well tolerated. It may be associated with acquired left heart disease. TR can be

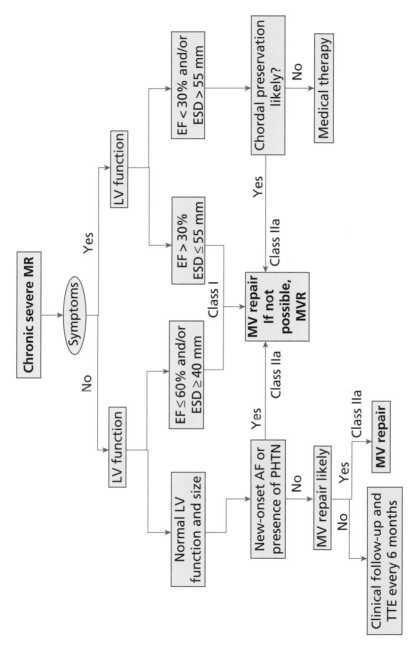

Figure 10.4 Management of patients with severe MR. ESD, end-systolic diameter; AF, atrial fibrillation; PHTN, portal hypertension

suspected on the basis of an early onset of right-sided heart failure and the characteristic jugular pulsation.

Diagnostic Tests
- ECG: RA enlargement, a tall R- or QR-wave in V1 (characteristic of RV hypertrophy).
- TTE: used to evaluate the severity of TR, valve morphology, RA and RV size, RV and LV function, septal flattening or paradoxical septal motion, and inferior vena cava engorgement and flow direction.

Treatment
- **Medical:**
  - TR is usually well tolerated and rarely requires treatment
  - Medical treatment of the primary causes (e.g. heart failure, endocarditis) is indicated
  - Diuresis and afterload reduction can decrease the severity of right heart failure in symptomatic patients with TR.
- **Surgical:**
  - Reserved for patients who have moderate-to-severe TR and a left-sided valve disorder (e.g. mitral stenosis) causing pulmonary hypertension and high RV pressures, and who also require mitral valve repair
  - May also be indicated for symptomatic patients with severe isolated TR to relieve hepatic and systemic venous congestion and prevent cardiac cirrhosis (Box 10.2).

Prosthetic Heart Valves

The patient's clinical situation should guide the selection of the prosthetic valve.
- **Mechanical valves:**
  - Three major groups: ball-in-cage (rarely used), tilting-disc, and bileaflet valves
  - Excellent durability, normally over 20 years
  - Regardless of design or site of placement, they all require life-long anticoagulation
  - Mitral and tricuspid valve prostheses are associated with higher risk of valve thrombosis than aortic valves
  - Valve dysfunction should be suspected from sudden appearance of dyspnea, muffled sounds, or new murmurs. If there is evidence of thrombus that interferes with valve function, surgical removal of the valve and thrombus is warranted.
- **Bioprosthetic valves:**
  - Bioprosthetic heterograft valves are composed of porcine valves or bovine pericardium; homograft valves are composed of preserved cadaveric human aortic valves

- Limited durability, normally <15 years.
- Depending on institutional practice, no anticoagulation is generally necessary, but Aspirin therapy is recommended.

Anticoagulation in Patients with Prosthetic Valves
- Goal INR in patients with mechanical valve prosthesis in the:
  - Aortic position: 2.0–3.0
  - Mitral position: 2.5–3.5.
- Certain centers recommend anticoagulation for the first 3 months in patients with biologic prosthetic atrial valve replacement (AVR) and MVR with a goal of 2.0–3.0 (Class IIa).
- All patients with MVR and AVR should be treated with Aspirin 75 mg daily.

Interruption of Anticoagulation Prior to an Invasive Procedure
- **Patients at low risk of thrombosis,** defined as those with a bileaflet mechanical AVR with no risk factors (i.e. AF, previous thromboembolism, LV dysfunction, hypercoagulable conditions, older-generation thrombogenic valves, mechanical tricuspid valves, or >1 mechanical valve) it is recommended that warfarin be stopped 48–72 h before the procedure (INR < 1.5) and restarted within 24 h after the procedure. Heparin is usually unnecessary.
- **Patients at high risk of thrombosis,** defined as those with any mechanical MVR or a mechanical AVR with any risk factor, therapeutic doses of intravenous UFH should be started when the INR falls below 2.0 (typically 48 h before surgery), stopped 4–6 h before the procedure, restarted as early after surgery as bleeding stability allows, and continued until the INR is again therapeutic with warfarin therapy.

Infective Endocarditis (IE)

Etiology
IE can be divided into four groups:
- **Native valve endocarditis:**
  - Acute endocarditis: normally due to highly pathogenic micro-organisms (i.e. *Staphylococcus aureus*) and the clinical course rapidly develops over 1–2 days
  - Subacute endocarditis: more indolent clinical course that can evolve over weeks to months. The pathogens are less virulent, i.e. *Streptococcus viridans*, or the HACEK group endocarditis: *Haemophilus aphrophilus*, *Actinobacillus actinomycetemcomitans*, *Cardiobacterium hominis*, *Eikenella corrodens*, and *Kingella kingae*.
- **Prosthetic valve endocarditis:**
  - Early onset: normally within the first 2 months, caused by coagulase-negative staphylococci or meticillin-resistant *Staphylococcus aureus* (MRSA) due to inoculation at time of surgery

- Late onset: normally after 6 months, caused by similar pathogens as in native valves with a higher incidence of fungi infection.
- **Intravenous drug use (IVDU)-associated endocarditis:**
  - Typically caused by skin flora, with *Staphylococcus aureus* being the most common pathogen. The tricuspid valve is usually affected.
- **Nosocomial endocarditis:**
  - Normally an entry portal serving as a source of bacteremia (i.e. hemodialysis catheters). The most common organisms are staphylococci, enterococci, *Candida* spp, and gram negative bacilla.

Clinical Assessment

- Hallmarks of IE are fever and a new murmur.
- Clinical manifestations of IE are highly variable:
  - Subacute IE can present with prolonged malaise
  - Acute IE can present rapidly with catastrophic symptoms.
  Complications from IE are listed in Box 10.3.

Diagnostics Tests

- ECG:
  - Conduction delay due to abscess formation (normally PR prolongation due to abscess around the aortic valve annulus)
  - Potential evidence of ischemia secondary to embolism to coronary arteries.
- CXR: to assess for septic emboli, especially in IVDU patients with IE.
- Labs:
  - Blood cultures from two different sites are of utmost importance
  - CBC may reveal leukocytosis, elevated platelets, and sometimes anemia in case of subacute IE. ESR, CRP, and rheumatoid factor may also be elevated
  - Urinalysis may reveal hematuria.

Box 10.3 Major complications from IE

Cardiac

Valvular destruction with or without CHF
Conduction system disruption from myocardial abscess
Purulent pericarditis from extension of myocardial abscess

Extracardiac

Septic pulmonary emboli resulting from tricuspid or pulmonary valve endocardtitis (right-sided IE)
Cerebral, renal, splenic, hepatic, or soft tissue emboli with concomitant abscess resulting from mitral or aortic valve endocarditis (left-sided IE)
Glomerulonephritis
Arthritis

- Echocardiography:
  - If there is clinical suspicion for IE, an echo should be obtained
  - TTE is highly specific if vegetation is detected and is typically the initial test of choice. However, TTE is reported to be 65% sensitive in native IE and 36% sensitive in prosthetic IE
  - If the TTE is nondiagnostic and clinical suspicion is high, transesophageal echocardiogram (TEE) should be performed, which has a sensitivity of 90–100% in native IE and 82–96% in prosthetic IE. TEE is also superior for detection of abscess.

  The modified Duke's criteria for diagnosis of IE are listed in Box 10.4.

Management
- **Medical:**
  - In case of acute IE, empiric antibiotic treatment (Box 10.5) must be initiated promptly, and later directed towards the causative agent once the organism is identified

---

Box 10.4 Modified Duke's criteria

Major criteria

- Positive blood culture for IE:
  - Typical micro-organisms consistent with IE from two separate blood cultures: *Viridans streptococci, Streptococcus bovis,* HACEK group, *Staphylococcus aureus;* or community-acquired enterococci in the absence of a primary focus
  - Persistently positive blood culture, defined as recovery of micro-organisms consistent with IE from two samples drawn ≥ 12 h apart; or all of three or a majority of >4 separate cultures of blood (with first and last sample drawn at least 1 h apart);
  - Single positive blood culture for *Coxlella burnetti* or antiphase 1 IgG antibody titer >1:800
- Evidence of endocardial involvement:
  - Echocardiogram positive for IE: oscillating intracardiac mass on valve or supporting structures, abscess, or new partial dehiscence of prosthetic valve
  - New valvular regurgitant (↑ or change in pre-existing murmur not sufficient)

Minor criteria

- Predisposing heart condition or injection drug use
- Fever >38°C
- Vascular phenomena, such as major arterial emboli, septic pulmonary infarcts, mycotic aneurysm, intracranial hemorrhage, conjunctival hemorrhages, and Janeway's lesions
- Immunologic phenomena, such as glomerulonephritis, Osler's nodes, Roth's spots, and rheumatoid factor
- Microbiologic evidence, such as positive blood culture that does not meet a major criterion, or serologic evidence of active infection with organism consistent with IE

Box 10.5 **Treatment for endocarditis**

Pathogen	Treatment	Duration (weeks)
Penicillin (PCN)-susceptible Viridans group streptococci and *Streptococcus bovis*	PCN 12–18 million U/24 h or ceftriaxone 2 g/24 h	4
	PCN 12–18 million U/24 h or ceftriaxone 2 g/24 h + gentamicin 3 mg/kg/24 h	2
	Vancomycin 30 mg/kg/24 h	4
PCN-intermediate resistant Viridans group streptococci and *Streptococcus bovis*	PCN 24 million U/24 h or ceftriaxone 2 g/24 h	4
	PCN 24 million U/24 h or ceftriaxone 2 g/24 h + gentamicin 3 mg/kg/24 h	4
	Vancomycin 30 mg/kg/24 h	4
Enterococcal susceptible to PCN, gentamicin, and vancomycin	Ampicillin 12 g/24 h or PCN 18–30 U/24 h + gentamicin 3 mg/kg/24 h (native valves)	4–6
	Ampicillin 12 g/24 h or PCN 18–30 U/24 h + gentamicin 3 mg/kg/24 h (prosthetic valves)	6
	Vancomycin 30 mg/kg/24 h + gentamicin 3 mg/kg/24 h	6
Methicillin-sensitive *Staphylococcus aureus*	*Native valves:*	
	Nafcillin or oxacillin 12 g/24 h (with option of adding gentamicin 3 mg/kg/24 h for first 3–5 days)	6
	Cefazolin 6 g/24 h (with option of adding gentamicin 3 mg/kg/24 h for first 3–5 days)	6
	Prosthetic valves:	
	Nafcillin or oxacillin 12 g/24 h plus rifampin 900 mg/24 h + gentamicin 3 mg/kg/24 h (for first 2 weeks)	At least 6
Methicillin-resistant *Staphylococcus aureus*	Vancomycin 30 mg/kg/24 h + gentamicin 3 mg/kg/24 h	6
	Vancomycin 30 mg/kg/24 h + rifampin 900 mg/24 h plus gentamicin 3 mg/kg/24 h (for first 2 weeks)	At least 6
HACEK group	Ceftriaxone 2 g/24 h	4
	Ampicillin–sulbactam 12 g/24 h	4
	Ciprofloxacin 1000 mg/24 h PO or 800 mg/24 h IV	4

- Therapy should cover for *Staphylococcus aureus*, streptococci, enterococci, and Gram-negative bacilli
- Pseudomonas and fungal IE may require both medical and surgical therapy.
- **Surgical:** for valve IE is indicated for the following:
  - Acute IE with valve stenosis or regurgitation leading to heart failure
  - Periannular or myocardial abscess, uncontrollable infection despite anti-biotic therapy
  - Large, hypermobile vegetation with potential for embolization
  - Aggressive IE caused by highly resistant micro-organisms, fungi, or *Pseudomonas aeruginosa*
  - Unstable prosthesis (i.e. dehiscence or valve dysfunction)
  - Relapse of IE after optimal therapy.

Prophylaxis

Recent guidelines for prevention of IE indicate that "only an extremely small number of cases of infective endocarditis might be prevented by antibiotic prophylaxis for dental procedures." Antibiotic prophylaxis to prevent endo-carditis is not recommended for genitourinary or gastrointestinal procedures. Conditions which require prophylaxis prior to dental procedures are:

- Prosthetic heart valves
- Previous history of IE
- Heart transplant patients who develop valvulopathy
- CHD including unrepaired cyanotic CHD, completely repaired CHD with prosthetic material or device for the first 6 months, and repaired CHD with residual defect.

CLINICAL PEARLS

- In a patient with a prosthetic aortic valve, only the mean gradient is assessed by TTE by measuring the continuous wave across the valve.
- In patients who undergo tricuspid valve replacement, generally bioprosthetic valves are preferred to mechanical valves due to the high risk of thrombosis, as the low pressure on the right side predisposes to thrombosis.
- The following groups of patients should receive bioprostheses valve replacement: those prone to bleeding; those noncompliant with anticoagulation; older patients who are unlikely to outlive their bioprosthesis; women wishing to bear children.
- Unexplained fever in a patient with a prosthetic valve should be presumed to be endocarditis until proven otherwise.
- If valve thrombosis is suspected in a patient, the hardware can be visualized with cinefluoroscopy. Best views for mitral prosthesis are RAO cranial projection and RAO caudal or LAO cranial for aortic valve prosthesis.

(Continued)

- The most commonly infected valve in IV drug users is the tricuspid (78%), followed by the mitral (24%) and aortic (8%) valves.
- The most common congenital heart anomalies predisposing to IE are: bicuspid AV, coarctation of aorta, patent ductus arteriosis, ventricular septal defect, and tetrology of Fallot.
- Antibiotic prophylaxis is indicated in all patients with a history of valve replacement for prevention of IE. The recommended treatment is amoxicillin 2 g PO 1 h prior to procedure. Patients with PCN allergies can be treated with cephalexin or cefadroxil (2 g), azithromycin (500 mg), or clindamycin (600 mg).

Recommended Reading

Clinical Trials and Meta-Analyses

Guidelines

Bonow RO, Carabello BA, Chatterjee K et al; American College of Cardiolgy/American Heart Association Task Force on Practice Guidelines. 2008 focused update incorporated into the ACC/AHA 2006 guidelines for the management of patients with valvular heart disease: a report of the American College of Cardiology/American Heart Association Task Force on Practice Guidelines (Writing Committee to revise the 1998 guidelines for the management of patients with valvular heart disease). Endorsed by the Society of Cardiovascular Anesthesiologists, Society for Cardiovascular Angiography and Interventions and the Society of Thoracic Surgeons. *J Am Coll Cardiol* 2008;**52**(13): e1–142.

Zoghbi WA, Enriquez-Sarano M, Foster E et al; American Society of Echocardiography. Recommendations for evaluation of the severity of native valvular regurgitation with two-dimensional and Doppler echocardiography. *J Am Soc Echocardiogr* 2003;**16**(7): 777–802.

Review Articles

Otto CM. Valvular aortic stenosis: disease severity and timing of intervention. *J Am Coll Cardiol* 2006;**47**(11):2141–2151.

Rahimtoola SH. The year in valvular heart disease. *J Am Coll Cardiol* 2007;**49**(3):361–674.

11 | Diseases of the Aorta

Michael Ho and David Liang
Department of Internal Medicine, Division of Cardiology, Stanford University School of Medicine, Stanford, CA, USA

Acute Aortic Syndrome

Acute aortic syndrome is a group of conditions that result in an abrupt compromise of the aortic wall, leading to chest and back pain, and are characterized by a high risk of morbidity and mortality. These conditions include aortic dissection, intramural hematoma, penetrating atherosclerotic ulcer, and unstable aortic aneurysms (Figure 11.1).

Aortic Dissections

Acute aortic dissections are relatively rare, with an incidence of 29 per million/year; approximately one-hundredth of the incidence of acute myocardial infarctions (MIs). However, an early mortality as high as 1–2%/h for dissection of the ascending aorta and a 10% inhospital mortality for descending aortic dissections makes recognition and proper management of aortic dissections important.

- An aortic dissection usually occurs as the result of a tear in the intimal layer that leads to the exposure of a weakened medial layer to the forces of the intraluminal blood.
- Force of the pulsatile blood flow then "dissects" the layers of the aortic wall, leading to the creation of a false lumen.
- Dissection is usually propagated in an antegrade fashion; however, retrograde propagation is also possible.
- Initial tear occurs within centimeters of the aortic valve in 65% of cases, leading to ascending aortic dissections, and just distal to the left subclavain artery in most of the remainder, leading to descending aortic dissections. Disposing factors for the development of aortic dissection are:
- Long-standing hypertension
- Atherosclerosis

A Practical Approach to Cardiovascular Medicine, First Edition. Edited by Reza Ardehali, Marco Perez, Paul Wang.
© 2011 Blackwell Publishing Ltd. Published 2011 by Blackwell Publishing Ltd.

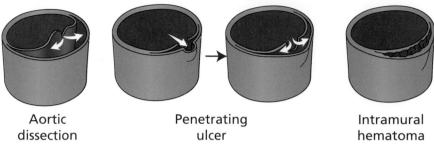

| Aortic dissection | Penetrating ulcer | Intramural hematoma |

Figure 11.1 Conditions of acute aortic syndrome

Box 11.1 Aortic dissection classification systems

Type	*Site of origin and extent of aortic involvement*
DeBakey (Figure 11.2)	
Type I	Originates in the ascending aorta, propagates at least to the aortic arch and often beyond it distally
Type II	Originates in and is confined to the ascending aorta
Type III	Originates in the descending aorta and extends distally down the aorta or, rarely, retrograde into the aortic arch and ascending aorta. Subtypes A – limited to above the diaphragm, B – extends beyond diaphragm
Stanford (Figure 11.2)	
Type A	All dissections involving the ascending aorta, regardless of the site of origin
Type B	All dissections not involving the ascending aorta

- Inherent weakness in the tissue of the aorta, such as occurs in bicuspid aortic valve disease
- Marfan syndrome.

Iatrogenic contributing factors are intra-aortic blood pump placement and cardiac surgery, particularly in those undergoing aortic valve replacement.

Outcomes and treatment of aortic dissections are dictated by their anatomic location and extent. Dissections are classified using either the Stanford or the DeBakey systems (Box 11.1 and Figure 11.2).

Diagnosis

Prompt diagnosis is dependent upon a high level of vigilance for features in the history and exam that should lead to definitive testing. Once the decision is made to proceed to definitive testing with CT, MRI, or transesophageal echocardiography (TEE), the sensitivity and specificity in detecting aortic

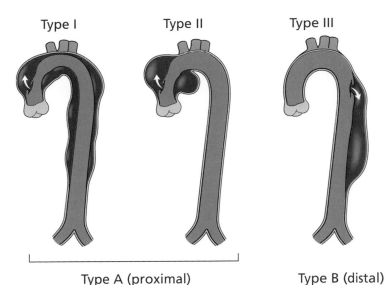

Figure 11.2 DeBakey and Stanford classifications

Table 11.1 Relative utility of symptoms/findings in diagnosis of aortic dissection

Symptom/findings	Sensitivity	Specificity
Abrupt onset of pain	++	+
Ripping/tearing pain	+	++
Migratory pain	–	++
Back pain	+	+
Pulse deficit	–	+++
Aortic insufficiency	+	++
Neurologic deficit	–	+++

dissection is excellent. Table 11.1 gives the relative utility of common symptoms and initial findings in the diagnosis of aortic dissection.

The presence of factors predisposing to aortic dissection must also be weighed in considering the diagnosis. These include:
- Family history of aortic aneurysm or dissection, particularly if it occurred at a young age (<55)
- Known or suspected connective tissue abnormality, e.g. Marfan syndrome, Loeys–Dietz syndrome, or Ehlers–Danlos syndrome – vascular type
- Bicuspid aortic valve
- Pre-existing aneurysm
- Hypertension and/or atherosclerosis – more important in older patients
- Recent cardiac surgery or intravascular procedure.

Chest X-ray findings may lend support in patients suspected of having aortic dissection, but the findings are nonspecific and rarely diagnostic. The most common abnormality seen is widening of the aortic and/or mediastinal silhouettes. ECG findings in patients with aortic dissection are nonspecific.

An abnormal D-dimer has been shown in small series to be highly sensitive for aortic dissection; however, its limited specificity and the limited size of the studies make its role in diagnosing aortic dissection unclear.

The high hourly mortality rate of aortic dissection, particularly ascending aortic dissection, mandates that when the suspicion is high enough to warrant definitive testing, it should be performed promptly:

- Echocardiography, MRI, and CT can all provide near perfect diagnostic accuracy when performed properly.
- **Computed tomography:**
  - Most commonly used diagnostic study due to its immediate availability in most emergency rooms and high degree of accuracy when performed properly
  - Optimum diagnostic accuracy is only achieved if rapid scanning is performed with a spiral sequence and a well-timed contrast injection
  - Noncontrast as well as contrast images should be obtained to improve the ability to discriminate intramural hematoma
  - Cardiac gating is necessary to freeze the motion of the aortic root
  - In cases where the diagnosis of aortic dissection is strongly suspected, e.g. in the presence of a pulse deficit, the abdomen and pelvis should be included in the scan to determine the effect of the dissection on the perfusion to the major branch vessels to the viscera and periphery
  - High dose of contrast and radiation involved in a CT angiogram, however, should be taken into consideration when the level of suspicion is lower.
- **Echocardiography:**
  - Can play an adjunctive role or a primary diagnostic role
  - **Transthoracic:**
    - Limited sensitivity for detecting aortic dissections
    - Can identify features that raise or lower the probability of aortic dissection in patients where the suspicion for dissection is not sufficient to warrant proceeding to more definitive testing, e.g. identification of an aortic root aneurysm or aortic insufficiency would raise the suspicion of an aortic dissection, whereas the finding of a segmental wall motion abnormality would direct attention toward coronary artery disease (CAD)
    - Additional information essential to the management of the patient with a dissection is also obtained, including aortic valve and left ventricular function
  - **Transesophageal:**
    - Sufficient accuracy to be a definitive tool in the diagnosis of thoracic aortic dissection
    - Due to its portability, particularly valuable when the patient is unstable, allowing the exam to be performed in the ICU or the operating room

- Due to the discomfort of the procedure, consideration should be given to elective intubation prior to the procedure in patients with a high suspicion of dissection
- Understanding of the dissection and its effect on peripheral perfusion is not as well characterized with TEE as it is with a CT scan.
- **Magnetic resonance imaging:**
  - Also highly accurate in the diagnosis of aortic dissection
  - Its role as an emergent diagnostic tool is limited by its availability, length of scan, and difficulty in monitoring the patient during the procedure
  - Primary role is in follow-up of dissections and in the few cases where the diagnosis remains in doubt after other forms of imaging.
- Aortography has no role as a primary tool in diagnosis of aortic dissection due to its invasive nature and limited accuracy. It should only be used as a component of a planned intervention or where dissection is suspected during an interventional procedure.

Treatment

Initial therapy for aortic dissection aims to halt progression of the dissection and should be started once dissection is suspected rather than waiting for definitive diagnosis. Acute dissections involving the ascending aorta are surgical emergencies. In contrast, dissections confined to the descending aorta are treated medically unless the patient demonstrates progression of dissection, organ or limb ischemia, or intractable pain.

Medical Management

- Heart rate and BP monitoring (consider arterial line placement).
- BP control with a goal of systolic BP (SBP) <110 mmHg or the lowest BP that maintains adequate end-organ perfusion:
  - Initial therapy should be with an intravenous beta-blocker to limit the rate of rise of the arterial pressure (dP/dt). A short-acting agent, such as esmolol, is preferred and should be titrated until the heart rate is <60 bpm or until no further effect is seen
  - Intravenous verapamil may be substituted in those patients intolerant of beta-blockers
  - A direct vasodilator, such as nitroprusside, may then be added to reach BP targets.
- Pain relief is important to reduce adrenergic stimulation and liberal use of intravenous narcotics is warranted.

Ascending Dissections

Surgery is the definitive treatment in acute ascending aortic dissection.

- Urgent intervention is required to prevent death due to tamponade or rupture.
- Surgery involves replacement of a portion of the ascending aorta and in some cases the aortic arch.

- False lumen is seldom obliterated distally; however, the interposed graft prevents retrograde extension of the dissection to the heart.
- In cases where the aortic root is significantly dilated, the root should be replaced and the coronary arteries reimplanted.

Operative mortality for ascending aortic dissections varies between 15% and 35%. Since the distal aorta frequently remains dissected following surgery, the issues associated with managing a descending aortic dissection should be kept in mind even after a successful surgery.

Descending Dissections
Currently most dissections limited to the descending aorta are managed medically.

- After BP and pain are controlled, the patient may be transitioned to oral antihypertensives and analgesics, and mobilized.
- When possible, a beta-blocker should remain a part of the medical regimen.
- Follow-up imaging should be performed prior to discharge or if pain persists.
- If features suggestive of imminent rupture are present, e.g. rapid false lumen expansion or contained blood in the periadventitial are present, the patient should be referred for surgery.

There are ongoing studies of the use of thoracic stent grafts to cover the primary intimal tear in acute descending aortic dissections, but for now these must be considered investigational.

Follow-up
- Dissected aorta following initial surgery and/or medical stabilization remains weakened and at risk for aneurysm formation.
- Close follow-up with imaging, such as CT or MRI, should be performed until the aorta stabilizes, typically at 1 month following dissection, and then at 3-month intervals until the aorta stabilizes.
- Thereafter, scanning should be performed annually in most cases.
- Until the aorta stabilizes isometric exercise and exercise beyond mild aerobic activities should be avoided.

Complications
- **Cardiac tamponade:**
  - Most common cause of death in ascending aortic dissections
  - Occurs as a consequence of retrograde extension of the dissection into the pericardium
  - In general, pericardial effusion when the patient has an adequate BP, even though features of tamponade are present, should be handled with emergent surgery
  - In rare cases pericardiocentesis may be needed as a temporizing step.
- **End-organ ischemia:**
  - Can occur in dissections due to their direct extension into the branch vessel occluding flow, or to collapse of the true lumen by increased pressure in the false lumen

- Peripheral pulses must be monitored closely and signs of visceral ischemia should not be overlooked
- Back pain, refractory hypertension, decreased urine output or rising creatinine should prompt concern for renal ischemia
- Abdominal pain (particularly post-prandial), nausea, anorexia, acidosis, and bloody stools may be indicative of bowel and or pancreatic ischemia
- If direct extension of the dissection is the cause of ischemia, stenting of the involved vessel is usually adequate for restoring flow
- If true lumen collapse is the cause of ischemia:
  - False lumen must be depressurized to allow the true lumen to expand
  - This may be done by allowing freer exit of blood from the false lumen by fenestrating the dissection flap beyond the area of collapse, either percutaneously or surgically
  - Alternatively, flow into the false lumen can be decreased by surgically replacing a segment of the aorta and oversewing the false lumen, or by covering the primary intimal tear with a stent graft
  - Use of a stent graft is relatively contraindicated in patients with connective tissue abnormalities, such as Marfan syndrome, due to the stiffness of current stent grafts and the fragility of the aorta in these cases.
- **Spinal cord ischemia:**
  - A rare complication of aortic dissection, but is particularly devastating
  - Neurologic symptoms should be taken very seriously in patients with dissections
  - Should evidence of cord ischemia occur, imaging should be undertaken to identify the cause; however, typically the involved intercostal spinal arteries are too small for direct intervention
  - BP control should be liberalized to some extent to improve perfusion from collaterals
  - Lumbar drain should also be placed to remove excessive CSF fluid which may impair circulation in an ischemic cord.

Intramural Hematoma (IMH)

- Aortic IMH may originate from rupture of the vasa vasorum in the medial wall and lack an intimal tear, or may represent a dissection with complete thromboses of the false lumen.
- It cannot be clinically distinguished from a true aortic dissection, as both have similar risk factors, signs, and symptoms.
- On imaging studies, IMH appears as a crescentic thickening of the aortic wall, with no evidence of flow within the hematoma. Aortography may often fail to make the diagnosis.

Penetrating Atherosclerotic Ulcer (PAU)

- PAU is an ulceration of an atherosclerotic plaque penetrating into the medial layer, which may lead to intramural hematoma, aneurysm formation, dissection, or rupture.

- Predominantly found in the descending thoracic aorta.
- Endovascular stent grafting is emerging as a therapeutic modality over conventional surgical repair.

Treatment strategies for IMH and PAU mirror those of true dissection: surgical intervention for proximal lesions and medical management for distal involvement. Serial imaging studies are necessary to monitor progression or regression. Medical management of ascending aortic IMH may be acceptable if the aorta is not excessively dilated, but close monitoring is essential.

Congenital Aortic Diseases

Coarctation of the Aorta

A defect of the aortic wall that results in a focal narrowing classically in the point immediately distal to the origin of the left subclavian artery (Figure 11.3). It accounts for 5–8% of all congenital heart defects. It may occur as an isolated defect or in association with various other lesions, most commonly bicuspid aortic valve, ventricular septal defect (VSD), and cerebral aneurysms. Coarctation of the aorta is a common cardiac defect associated with Turner's syndrome.

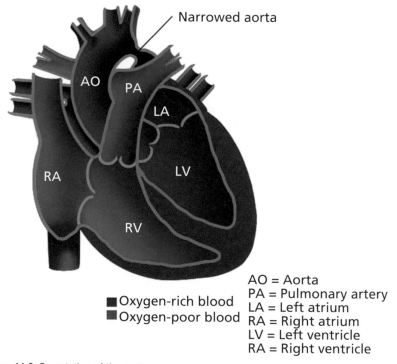

Figure 11.3 Coarctation of the aorta

Autopsy studies suggest that the mortality rate in patients who do not undergo surgical repair is 90% by age 50 years, with a mean lifespan of 35 years. Associated problems that may contribute to death or morbidity include hypertension, intracranial hemorrhage, aortic aneursym or dissection, endocarditis, and congestive heart failure (CHF).

Diagnosis
- **Physical exam:**
  - Classic finding is elevated BP in the upper extremities with diminished or delayed femoral pulses
  - A systolic murmur may be heard over the back, as well as a continuous murmur in the precordium secondary to collateral vessels.
- **Echocardiography:**
  - Primary diagnostic tool in infants and children
  - In adults, clear visualization of the descending aorta and accurate Doppler velocities may be difficult to obtain
  - A full echo study is important for evaluation of valvular function and ruling out structural defects.
- **CT/MRI:**
  - Offers full anatomic detail of the region of coarctation, as well as involvement of branch vessels and formation of collaterals.
- **Angiography:**
  - Allows for direct hemodynamic assessment of the gradient across the coarctation
  - Intervention is typically considered when the peak gradient is >20 mmHg.

Treatment
Treatment depends upon age, clinical presentation, and morphology of the lesion. Medical management is warranted in asymptomatic patients without arterial hypertension.

Indications for intervention are:
- Refractory hypertension
- Development of heart failure
- Hemodynamically significant aortic stenosis (peak gradient >20 mmHg)
- Female patients contemplating pregnancy.

Corrective interventions include surgery and balloon angioplasty with or without stent placement.
- **Surgical repair:**
  - Involves resection of the area of coarctation with either end-to-end anastomosis or placement of a bypass graft
  - Preferred option for neonates.
- **Balloon angioplasty:**
  - Recommended as the preferred treatment for children and adults with native coarctation or recoarctation after surgery

- Initial success rate, defined as a gradient <20 mmHg across the coarctation, is approximately 80–90%
- Long-term complications include recoarctation and development of aortic aneurysm
- Due to high recurrence rates, balloon angioplasty is not optimal for infants <6 months of age
- Stent implantation following balloon angioplasty improves luminal diameter and results in a minimal residual gradient. The stent can be dilated as the child grows.

Acquired Aortic Diseases

Aortic Aneurysm

Aortic aneurysm refers to a pathologic dilatation of the aortic lumen >50% of the expected normal diameter for the given aortic segment. The etiology is multifactorial and the condition occurs in individuals with multiple risk factors. Aneurysms are more common in men than in women. Management includes serial monitoring to prevent catastrophic rupture.

Abdominal Aortic Aneurysm

Abdominal aortic aneurysms (AAA) are much more common (up to 75% of aneurysms) than thoracic aortic aneurysms. Incidence increases dramatically after age 55 in men and 70 in women. Approximately 15 000 deaths annually in the United States are attributed to AAAs.

Atherosclerosis is the underlying cause of AAAs. Associated risk factors are tobacco use, age, hypertension, and hyperlipidemia.

- Majority of AAAs arise below the renal arteries and are known as infrarenal aneurysms; aneurysms that arise between the level of the diaphragm and the renal arteries are termed suprarenal aneurysms.
- Over 80% of AAAs expand over time, at a mean rate of ~0.4 cm/year. Increasing aneurysmal size is proportional to the risk of rupture. Aneurysms >7 cm have a 20%/year risk of rupture.
- When rupture does occur, 80% open into the left retroperitoneum, which may contain the bleeding. The remainder tend to rupture into the peritoneal cavity, leading to exsanguination and rapid cardiovascular collapse.
- Operative mortality for emergent surgery is 50%.

Clinical Manifestations
- Majority of AAAs are asymptomatic and discovered incidentally on routine physical examination or on imaging studies ordered for other indications.
- In cases of rapid enlargement or impending rupture, severe pain may be reported in the hypogastrium, flank, or lower back.
- On examination, a pulsatile mass may be palpated in the periumbilical region.
- Accurate assessment of size cannot be done by exam alone.

- Associated vascular disease may manifest as abdominal or femoral bruits, as well as diminished distal pulses.

Diagnosis
- **Abdominal ultrasound:**
  - Most practical method of AAA screening
  - Accurately defines aneurysm size to within ±0.3 cm
  - Ultrasonography is limited in its ability to visualize the entire length of aorta and define the anatomy of branch vessels; insufficient for surgical planning
  - The US Preventive Services Task Force recommends one-time screening for AAA by ultrasound in men aged 65–75 years who have ever smoked.
- **CT/MR angiography:**
  - Allows accurate assessment of aneurysm size (to within 0.2 cm) and morphology
  - Both routinely used for serial monitoring of aneurysm size and provide comprehensive anatomic detail of branch vessels for preoperative evaluation.
- **Aortography:**
  - Used for preoperative evaluation in limited cases.

Treatment
- **Medical treatment:**
  - Aimed at slowing the progression of expansion and decreasing the risk of rupture
  - Beta-blockers are first-line agents that decrease BP and dP/dt of the aortic wall
  - Risk factor management with smoking cessation, antihypertensive therapy, and lipid-lowering agents
  - Serial screening by CT or MRA is warranted every 6 months and more frequently in higher risk patients
  - Half of all perioperative deaths from aneurysm repair result from acute MI. Therefore, all patients being considered for AAA repair need preoperative risk assessment with evaluation for presence and severity of CAD.
- **Surgical repair:**
  - Involves placement of a synthetic Dacron graft in the area of aneurysm with reimplantation of branch vessels
  - Timing of surgery is not definitively defined, though aneurysm size remains the primary indicator for repair
  - Generally, elective repair is recommended for aneurysms ≥5.5 cm in diameter and for those enlarging >0.5 cm/year or in symptomatic patients. A smaller threshold diameter for surgery may be appropriate in women due to a higher rupture rate among women at any given aneurysm size.

- **Percutaneous endovascular stent-graft placement:**
  - Less invasive alternative to open surgery for aneurysms with suitable anatomy
  - Major complication is the frequent occurrence of endoleaks into aneurysm sac, which may lead to further aneurysm expansion or rupture
  - Randomized trials comparing surgery to stent grafting have shown decreased initial mortality and morbidity with stent grafting at the cost of increased need for revision of the repair during follow-up (9% vs 1.7% at 4 years). Long-term outcomes compared to conventional surgical repair suggest similar survival rates.

Thoracic Aortic Aneurysms

Thoracic aortic aneurysms (TAAs) are much less common than AAAs and are classified by the segment of aorta involved:
- Ascending aorta (60%)
- Descending thoracic aorta (40%)
- Arch (10%).

Etiology
- Cystic medial degeneration
- Atherosclerosis
- Traumatic injury
- Chronic infection (syphilis, tuberculosis)
- Connective tissue disorders (Marfan syndrome, Ehlers–Danlos)
- Inflammatory disorders (Takayasu, giant cell arteritis)

Clinical Manifestations
- More than half of patients with thoracic aortic aneurysms are asymptomatic at the time of diagnosis.
- Most are identified as incidental findings on physical exam, chest radiograph, or CT scan.
- Development of symptoms often occur secondary to vascular consequence or compressive mass effect.
- Vascular consequences include:
  - Aortic regurgitation from dilatation of the aortic root
  - Thromboembolism causing stroke
  - Peripheral ischemia.
- Local mass effect from an ascending or arch aneurysm may cause compression of the superior vena cava (SVC), trachea, esophagus, and recurrent laryngeal nerve.
- Most serious consequence is dissection, leakage, or rupture, which can be associated with acute onset of severe pain.
- Rupture occurs into:
  - Left intrapleural space or the mediastinum (most common)
  - Esophagus, forming an aortoesophageal fistula which manifests with massive hematemesis.

Diagnosis
- Chest radiograph: large TAA may exhibit widening of the mediastinal silhouette, enlargement of the aortic knob, or displacement of the trachea from the midline.
- Transthoracic echocardiography (TTE): excellent modality for imaging the aortic root, which is important for patients with Marfan syndrome, but does not offer reliable views of the remainder of the ascending, arch, or descending aorta.
- TEE: can visualize the entire thoracic aorta
- CT and MRI: preferred imaging techniques to detect a TAA, determine its size, and clearly evaluate morphology and branch vessel anatomy. MRI is preferred for aneurysms involving the aortic root
- Aortography: reserved for preoperative evaluation in a limited number of cases.

Treatment
Surgical therapy is often recommended prophylactically to prevent the morbidity and mortality associated with aneurysm rupture. For aneurysms <5 cm, the optimal timing of surgery is uncertain since the natural history is variable

Indications for surgery:
- Presence of aneurysm-related symptoms
- Diameter of 5–6 cm for an ascending aortic aneurysm and 6–7 cm for a descending aortic aneurysm
- In patients with Marfan syndrome, bicuspid aortic valve, or a familial thoracic aortic aneurysm syndrome, surgical repair is recommended earlier (at 5 cm) due to higher risk of dissection and rupture
- Replacement before aortic size index [aortic diameter (cm) ÷ body surface area (m^2)] for the ascending aorta is 2.75 cm/m^2
- Accelerated growth rate (≥10 mm/year) in aneurysms <5 cm in diameter
- Evidence of dissection.

Takayasu Arteritis

Takayasu arteritis (TA) is a large-vessel vasculitis of young individuals that commonly affects the aorta and its major branches. Women are affected about 10 times more often than men. The median age at onset is 25 years.

It causes intimal fibroproliferation which can lead to aortic stenosis and occlusion. The pathogenesis is not clearly understood.

TA is divided into early and late phases, which may be separated by a 5–20-year interval:
- **Early phase** involves vessel inflammation that is associated with fevers, fatigue, and arthralgias
- **Late or "pulseless," phase** is characterized by arterial occlusions of various branch vessels off the proximal and distal aorta, commonly involving the left subclavian artery (50%), left common carotid artery (20%), brachiocephalic trunk, celiac, mesenteric, and renal arteries.

Aneurysm formation may occur and is most common in the aortic root, which can result in aortic insufficiency. Hypertension can be present in 40–90% of patients and is often secondary to renal artery stenosis. Cardiac, renal, and cerebrovascular diseases are the principal causes of severe morbidity and mortality.

Diagnosis

There are no specific diagnostic tests for TA. Diagnosis is based on clinical features in conjunction with vascular imaging abnormalities, both noninvasively with CT and MRI, or by catheter-based angiography.

The American College of Rheumatology has established classification criteria for TA to distinguish it from other forms of vasculitis:
- Age at disease onset <40 years
- Claudication of the extremities
- Decreased pulsation of one or both brachial arteries
- Difference of at least 10 mmHg in SBP between the arms
- Bruit over one or both subclavian arteries or the abdominal aorta
- Arteriographic narrowing or occlusion of the entire aorta, its primary branches, or large arteries in the proximal upper or lower extremities, not due to arteriosclerosis, fibromuscular dysplasia, or other causes.

Fulfillment of at least three of these criteria is suggestive of TA. Diagnosis is confirmed by histopathology, but in general biopsy is not a safe or feasible option.

Treatment
- Mainstay of treatment is corticosteroid therapy, which can improve the clinical findings and symptoms in about 50% of cases. However, remission may occur in ~40% of cases.
- Other medications in steroid-refractive cases include cyclophosphamide, methotrexate, and anti-TNF therapy.
- Angioplasty is a therapeutic option in the late phase of disease, particularly for treatment of focal stenoses.
- Stent placement may be appropriate in a small proportion of cases that are high risk for renarrowing.

CLINICAL PEARLS

- Pain of aortic dissection typically is distinguished from pain of acute MI by its abrupt onset, and is often described as ripping or tearing. A family history of aortic aneurysm or dissection is present in up to 20% of cases, even in the absence of obvious inherited syndromes; thus, a positive family history should raise the level of suspicion for aortic disease in patients presenting with suitable symptoms, and relatives of patients with aortic disease should be screened appropriately.

- A bicuspid aortic valve is a well-established risk factor for proximal aortic dissection and occurs in 5–7% of aortic dissections.
- About half of all aortic dissections in women younger than 40 years occur during pregnancy, typically in the third trimester and also occasionally in the early postpartum period.
- In the International Registry of Acute Aortic Dissection (IRAD), >12% of chest radiographs of patients with aortic dissection were read as normal.
- Proximal or type A dissections occur in about two-thirds of cases, with distal dissections comprising the remaining one-third.
- Mortality rate of patients with acute ascending aortic dissection is 1–2%/h for the first 24–48 h.
- Emergent surgery is indicated for dissections involving the ascending aorta (Stanford type A).
- Medical management, consisting of beta-blocker therapy and aggressive BP control, is preferred treatment for descending aortic dissections (Stanford type B).

Recommended Reading

Clinical Trials and Meta-Analyses

Lacro RV, Dietz HC, Wruck LM; Pediatric Heart Network Investigators. Rationale and design of a randomized clinical trial of beta-blocker therapy (atenolol) versus angiotensin II receptor blocker therapy (losartan) in individuals with Marfan syndrome. *Am Heart J* 2007;**154**:624–631.

Nienaber CA, Rousseau H, Eggebrecht H et al.; INSTEAD Trial. Randomized comparison of strategies for type B aortic dissection: the INvestigation of STEnt Grafts in Aortic Dissection (INSTEAD) trial. *Circulation* 2009;**120**:2519–2528.

Guidelines

Bonow RO, Carabello BA, Kanu C et al. American College of Cardiology/American Heart Association Task Force on Practice Guidelines; Society of Cardiovascular Anesthesiologists; Society for Cardiovascular Angiography and Interventions; Society of Thoracic Surgeons, ACC/AHA 2006 guidelines for the management of patients with valvular heart disease: a report of the American College of Cardiology/American Heart Association Task Force on Practice Guidelines: developed in collaboration with the Society of Cardiovascular Anesthesiologists: endorsed by the Society for Cardiovascular Angiography and Interventions and the Society of Thoracic Surgeons. *Circulation* 2006;**114**:e84–231.

Review Articles

Golledge J, Eagle KA. Acute aortic dissection. *Lancet* 2008;**372**:55–66.

Lederle FA. In the clinic. Abdominal aortic aneurysm. *Ann Intern Med* 2009;**150**: ITC5-1–15.

Weyand CM, Goronzy JJ. Medium- and large-vessel vasculitis. *N Engl J Med* 2003;**349**: 160–169.

12 Peripheral Vascular Disease

Andrew Wilson, Reza Ardehali, and John Cooke
Department of Internal Medicine, Division of Cardiology, Stanford
University School of Medicine, Stanford, CA, USA

Etiology

Peripheral artery disease (PAD) is any pathologic process causing obstruction to blood flow and its consequences in the arteries of the noncoronary and noncerebral beds.

Lower extremity PAD is chronic obstructive disease of the lower extremities, including the aorta and its terminal branches in the lower limbs. This is primarily caused by atherosclerosis (Box 12.1).

At-risk Groups
- Leg symptoms with exertion (suggestive of claudication) or ischemic rest pain (although only 10–30% of patients have classical intermittent claudication)
- Abnormal lower extremity pulse examination
- Known atherosclerotic coronary, carotid, or renal artery disease
- Age <50 years plus diabetes, and one additional risk factor (smoking, dyslipidemia, and/or hypertension)
- Age 50–69 years and history of smoking or diabetes
- Age 70 years and older

Clinical Assessment

Clinical Syndromes
Patients with PAD often present with leg discomfort. However, distribution of symptoms can vary:
- 50% asymptomatic (may or may not have functional impairment)
- 15% intermittent claudication

A Practical Approach to Cardiovascular Medicine, First Edition. Edited by Reza Ardehali,
Marco Perez, Paul Wang.
© 2011 Blackwell Publishing Ltd. Published 2011 by Blackwell Publishing Ltd.

- 33% atypical symptoms
- 2% chronic limb ischemia

Symptoms

- **Classic claudication:** lower extremity symptoms confined to the muscles with a consistent (reproducible) onset with exercise and relief with rest. The usual association between the location of pain/claudication and site of arterial lesion is given in Box 12.2.
- **"Atypical" leg pain:** lower extremity discomfort that is exertional but does not consistently resolve with rest, consistently limits exercise at a reproducible distance, or meets all "Rose questionnaire" criteria.
- **Critical limb ischemia:** ischemic rest pain (typically noted as an aching in the foot, occurring at night or with legs elevated, relieved by dependency), nonhealing wound, or gangrene.
- **Acute limb ischemia:** the five "Ps" (pain, pulselessness, pallor, paresthesias, and paralysis) are markers of the limb in jeopardy.

Box 12.1 Causes of lower limb arterial insufficiency

Large artery pathology	Small vessel pathology
Atherosclerotic disease	Diabetic or hypertensive microangiopathies
Embolic: cardiac sources, aortic aneurysm/thrombus	Vasculitis: connective tissue disease, drug related, infection (endocarditis)
Thromboangiitis obliterans (Buerger's disease)	Cholesterol emboli (e.g. postaortic instrumentation, aortic atheroembolic disease)
Rare causes: trauma, radiation, popliteal artery diseases (aneurysm, entrapment), aortic dissection, vascular malignancy	Hyperviscosity, e.g. sickle cell anemia, myeloproliferative diseases – polycythemia, thrombocytosis, cold agglutinin disease, cryoglobulinemia

---

Box 12.2 Location of pain and site of arterial lesion

Location of claudication	Common site of arterial lesion
Buttock and hip	Aortoiliac artery
Thigh	Common femoral artery
	Aortoiliac artery
Calf	Superficial femoral artery
	Popliteal artery
Foot	Tibial artery
	Peroneal artery

Box 12.3 Features of claudication and pseudoclaudication

	Claudication	Pseudoclaudication
Cause of pain	Impaired blood flow to muscles	Compression of spinal root nerves
Characteristic of discomfort	Cramping, tightness, aching, fatigue	Associated neural symptoms more common (e.g tingling, burning, numbness)
Location of discomfort	Calf buttock, hip, thigh, foot	More commonly bilateral, associated with back and/or hip pain
Exercise induced	++	±
Claudication distance	Consistent	Variable
Positional	No	Yes, sitting or bending forward at the waist may relieve pain
Relief with rest	++	±
Time to relief	<5 min	≤30 min

Clinical Features Suggesting Acute Limb Ischemia (Box 12.3)
- Sudden onset of constant pain, rest pain
- History of embolic source – atrial fibrillation, prosthetic cardiac valve
- No past history of claudication or lower limb
- Normal arterial pulses and Doppler systolic BP (SBP) in the contralateral limb

Neurologic claudication, also referred to as pseudoclaudication, is generally a result of spinal stenosis and causes similar symptoms when compared to claudication from PAD.

Assessment of the Patient with Known or Suspected PAD

History
- History suggestive of lower limb vascular insufficiency
- Cardiovascular risk factors:
  - Smoking history
  - Diabetes
  - Hypertension
  - Hyperlipidemia
- Past history:
  - Atrial fibrillation
  - Previous myocardial infarction (MI)
  - Abdominal aortic aneurysm (AAA)

- Other relevant history:
  - Connective tissue disease
  - Recent vascular instrumentation
  - Risk factors for subacute bacterial endocarditis (SBE), history of hematologic malignancy, etc.

Physical Exam
- Examination of peripheries:
  - Nail beds, capillary return, ulceration, vasculitic lesions, etc.
  - Emphasis must be placed on the inspection of peripheral pulses, including carotid, radial/ulnar, femoral, popliteal, dorsalis pedis, and posterior tibia
  - Pulse description scale: 0 = absent, 1 = diminished, 2 = normal, 3 = ectatic
- Bilateral arm BP:
  - Difference between the arm pressures of >20 mmHg is abnormal, and is usually associated with subclavian artery stenosis
  - Difference of 10–20 mmHg is suspicious for disease
- Cardiac examination:
  - Check for presence of cardiac murmurs and arrhythmias, including atrial fibrillation
  - Before palpating the carotid pulse, listen for bruits which may indicate carotid artery stenosis
  - Important to perform auscultation and palpation of the abdominal aorta to evaluate for aneurysm, as well as palpation of the popliteal space to detect aneurysm.

Noninvasive Diagnostic Tests
- Resting ankle brachial index (ABI):
  - Defined as the ratio of ankle to brachial artery SBP, with a normal value ranging between 1.0 and 1.3 (Table 12.1)
  - Simple method to confirm the presence of arterial occlusive disease
  - 85–95% sensitive and 95–99% specific for PAD
  - To calculate the ABI, SBPs are obtained using a hand-held Doppler at the brachial, posterior tibial, and dorsalis pedis arteries bilaterally. Typically,

Table 12.1 Interpretation of ABI

ABI	Interpretation
1.00–1.29	Normal
0.91–0.99	Borderline
0.50–0.90	Mild-to-moderate disease
≤0.50	Severe disease
≥1.30	Noncompressible

the ABI is calculated for a leg by using the higher of the two pedal pressures, divided by the higher of the two arm pressures.

- Measurement of ABI after treadmill testing is indicated when the resting ABI is normal or borderline but symptoms are suggestive of PAD. A fall of 20% or more in the ABI after exercise supports a PAD diagnosis
- Once the diagnosis of PAD is established, segmental limb pressures can be used to assess the extent of disease. A pressure gradient of >20 mmHg between two segments of the same limb or same levels in opposite limbs can identify the position of the occlusion as well as estimate the severity of disease.
- Duplex ultrasound:
  - Generally the first-line imaging test
  - Can confirm diagnosis and is useful for assessment of functional severity by measuring hemodynamics (Doppler velocities) across the lesion
  - Normal peripheral arterial velocity waveform consists of three phases: systolic peak forward flow; early diastolic reversal flow; late diastolic forward flow
  - As PAD worsens, there is a decrease in systolic peak flow, elimination of reversal flow in early diastole, and an increase of forward flow in late diastole.
- MR/CT angiography:
  - Give detailed anatomic information, including for the aorta, brachial, iliac, and femoral artery
  - Useful for planning therapy
  - Care must be taken in patients with impaired renal function.

Therapy

The goals of therapy include reducing the risk of major adverse cardiovascular events; alleviation of pain, improvement in perfusion, healing of ulcers, reduction of progression to chronic limb ischemia or amputation, and improvement or preservation of leg function.

Management of patients with PAD may involve medical therapy or revascularization via percutaneous or surgical approaches.

Medical therapy
- **Cardiovascular risk reduction:**
  - Smoking cessation
  - Lipid lowering
  - BP control [target 140/90 or lower in presence of comorbidity such as diabetes mellitus (DM). Reduced leg perfusion only seen with extreme BP lowering]
  - DM control [although evidence is less strong, there is reasonable evidence from the Diabetic Control and Complications Trial (DCCT) and the United Kingdom Prospective Diabetes Study (UKPDS) studies].

EVIDENCE-BASED PRACTICE

Heart Outcomes Protection Evaluation (HOPE)
Context: Substudy in PAD patients. Use of angiotensin-converting enzyme inhibitor (ACE-I) in high-risk patients.
Goal: To reduce cardiovascular disease (CVD) endpoints.
Methods: Multicenter, RCT. 4051 patients with PAD. Ramipril 10 mg daily versus placebo.
Results: 25% relative risk reduction for CVD endpoints.
Take-home message: PAD patients appear to benefit from addition of ACE-I to existing medical regimen.

- **Exercise training:**
  - Supervised and structured exercise programs beneficial in improving walking distance in patients with PAD (home-based programs are not effective)
  - Involvement in structured exercise programs associated with 100–150% improvement in maximal walking distance and improvement in quality of life
  - Guidelines for exercise programs in patients with PAD:
    - Frequency: 3–5 supervised sessions/week
    - Duration: 35–50 min of exercise
    - Type of exercise: walking to onset of pain
    - Program length: ≥6 months.
- **Pharmacotherapy:**
  - Statins improve walking distance as well reduce overall major cardiovascular events in patients with PAD
  - Cilostazol (phosphodiesterase III inhibitor; 100 mg bid) inhibits platelet aggregation and acts as an arterial vasodilator
  - Pentoxifylline (methylxanthine, 400 mg tid) decreases platelet adhesion and whole-blood viscosity. There are some conflicting data regarding its efficacy, but may be used as a second-line drug to cilostazol to improve walking distance.

EVIDENCE-BASED PRACTICE

Effect of cilostazol on patients with intermittent claudication
Context: Meta-analysis of eight studies of cilostazol in claudication.
Goal: To improve walking distance.
Methods: Meta-analysis of cilostazol therapy versus placebo of 12–24 weeks' duration.
Results: Maximal walking distance improved by 50%. Note significant placebo effects.
Take-home message: Cilostazol therapy modestly improves walking distance versus placebo in patients with claudication.

- Antiplatelet therapy – Aspirin, clopidogrel. No evidence exists regarding improvement of claudication. Clopidogrel has been shown to reduce vascular events in PAD patients versus Aspirin alone.

EVIDENCE-BASED PRACTICE

Antithrombotic Trialist's Collaboration
Context: Meta-analysis (substudy in PAD patients).
Goal: To reduce CVD endpoints
Methods: Meta-analysis of antiplatelet therapy versus placebo.
Results: 23% odds reduction for CVD endpoints.
Take-home: PAD patients should be treated with antiplatelet therapy unless contraindicated.

Revascularization

There is no evidence for therapy in asymptomatic patients. Indications include claudication but also proximal partial revascularization to facilitate healing of ulceration or relief of distal gangrene. Benefits depend on site of disease treated.

- **Aortoiliac disease:**
  - Angioplasty + vascular stenting:
    - High procedural success rates (90%)
    - Excellent long-term patency (>70% at 5 years)
    - Factors associated with a poor outcome: long segment occlusion, multifocal stenoses, eccentric calcification, poor distal run-off
  - Surgery:
    - Excellent long-term patency rate (85–90% at 5 years)
    - Requires general anesthesia
    - 1–3% mortality rate.
- **Femoropopliteal disease:**
  - Angioplasty:
    - Excellent initial procedural success
    - Reported patency varies widely (30–80% at 1 year)
    - Role of stenting less clear than in aortoiliac lesions
    - Percutaneous therapy recommended for short segment (<3 cm) disease
  - Surgery:
    - 60–80% 5-year patency rate
    - Limb salvage rates are 70% at 5 years
    - 1–3% mortality rate.
- **Acute limb ischemia:**
  - Urgent assessment indicated to identify level of lesion, extent of ischemia, and salvageable viable tissue
  - Consider endovascular therapy including lysis in the acute setting.

For critical limb ischemia not amenable or responsive to revascularization, intermittent pneumatic compression has proven useful to heal ulcers and relieve rest pain. Hyperbaric oxygen may provide modest benefit for non-healing wounds.

CLINICAL PEARLS

- Diagnosis of PAD is associated with adverse prognosis from all CVD endpoints.
- Observational studies have revealed higher prevalence of PAD in blacks and non-Hispanic whites compared to Asians and Hispanics.
- CVD endpoints can be reduced with smoking cessation, statins, ACE-I, beta-blockers, and clopidogrel therapy.
- Cornerstone of therapy in the asymptomatic patient with PAD is CVD risk reduction.
- ABI and segmental pressure measurements can be artificially elevated in patients with noncompressible vessels; most commonly observed in elderly diabetic patients.
- Cilostazol should be taken 30 min before or 2 h after a meal. This is due to an increased absorption in the presence of fatty meals.
- Revascularization for claudication is indicated only if exercise programs and medical therapy provide insufficient relief. It must be assessed on a case-by-case basis.
- Endovascular therapy is very effective for aortoiliac and short-segment femoropopliteal disease.
- Atheroembolic disease usually presents with bilateral painful ischemic toes and feet. A history of abdominal aortic aneurysm or recent arterial procedures is common. Pulses may be normal.

Recommended Reading

Clinical Trials and Meta-Analyses

McDermott MM, Ades P, Guralnik JM et al. Treadmill exercise and resistance training in patients with peripheral arterial disease with and without intermittent claudication: a randomized controlled trial. *JAMA* 2009;**301**(2):165–174.

Guidelines

Hirsch AT, Haskal ZJ, Hertzer NR et al.; American Association for Vascular Surgery; Society for Vascular Surgery; Society for Cardiovascular Agniography and Interventions; Society for Vascular Medicine and Biology; Society for Interventional Radiology; ACC/AHA Task Force on Practice Guidelines Writing Committee to Develop Guidelines for the Management of Patients with Peripheral Arterial Disease; American Association for Cardiovascular and Pulmonary Rehabilitation; National Heart, Lung, and Blood Institute; Society for Vascular Nursing; TransAtlantic Inter-Society Consensus; Vascular Disease Foundation. ACC/AHA 2005 Practice Guidelines for the management of patients with peripheral arterial disease (lower extremity, renal, mesenteric, and abdominal aortic). *Circulation* 2006;**113**(11) e463–654.

Review Articles

Hankey GJ, Norman PE, Eikelboom JW. Medical treatment of peripheral arterial disease. *JAMA* 2006;**295**:547–553.

Hirsch AT, Criqui MH, Treat-Jacobsen D et al. Peripheral arterial disease detection, awareness and management in primary care. *JAMA* 2001;**286**:1317–1324.

Stewart KJ, Hiatt WR, Regensteiner JG. Exercise training for claudication. *N Engl J Med* 2002; **347**:1941–1951.

V Arrhythmias and Sudden Cardiac Death

13 Atrial Fibrillation and Flutter

Marco Perez and Amin Al-Ahmad

Department of Internal Medicine, Division of Cardiology, Stanford
University School of Medicine, Stanford, CA, USA

Atrial Fibrillation

- Atrial fibrillation (AF) is characterized by disorganized electrical activity in the atrium leading to loss of effective atrial contraction (Figures 13.1 and 13.2).
- Most common arrhythmia, affecting 1% of the United States population.
- Associated with an increased risk of stroke (up to 5% per person/year in the elderly) and death.

Classification

- **Paroxysmal:** recurrent episodes lasting <7 days
- **Persistent:** recurrent episodes lasting >7 days, often requiring cardioversion
- **Permanent:** episodes lasting >1 year
  Other terminology used:
- Lone AF:
  - No associated hypertension or evidence of cardiopulmonary disease
  - Usually applies to younger patients, with a stronger genetic link
  - Implies a lower risk of thromboembolism
  - Can be paroxysmal, persistent, or permanent
- Acquired AF: not lone AF
- Chronic AF: term formerly used to refer to permanent AF
- Familial AF: AF that runs in families with a Mendelian pattern of inheritance.

Work-up of New-Onset AF

- Assess for associated conditions: hypertension, heart failure, valvular disease, chronic obstructive pulmonary disease (COPD), pulmonary embolism, hypertrophic cardiomyopathy, myocardial infarction (MI),

---

A Practical Approach to Cardiovascular Medicine, First Edition. Edited by Reza Ardehali, Marco Perez, Paul Wang.

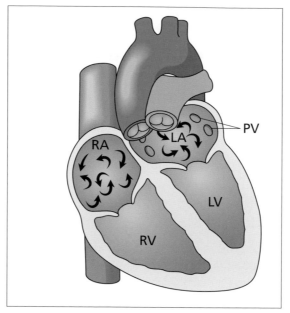

Figure 13.1 Disorganized electrical activity in atrial fibrillation. PV, pulmonary vein

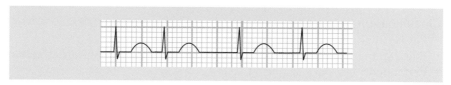

Figure 13.2 Characteristic ECG hallmarks of AF: irregular rhythm and poorly defined P-waves

hyperthyroidism, endocarditis, binge drinking, excessive caffeine, diabetes mellitus (DM).
- **Routine tests** to consider:
  - Echo:
    - Consider in all patients
    - High yield for younger patients or undiagnosed cardiopulmonary disease
  - TSH: low yield (<1% of new AF have hyperthyroidism), but routinely done
  - Fasting glucose: if DM not already established.
- **Hospitalization:** consider if:
  - Rate control and hemodynamic stability are not achieved
  - MI is suspected (ST abnormalities, chest pain)
  - Evidence of heart failure.
- **Acute cardioversion:** consider if:
  - Hemodynamically unstable
  - Heart failure believed to be secondary to or worsened by AF
  - Signs of end-organ damage: chest pain, altered mental status, renal failure.

Rate and Rhythm Control

In older, asymptomatic patients, who account for the vast majority of patients with AF, **rate control** is the first-line therapy.

Consider **rhythm control** if:
- Patient is symptomatic
- Adequate rate control cannot be achieved or drop in ejection fraction (EF) is attributed to tachycardia
- Patient is young or has their first episode of AF.

EVIDENCE-BASED PRACTICE

Atrial Fibrillation Follow-up Investigation of Rhythm Management (AFFIRM)

Context: Debate as to whether or not aggressive rhythm control is warranted in asymptomatic patients.

Goal: To compare outcomes in patients randomized to rate versus rhythm control.

Methods: Multicenter, RCT. 4060 patients >65 years old or risk factors; symptomatic patients excluded.

Results: No significant difference in mortality or stroke between groups.

Take-home message: Recommend rate control if patient is truly asymptomatic.

Controlling Heart Rate

Target heart rate (HR) is <80bpm at rest and <110bpm during normal activities.
- Beta-blockers:
  - Older patients, concomitant cardiovascular disease
  - Success is only slightly higher compared with calcium channel blockers (CCBs) or digoxin
- CCBs:
  - Younger, more active patients; side effects from beta-blockers
- Digoxin:
  - Good as a second agent when beta-blocker or CCB are insufficient
  - Alone is generally not preferred because of the associated toxicities and need for monitoring.

Achieving Sinus Rhythm

The choice of drugs versus electric shock is guided by patient and physician preference.
- **Drugs:**
  - Pharmacologic conversion is less efficacious and carries a higher risk of ventricular arrhythmia
  - Does not require sedation
  - Ibutilide is most efficacious, closely followed by flecainide and dofetilide
  - Amiodarone and propafenone are moderately effective

- Sotalol is generally not effective
- Class Ic agents are contraindicated in those with structural heart disease.
- **Electric shock:**
  - Sedation is necessary if nonemergent
  - Anterior (sternum) and posterior (left scapula) placement of pads is most effective
  - **Biphasic:** 50 J for <48 h, 100 J for <7 days, 150 J for >7 days. Titrate to max 200 J
  - **Monophasic:** 100 J for <48 h, 150 J for <7 days, 200 J for >7 days. Titrate to max 360 J
  - Biphasic more efficacious. Patients with a permanent pacemaker (PPM)/ implantable cardioverter defibrillator (ICD) should have these devices interrogated. Higher energy should be considered in obese or large individuals.
- Anticoagulation:
  - Periprocedural stroke rates are as high as 7% in those who are not anticoagulated
  - Therapeutic anticoagulation (INR 2–3) must be documented for 3 weeks prior to cardioversion, otherwise transesophageal echocardiography (TEE) should be performed
  - Continue anticoagulation for 4 weeks.

Maintaining Sinus Rhythm
- Goal is to select an effective agent with minimal risk and toxicity (Figures 13.3 and 13.4).
- Amiodarone has the lowest risk of ventricular arrhythmia, but has several associated toxicities and is reserved for those with structural heart disease.

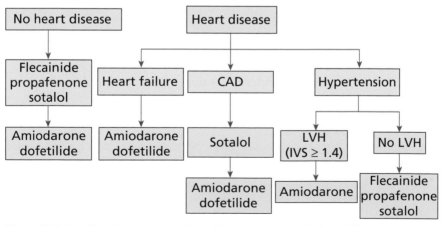

Figure 13.3 Algorithm for pharmacologic maintenance of sinus rhythm. CAD, coronary artery disease; LVH, left ventricular hypertrophy; IVS, intraventricular septal thickness

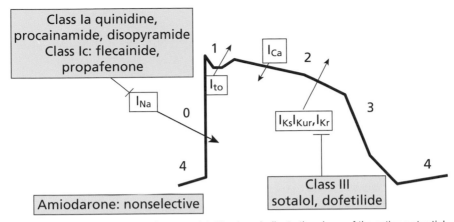

Figure 13.4 Myocardial cell action potential. Numbers indicate the phase of the action potential. Arrows pointing towards the center depict a net cellular influx of ions throughout the corresponding ion channels

---

Box 13.1 Dosing recommendations in AF

- **Amiodarone:** Goal = 8 g load, regimens vary. Suggest 1 mg/h x 6 h IV, then 0.5 mg/h, or 400 mg PO bid. After loading, most patients can be maintained on 200 mg qd
- **Sotalol:** Dose calculated based on age, weight, and creatinine (www.betapaceaf.com)
- **Flecainide:** Start 50 mg bid, increase by 50 mg bid q4d to 150 mg bid. Sustained-release formulation is available. Should be given with an AV nodal blocking agent
- **Propafenone:** 150 mg q8h, then titrate to max 300 mg q8h. Should be given with an AV nodal blocking agent
- **Dofetilide:** Dose depends on creatinine and QTc. Patient must be monitored during load. The following medications must be discontinued: cimetidine, CCB, trimethoprim, ketoconazole, hydrochlorothiazide, prochlorperazine, megestrol

Each antiarrhythmic agent carries risk of VT or torsades; monitor QTc closely

---

- Class Ic agents (flecainide and propafenone) are first-line agents for those with no structural heart disease.
- Class III agents (sotalol, dofetilide) are effective but carry a higher risk of torsades, and inpatient loading is recommended.
- Class Ia agents are generally not as effective and generally are not used. Dosing recommendations are given in Box 13.1.

Second-Line Management
- **AV node ablation + pacemaker:**
  - For patients in whom rate control is desired but cannot be achieved with medications alone
  - Usually performed in the older, less active population
  - No evidence of survival advantage but may be associated with improved resting symptoms.
- **Pill-in-the-pocket:**
  - Reserved for patients who rarely have paroxysms (once or twice a year) and prefer not to take daily medication
  - Propafenone (450 mg for <70 kg, 600 mg for >70 kg) after successful inpatient conversion and observation has been studied.
- **Catheter ablation (Figure 13.5):**
  - Consider in patients who have symptomatic AF and have failed antiarrhythmic agents
  - Techniques vary, but all involve electrically isolating pulmonary vein potentials and ablating fractionated electric signals
  - Majority of experience is in young patients with paroxysmal AF where success rates are of the order of 80% and major complications about 1%
  - Ablation in patients with permanent AF is less well studied, but success is of the order of 50%

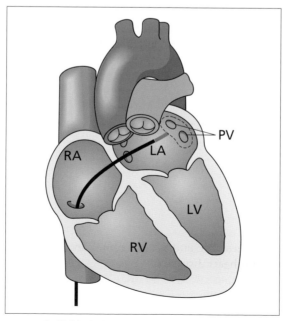

Figure 13.5 Pulmonary vein (PV) isolation via a transseptal catheter ablation approach

- Repeat ablations are often necessary
- Need for long-term anticoagulation after successful ablation is still controversial.
- **MAZE procedure**:
  - Consider in patients who undergo thoracic surgery for other indications, such as coronary artery bypass graft (CABG) or valvular surgery
  - Original MAZE procedure involved elaborate and time-consuming cutting and suturing around critical structures, resulting in success rates >90%
  - Modified techniques use ablative therapy thereby saving time, but do result in a slightly lower success rates.
- **Adjuvant therapies**:
  - AF can be thought of as a manifestation of diseased atrial tissue
  - As in ventricular heart failure, several medications such as angiotensin-converting enzyme inhibitors (ACE-Is), angiotensin receptor II blockers (ARBs), and statins may reduce AF burden; randomized trials designed to demonstrate this are ongoing.

Stroke Prophylaxis

- Stroke remains the most devastating consequence of AF.
- Risk of thromboembolism rises with age and associated risk factors.
- Patients with lone AF, younger than 60 years of age without any risk factors, have stroke rates of 1% per year and can be treated with Aspirin (ASA) alone (Figure 13.6).
- Most other patients should be placed on warfarin with a goal INR of 2–3.
- Plavix + ASA is not as effective as coumadin, but is more effective than ASA alone.

  CHADS2 scores are often used to help determine risk of stroke (Figure 13.6):
- 0: low risk and may be treated with ASA alone
- ≥3 or prior stroke/transient ischemic attack (TIA): high risk and benefit most from anticoagulation
- 1–2: intermediate risk and choice of anticoagulation is individualized.

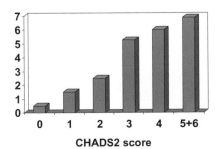

Adjusted stroke rate (%/year)

Criteria	score
Prior stroke/TIA	2
Age > 75 years	1
Hypertension	1
Diabetes	1
Heart failure	1

CHADS2 score

Figure 13.6 CHADS2 score for prediction of rate of stroke

Managing Special Situations

Symptomatic Rapid Ventricular Response (RVR)

Hemodynamically unstable patients should undergo immediate cardioversion. Stable patients may receive intravenous beta-blockers or CCB for quick and effective rate control.

Suggested regimens:
- Metoprolol:
  - 1.25–5 mg IV, titrate initial dose to response, max 15 mg q3–6h.
- Diltiazem:
  - 0.25 mg/kg initial bolus; 0.35 mg/kg repeat bolus in 15 min if needed
  - Drip 10 mg/h, then titrate to effect with max 15 mg/h.

Start comparable oral agent early and quickly titrate off IV formulation. Consider cardioversion if rate control is inadequate and symptoms persist.

Postoperative AF

- Highest incidence (up to 40%) after cardiothoracic surgery.
- Unstable patients should be cardioverted.
- Patients with permanent AF can be managed with rate control.
- Stable patients with new AF can be cardioverted (see above).
- It is reasonable to continue antiarrhythmic use for 4 weeks after cardioversion.
- Long-term anticoagulation usually not indicated if sinus rhythm is maintained.
- Routine prophylaxis with statins, steroids, or antiarrhythmics is under investigation.

CLINICAL PEARLS

- Holter monitor may help assess adequacy of rate control.
- Adding digoxin to a beta-blocker or CCB can result in better rate control.
- Patients undergoing electrical cardioversion should have an antiarrhythmic started beforehand.
- Consider MAZE procedure in patients with AF undergoing other cardiac surgeries.

Atrial Flutter

- Atrial flutter (AFL) refers to a macro-re-entrant atrial tachyarrhythmia (Figure 13.7).
- Risk of AFL increases with age, is often associated with AF, and is almost always associated with structural heart disease.

Classification

The distinction between typical and atypical AFL has important therapeutic implications and can often be made on surface ECG analysis.

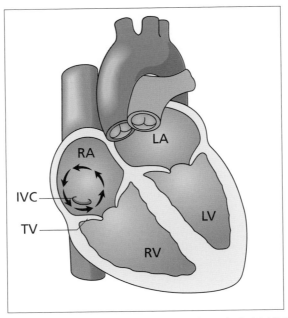

Figure 13.7 Circuit depicting counter-clockwise, isthmus-dependent atrial flutter. TV, tricuspid valve; IVC, inferior vena cava

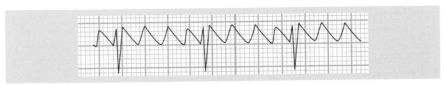

Figure 13.8 Characteristic ECG hallmarks of Type I (typical) atrial flutter: "saw tooth" flutter (F)-waves; no isoelectric interval in II, III, aVF; atrial rate usually 300 bpm; 2:1 or higher AV block (in this example 4:1)

- **Typical (Type I)** (Figure 13.8):
  - Wave of depolarizing myocardium that travels around the tricuspid valve and passes through the isthmus, the area between the inferior vena cava (IVC) and tricuspid valve (see Figure 13.7)
  - Common form of AFL involves a counterclockwise circuit around the tricuspid valve and is usually associated with positive P-waves in lead V1
  - "Reverse" typical AFL is also isthmus-dependent but travels in a clockwise direction around the tricuspid valve
  - On electrophysiology testing, the rhythm is characterized by the presence of an excitable gap and its ability to be entrained in the isthmus.

- **Atypical (Type II):**
  - Defined as an atrial tachycardia resulting in an undulating ECG pattern that does not fulfill the classic criteria of typical AFL
  - Much less common and less-well understood than Type I flutter, though it is usually associated with atrial scarring, surgical incisions, or ablative lines, and is commonly seen after AF ablation.

Management

The evaluation and management of AFL is very similar to that of AF with a few notable exceptions: AFL is uncommon in the structurally normal heart, is less likely to persist, and ablative cure is much more feasible in typical AFL. Patients with AFL are at risk for thromboembolic stroke.

Young Patients with AFL

- Should raise suspicion for underlying structural disease such as rheumatic heart disease, left ventricular dysfunction and congenital heart disease, particularly atrial septal defects.
- Echocardiograms should be performed.

Rate versus Rhythm Control

- AFL is normally not sustained longer than a few weeks and conservative management with rate control is a very reasonable initial therapeutic approach, unless the patient is hemodynamically unstable, highly symptomatic, or has inadequate rate control.
- Since AFL is often associated with structural heart disease, electrical cardioverion is usually preferred over pharmacologic intervention if early reversion to normal sinus rhythm is desired.
- Relatively low energies (50 J) are usually sufficient.

Maintenance of Normal Sinus Rhythm

- Those with recurrent episodes of symptomatic AFL may require more aggressive means of maintaining normal sinus rhythm.
- Again, the frequent association with structural heart disease make Class III agents, particularly amiodarone, the drugs of choice.
- Given the ease and low complication rates of AFL ablation, there should be a low threshold to refer for isthmus ablation when typical AFL is present.

Ablation

The macro-re-entrant circuit in typical AFL traverses the isthmus between the IVC and tricuspid annulus. An ablation line between these two structures effectively interrupts the circuit (Figure 13.9). Success rates as high as 86% and low complication rates make this an attractive alternative to long-term antiarrhythmic therapy, even in the elderly population.

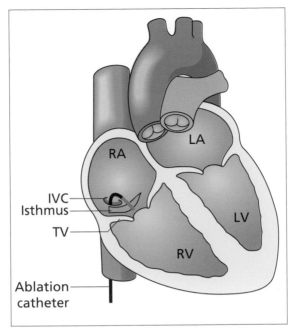

Figure 13.9 Catheter position in a cavotricuspid isthmus ablation. TV, tricuspid valve; IVC, inferior vena cava

Stroke Prophylaxis

AFL is associated with an augmented risk of thromboembolic events, including strokes. Although the efficacy of anticoagulation has not been as well studied as in AF, current guidelines recommend an anticoagulant approach similar to that for AF.

CLINICAL PEARLS

- When treating patients with antiarrhythmic medications, particularly Class Ic and III agents, concomitant AV nodal blockade is necessary to prevent slowing of AFL and 1:1 AV conduction.
- Young patients with AFL should be carefully evaluated for structural heart disease.

Recommended Reading

Clinical Trials and Meta-Analyses

Gage BF, Waterman AD, Shannon W, Boechler M, Rich MW, Radford MJ. Validation of clinical classification schemes for predicting stroke: results from the National Registry of Atrial Fibrillation. *JAMA* 2001;**285**:2864–2870.

Wyse DG, Waldo AL, DiMarco JP et al. A comparison of rate control and rhythm control in patients with atrial fibrillation. *N Engl J Med* 2002;**347**:1825–1823.

Guidelines

ACC/AHA/ESC 2006 guidelines for the management of patients with atrial fibrillation. *J Am Coll Cardiol* 2006;**48**:e149.

Review Articles

Falk RH. Atrial fibrillation. *N Engl J Med* 2001;**344**:1067–1078.

Lee KW, Yang Y, Scheinman MM; University of California-San Francisco. Atrial flutter: a review of its history, mechanisms, clinical features, and current therapy. *Curr Probl Cardiol* 2005;**30**(3):121–167.

14 | Supraventricular Tachycardia

Marco Perez and Paul Zei

Department of Internal Medicine, Division of Cardiology, Stanford
University School of Medicine, Stanford, CA, USA

- Supraventricular tachycardia (SVT) refers to the group of tachyarrhythmias whose mechanisms are critically dependent on the atrium or AV node, above the His–Purkinje system.
- Although atrial fibrillation (AF) and atrial flutter (AFL) meet this definition of SVT, the term is often reserved for the remaining tachyarrhythmias.
- These arrhythmias are usually paroxysmal, i.e. the attacks are sudden and often recurrent.

Differential Diagnosis

Once hemodynamically stable, the initial step in managing a patient with SVT is determining the likely rhythm based on the surface ECG. It is essential to distinguish a tachyarrhythmia requiring intervention from sinus tachycardia or premature atrial contractions (PACs).

The key features in determining the rhythm are (Figure 14.1):
- Narrow (QRS <120 ms) versus wide complex
- Regular versus irregular
- P-wave morphology.

The last feature will help narrow the differential further. There are a few other causes of SVT, such as sinus node re-entry tachycardia and junctional tachycardia; however, the diagnoses in Figure 14.1 include the vast majority of SVTs that will be encountered in the adult patient.

ECG Distinction

A better understanding of the physiology and anatomic pathways of these arrhythmias allows them to be better distinguished on surface ECG. The fundamental mechanisms that cause SVT are:

A Practical Approach to Cardiovascular Medicine, First Edition. Edited by Reza Ardehali,
Marco Perez, Paul Wang.
© 2011 Blackwell Publishing Ltd. Published 2011 by Blackwell Publishing Ltd.

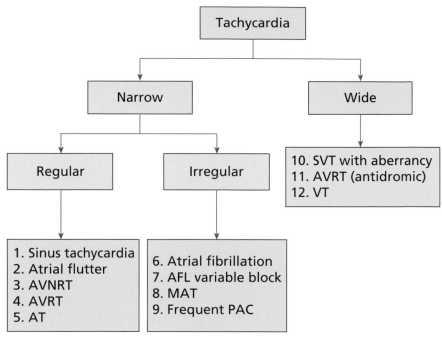

Figure 14.1 Differential diagnosis of SVTs. AVNRT, atrioventricular nodal re-entrant tachycardia; AVRT, atrioventricular re-entrant tachycardia; AT, atrial tachycardia; AFL, atrial flutter; MAT, multifocal atrial tachycardia; PAC, premature atrial contraction

- Enhanced automaticity
- Triggered activity
- Re-entrant circuits.
  These mechanisms will be discussed under the relevant SVT.

Types of Tachyarrythmia

Sinus Tachycardia
- The normal sinus impulse initiates in the sinoatrial (SA) node, travels down atrial-specific fibers to the AV node, where, after a slow conductive period, it then travels down to the bundle of His and Purkinje fibers, and finally spreads to the ventricle (Figure 14.2).
- Sinus tachycardia on an ECG is defined by a rate >100 with a P-wave preceding every QRS complex and a QRS complex following every P-wave, as well as positive P-waves in lead II and biphasic P-waves in V1 (Figure 14.2).
- Sinus tachycardia at rest can reach rates up to 180 bpm in adults, particularly during critical volume depletion or septic shock.

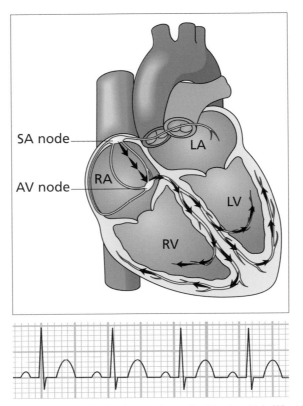

Figure 14.2 Sinus impulse and ECG for sinus tachycardia. SA, sinoatrial; AV, atrioventricular

Atrial Flutter
- **Typical (Type I):**
  - A macro-re-entrant circuit that travels around the tricuspid valve and passes through the cavotricusgh isthmus, the area between the IVC and tricuspid valve, an anatomically narrow region critical to maintenance of the arrhythmia (Figure 14.3; see Chapter 15)
  - Characterized by a "saw tooth" pattern, with absence of an isoelectric interval (flat line) seen in II, III, aVF (Figure 14.3)
  - Flutter rate is typically 300 bpm, but can vary, depending on underlying structural disease or presence of antiarrhythmic medications
  - Due to the refractory period of the AV node, there is usually 2:1 AV block, resulting in a ventricular rate of 150 bpm, though higher degree and variable blocks are also seen, particularly when AV nodal blocking agents are used.
- **Atypical (Type II):**
  - Usually due to a circuit that travels around other anatomic barriers, such as a surgical scar or ablation line, and does not pass through the cavotricuspid isthmus

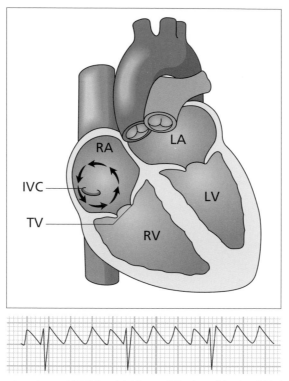

Figure 14.3 Sinus impulse and ECG for atrial flutter. TV, tricuspid valve; IVC, inferior vena cava

- Rate and P-wave morphology on ECG depends on the size and location of the circuit and can mimic atrial tachycardia.

Atrioventricular Nodal Re-entrant Tachycardia

AVNRT (Figure 14.4) is due to a re-entrant circuit contained predominantly within the AV nodal and perinodal areas:
- Re-entrant circuit consists of a loop of tissue with a region of slow conduction critical to sustaining reentry.
- Thus, in AVNRT an abnormal "slow pathway" is present in addition to the normal "fast pathway".
- An impulse is initially propagated down both pathways simultaneously.
- However, retrograde conduction via the slow pathway usually terminates as it collides with antegrade (forward) slow conduction (Figure 14.5).
  In this setting, a PAC can initiate the re-entrant tachycardia:
- A PAC initially conducts down the slow and fast pathways; however, only the fast pathway encounters a refractory phase.
- Slow pathway conduction continues until it reaches the fast pathway.
- By the time the impulse begins to conduct in a retrograde direction up the fast pathway, the refractory period has ended.
- What follows is a self-maintained circulation of the electrical impulse around both pathways (Figure 14.6).

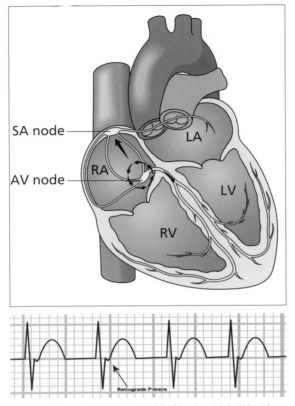

Figure 14.4 Electrical impulse and ECG for AVNRT. SA, sinoatrial; AV, atrioventricular

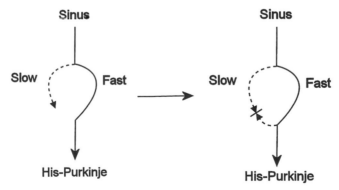

Figure 14.5 Normal conduction down AV node with dual pathways (left), followed by collision with retrograde conduction in the slow pathway (right)

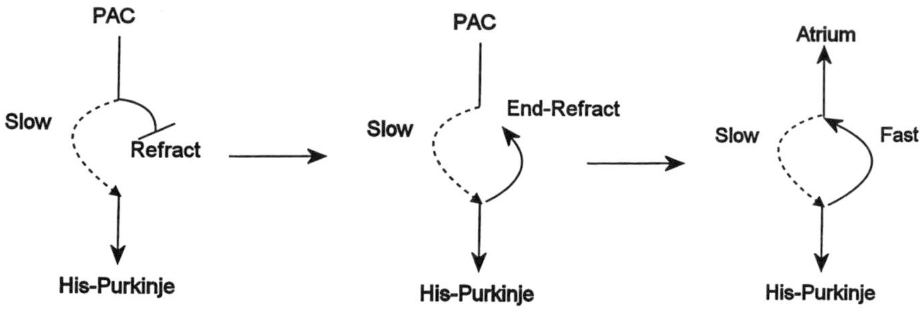

Figure 14.6 Development of re-entrant tachycardia

In typical AVNRT, the atrium and the ventricle are both depolarized at almost the same time; because of this, typical AVNRT is often called a "short RP" tachycardia. On the ECG, the ventricular rate is usually 150–180 bpm. Since the P-wave is much smaller, it is usually buried within the QRS complex but an inverted P-wave can sometimes be seen immediately after the QRS complex (Figure 14.4).

Atypical AVNRT, accounting for 20% of cases, involves reverse flow through such a circuit.

Atrioventricular Re-entrant Tachycardia

AVRT is due to a reentry circuit that passes through the AV node and an accessory pathway (an abnormal electrical connection between the atrium and ventricle outside the AV node, which can be present on the left or right side) (Figures 14.7 and 14.8).

A delta wave results from the early depolarization of the ventricle during normal sinus propagation through an accessory pathway (Figures 14.7 and 14.9):

- Shape and direction depend on the location of the accessory pathway
- Presence with a short P–R interval, a wide QRS, and either symptoms of palpitation or a documented arrhythmia, are diagnostic of the Wolff–Parkinson–White syndrome.

In a mechanism similar to that of AVNRT, a PAC or PVC can trigger re-entrant arrhythmia and the ECG appearance depends on the direction of the circuit:

- When the direction of the macro-re-entrant circuit is antegrade down the AV node and retrograde up the accessory pathway, the tachycardia that results is called **orthodromic**. The His-Purkinje system is activated first, resulting in a narrow QRS with an inverted P-wave usually seen between the QRS and T-wave (short RP). (Figure 14.10).
- When the circuit travels antegrade down the accessory pathway and retrograde up the AV node, it is called **antidromic**. The ventricle is activated directly, resulting in a wide QRS and an ECG that resembles VT (Figure 14.11).

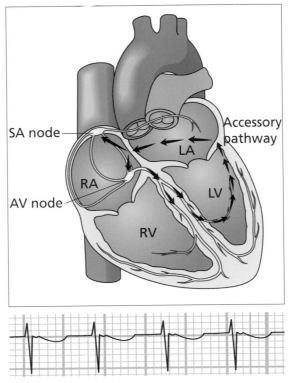

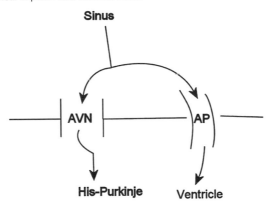

Figure 14.7 Electrical impulse and ECG for AVRT

Sinus

AVN

AP

His-Purkinje   **Ventricle**

Figure 14.8 Accessory pathway

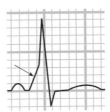

Figure 14.9 Delta wave

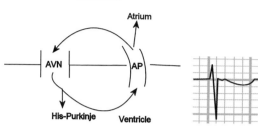

Figure 14.10 Orthodromic AVRT

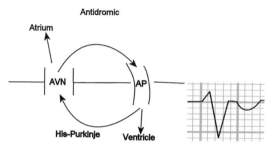

Figure 14.11 Antidromic AVRT

Atrial Tachycardia

AT refers to a rapid rhythm originating from a single, focal area in the atrium, outside the sinus node (Figure 14.12). Although the primary mechanism is believed to be enhanced automaticity, triggered and micro-re-entrant etiologies are also possible. The morphology of the P-wave on ECG depends primarily on the location of the focus. A focus close to the SA node may resemble a sinus P-wave.

As with AFL, the ratio of ventricular beats to atrial beats depends on the refractory period of the AV node. The atrial rate is typically 130–250 bpm, slightly slower than typical AFL (Figure 14.12). Most AT conducts 1:1; however, patients with very fast atrial rates, on nodal blocking agents or with AV nodal disease can have higher degrees of block.

Atrial Fibrillation (Figure 14.13)

AF is characterized by disorganized electrical activity in the atrium leading to loss of effective atrial contraction. Although its mechanism is not entirely understood, in many patients it is thought to be triggered by pulmonary vein potentials and maintained by multiple wavelets in diseased, often dilated, atria.

The hallmarks of the ECG include:
- Irregular ventricular rhythm
- Absence of clearly defined P-waves
- Occasionally, very low amplitude atrial waves are noted; however, these are often high frequency and highly irregular.

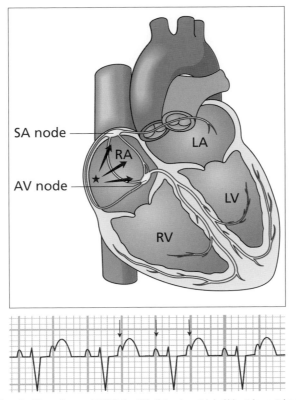

Figure 14.12 Electrical impulse and ECG for AT. SA, sinoatrial; AV, atrioventricular

Atrial Flutter with Variable Block

Although most AFL conducts 2:1, patients can have higher degrees of AV block, particularly when AV nodal blocking agents are used or when AV nodal disease is present. The degree of block can also vary from one ventricular beat to the next, resulting in "variable block" and an irregular rhythm.

Multifocal Atrial Tachycardia

MAT results when at least two different foci in the atrium compete with the SA node for atrial depolarization and conduction down through the AV node (Figure 14.14). The finding of MAT suggests severe atrial disease and is often associated with chronic obstructive pulmonary disease (COPD).

By definition, the ECG must reveal a fast, irregular rhythm with at least three different P-wave morphologies (Figure 14.14). This latter characteristic also distinguishes this rhythm from frequent PACs coming from a single focus.

Frequent PACs (Figure 14.15)

PACs are often mistaken for an SVT, particularly when they are frequent or when nonconducted PACs and post-PAC compensatory pauses result in a

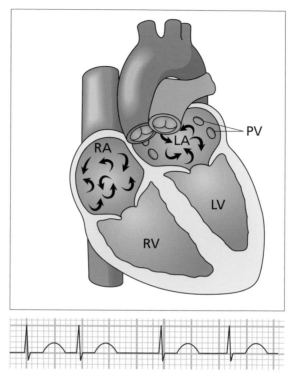

Figure 14.13 Electrical impulse and ECG for AF

highly irregular rhythm. Frequent PACs are also a sign of diseased, often dilated, atria and can be a prelude to AF or AFL. The PACs can originate from a single focus or multiple foci and can be mistaken for MAT. However, if the majority of beats are of sinus origin, then the diagnosis of MAT is avoided.

SVT with Aberrancy
Most SVTs conduct down the AV node and result in a narrow complex ventricular complex. However, if there is an underlying bundle branch block (BBB) or a bystander accessory pathway, then the ECG will reveal a wide complex tachycardia. In some patients without BBB; however, a fast rate of conduction can lead to a preferential prolongation of the refractory period of a single bundle branch (usually the right bundle) and result in a wide complex tachycardia. In these cases, the BBB tends to disappear once the rate slows down. It is often difficult to distinguish SVT with aberrancy from VT (see Chapter 15).

Antidromic AVRT
Antidromic AVRT results in a regular, wide complex tachycardia often confused with VT (see above).

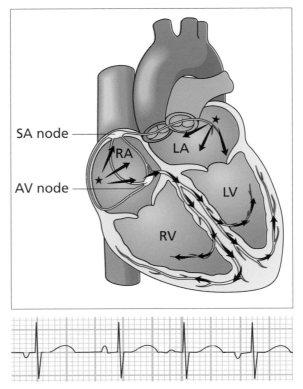

Figure 14.14 Electrical impulse and ECG for MAT

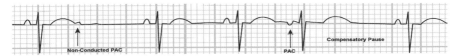

Figure 14.15 Electrical impulse and ECG for frequent PACs

Ventricular Tachycardia (VT)
See Chapter 15 for a detailed discussion of VT and instructions on how to distinguish VT from SVT with aberrancy.

Management

Unstable Patients
Initial management of a patient with SVT depends on the stability of the patient. Any signs of hemodynamic compromise or end-organ damage *that are attributed to the SVT* are grounds for urgent management of the SVT:
• Hypotension
• Unresponsiveness

Table 14.1 Suggested titration for SVT of very recent onset

Shock sequence	Monophasic (J)	Biphasic (J)
First[t]	50	50
Second	100	100
Third	200	150
Fourth	300	200
Subsequent	360	200

- Chest pain
- Lethargy or other mental status changes
- New-onset or worsened heart failure

If any of these are present, then cardioversion should be attempted urgently. If the patient is still responsive, this must be done under sedation. Many of the SVTs, especially when short-lived, will respond to low levels of cardioversion energy and it is very reasonable to start low and titrate as needed, unless the patient is obese. Always remember to perform *synchronized* cardioversion with SVT. Table 14.1 shows a suggested titration that can be used if the SVT is of very recent onset.

Sinus tachycardia, of course, should be carefully excluded and if found, all efforts should be made to identify the underlying etiology. Lack of a pulse should lead straight to the pulseless electrical activity (PEA) algorithm (see Chapter 21), regardless of which SVT is diagnosed.

Borderline Unstable Patients

Many patients present with "borderline" hypotension, or mild symptoms, making it difficult to categorize them as stable or unstable. Another complicating factor is that the SVT may be secondary and the presenting symptoms may be due to a different cause. Primary coronary events or heart failure exacerbations that precede the arrhythmia are frequent confounders. A careful history and diagnostic work-up is indicated.

- Treat borderline patients with adenosine or nodal agents initially, with careful attention to BP and other clinical parameters.
- Breaking the SVT in this manner often improves the BP.
- Electrical cardioversion should be readily available if the hemodynamic or symptomatic state worsens.

Stable Patients

Patients with a normal BP, a clear mental state, and no symptoms are considered stable. The next step in the management of these patients is to determine the precise rhythm.

Patients with regular, narrow complex rhythms can be very difficult and often impossible to distinguish because at fast heart rates, the P-waves may be buried in the T-waves. In this situation, vagal maneuvers or adenosine administration are indicated to make the diagnosis (Box 14.1) and potentially break the rhythm. Avoid carotid massage in older patients.

Box 14.1 Interpreting the adenosine response

Condition	Response
Sinus tachycardia	Sinus rate slows, revealing sinus P-waves
	Sinus arrest is also possible
	Varying degrees of AV block are observed
	Changes are gradual and transient
AVNRT and AVRT	Usually sudden break into sinus rhythm
	Successful in 90–95% of patients
Atrial tachycardia	Ventricular rate slows down revealing P-waves
	A few ATs can also break with adenosine
Atrial flutter	Ventricular rate slows revealing F-waves
	AFL does *not* break with adenosine

Adenosine Administration

- Check for contraindications: second- or third-degree AV block, sick sinus syndrome, COPD, or asthma.
- Check BP at baseline and between doses; avoid in hypotensive patients.
- Have atropine and pacing pads at the bedside.
- Place patient on monitor and *print* a continuous ECG during administration.
- Adenosine has a half-life of seconds, so administration must be with a quick push (1–2 s), followed quickly by a saline flush.
- Transient sinus arrest, AV block, hypotension, dizziness, and flushing are normal and the patient should be warned beforehand.
- Recommended dosing:
  - 6 mg initially, followed by max 12 mg if not effective within 2 min
  - May repeat 12 mg if necessary
  - Give 3 mg as initial dose if central line is used.

It is important to note that adenosine acts on *both* the sinus node and AV node even in normal patients, and can result in a spectrum from bradycardia to complete heart block.

Once converted to sinus rhythm, a few patients revert back to their dysrhythmia within seconds. The adenosine may be repeated, however, appropriate maintenance therapy should be started immediately in all patients. Adenosine may, in some cases, also induce AF.

Alternative Acute Termination

If the SVT is refractory to adenosine or if adenosine is contraindicated, there are a few alternative approaches. Always remember that sinus tachycardia, which can be as fast as 180 bpm at rest in adult patients, should be excluded. Also note that the irregular SVTs (AF, AFL with variable block, MAT) will not respond to adenosine.

Choice of acute therapy will depend on whether or not the patient is known to have heart failure. Beta-blockers and calcium channel blockers (CCBs) would be a poor choice in breaking an SVT in someone with known, or suspected, depressed LV function.

- **Normal LV function:**
  - Verapamil 5 mg IV, then 10 mg IV after 15 min if no response
  - Diltiazem 10 mg IV, then 20 mg IV after 15 min if no response
  - Metoprolol 5 mg IV every 10 min as needed, max 3 doses.
- **Depressed LV function:**
  - Digoxin 0.25 mg IV every 15 min, maximum 1 mg
  - Amiodarone 150 mg IV, then another 150 mg IV after 15 min if needed

If there is still no response, then consider cardioversion or continuous diltiazem (10 mg/h) or amiodarone (1 mg/min) infusion.

Maintenance Therapy

Once the SVT has broken, early administration of maintenance therapy will be important in order to avoid reversion of the arrhythmia. The choice of maintenance therapy depends highly on the type of SVT identified and the patient's LV function.

AF/AFL

See Chapter 13 for details of maintenance therapy.

AVNRT and AVRT

Treatment choice depends substantially on severity of symptoms and patient preference.

- Patients with infrequent, self-contained episodes may opt for:
  - No chronic therapy, particularly when they can break the episodes with safe vagotonic maneuvers, such as a valsalva maneuver
  - A "pill-in-the pocket" approach with verapamil (40–160 mg), beta-blockers, flecainide (100–300 mg) or propafenone (150–450 mg). Initial dose should be made under observation to assess tolerance. Class Ic agents should only be used in patients without structural heart disease.
- First-line therapies for patients with more frequent symptoms are:
  - AV nodal blocking agents including beta-blockers, CCBs, or digoxin
  - In patients refractory to these agents, antiarrhythmic drug therapy is an option (either Class Ic for those with structurally normal hearts or amiodarone in those with LV dysfunction).
- Given the relative ease of the procedure and high success rates, there should be a very low threshold for referral to catheter ablation:
  - **AVNRT:**
    – Usually the slow pathway is targeted for ablation and success rates are of the order of 95%
    – Most common serious complication is AV block, occurring in <1% of patients

- **AVRT:**
  - Accessory pathway is also ablated with an approximately 95% success rate
  - Risk of AV block is not nearly as high
  - Because of the need to perform either retrograde or trans-septal approach to access left-sided pathways, there are small risks of perforation and systemic thromboembolism (<1%)
  - Successful procedures obviate the need for chronic therapy and are often preferred by patients.

Atrial Tachycardia

The goals in maintenance therapy are to suppress atrial foci and prevent a rapid ventricular response during the arrhythmia.

- Those with rare, self-limited episodes and mild symptoms may opt for no chronic therapy.
- First-line therapy for those with more frequent or symptomatic cases includes a beta-blocker or CCB.
- For patients refractory to AV nodal agents:
  - Catheter ablation is a reasonable next step, particularly in younger patients or those with a right atrial focus
  - Success rate depends on the location of the atrial focus, but overall cure rates of approximately 85% have been reported
  - As with AVRT, the complication rates depend on the site of ablation and left-sided ablations carry a small thromboembolic risk (<1%).
- In elderly patients or those otherwise not good candidates for ablation therapy:
  - Antiarrhythmic therapy may be considered
  - Class Ic agents are reasonable in those without structural heart disease and amiodarone in those with known or suspected structural heart disease.

Multifocal Atrial Tachycardia

Therapy of the underlying associated disease, usually pulmonary disease or sepsis, typically results in improvement of MAT.

- Treatment with AV nodal agents is first-line therapy and often results in adequate rate control or conversion to sinus rhythm.
- Although beta-blockers are more effective, associated bronchospasm may be a contraindication in many of these patients, and verapamil is a good alternative.
- Antiarrhythmic drug use has overall been disappointing and is generally avoided.
- Small studies suggest that magnesium infusion may also help control the heart rate.
- In patients refractory to AV nodal agents alone, catheter-based AV node modification may be considered. The goal is to limit the rapid conduction

of atrial impulses to the ventricle by partially burning the AV node. This technique is still somewhat unreliable.

- Alternative to complete AV nodal ablation is permanent pacemaker implantation and this may be the better option in patients who do not respond to drug therapy.

Frequent PACs

Frequent PACs alone generally do not require therapy. However, if the PACs are frequent enough, they may cause symptoms or tachycardia-induced cardiomyopathy.

- AV nodal agents are reasonable agents to use for rate control.
- Rarely, catheter ablation of the PAC focus can be considered in refractory cases, especially if LV dysfunction is thought to be secondary to the frequent PACs.

SVTs and Accessory Pathways

Approximately 10–30% of patients with accessory pathways also develop AF or other atrial tachyarrhythmias. Unlike the AV node, accessory pathways do not have protective refractory periods and can allow unfettered conduction from the atrium to the ventricle. AF can therefore result in a rapid, irregular, wide-complex tachycardia (Figure 14.16), which can degenerate into ventricular fibrillation.

- Acute therapy usually requires electrical cardioversion as many of these patients will be unstable.
- In hemodynamically stable patients, IV procainamide has traditionally been the drug of choice, however, if structural heart disease is suspected, amiodarone may be a reasonable alternative.
- Stable patients should all be referred for catheter ablation of the accessory pathway. Successful ablation often also results in cure of the AF.
- AV nodal blocking agents, such as CCBs, digoxin, and beta-blockers, should generally be avoided in patients with evidence of accessory pathways on ECG (Wolff–Parkinson–White syndrome).

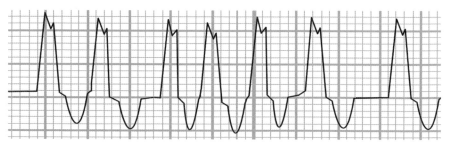

Figure 14.16 Wide-complex tachycardia resulting from rapid conduction via an accessory pathway during atrial fibrillation

CLINICAL PEARLS

- Always rule out sinus tachycardia or frequent PACs.
- In a regular, narrow complex tachycardia with no clear sign of P-waves, adenosine may be necessary to make the diagnosis.
- Digoxin toxicity may cause just about *any* arrhythmia and should be considered especially in those with atrial tachycardia and AV block, or junctional tachycardia.
- Effective administration of adenosine depends on its rapid infusion.
- Check the 12-lead ECG after cardioversion for presence of delta waves.

Recommended Reading

Clinical Trials and Meta-Analyses

Kay GN, Epstein AE, Dailey SM, Plumb VJ. Role of radiofrequency ablation in management of supraventricular arrhythmias: experience in 760 consecutive patients. *J Cardiovasc Electrophysiol* 1993;**4**:371–392.

Guidelines

ECC Committee, Subcommittees and Task Forces of the American Heart Association. 2005 American Heart Association Guidelines for Cardiopulmonary Resuscitation and Emergency Cardiovascular Care. *Circulation* 2005;**112**:IV1–203.

Review Articles

Delacretaz E. Clinical practice. Supraventricular tachycardia. *N Engl J Med* 2006;**354**: 1039–1051.

15 Ventricular Tachycardia

Jeffrey Hsing and Henry Hsia
Department of Internal Medicine, Division of Cardiology, Stanford University School of Medicine, Stanford, CA, USA

- Ventricular tachycardia (VT) is a rapid rhythm that originates in the ventricle (Figure 15.1).
- Mechanism of VT can be re-entry, automaticity, or triggered activity.
- Vast majority of VT is observed in the setting of cardiomyopathy and/or coronary disease, and is associated with either scar or ongoing ischemia.
- Several less common VT syndromes, some of which can have a benign clinical course, can occur in the setting of structurally normal hearts.

Describing VTs

- Premature ventricular contraction/depolarization (PVC/PVD): single beat originating in the ventricle
- Couplet: two consecutive beats originating in the ventricle
- Nonsustained VT: three or more beats in duration, terminating spontaneously in <30 seconds in duration
- Sustained VT: VT longer than 30s in duration and/or requiring termination due to hemodynamic compromise
- Monomorphic VT: single stable QRS morphology
- Polymorphic VT: changing QRS morphologies
- Ventricular fibrillation (VF): extremely rapid (>300 beats/min), erratic ventricular rhythms with marked variability in QRS cycle length, morphology, and amplitude due to disorganized ventricular activity
- Torsades de pointes: French term literally meaning "twisting of the points," sometimes preceded by long QT intervals and characterized by twisting of the peaks of the QRS complexes around the isoelectric line during the arrhythmia

A Practical Approach to Cardiovascular Medicine, First Edition. Edited by Reza Ardehali, Marco Perez, Paul Wang.
© 2011 Blackwell Publishing Ltd. Published 2011 by Blackwell Publishing Ltd.

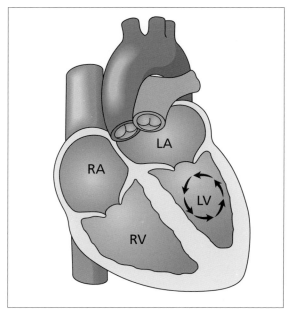

Figure 15.1 Re-entrant circuit in ventricular tachycardia

Diagnosis

Nearly all VTs are wide complex (QRS >120 ms), with the rare exception of VTs originating near or in the His–Purkinje system. However, not all wide complex tachycardia (WCT) is VT. The clinical diagnostic challenge is distinguishing VT from other causes of WCT based on ECG and clinical findings:

- Supraventricular tachycardia (SVT) with aberrant conduction or pre-excitation (accessory pathway)
- Antidromic atrioventricular re-entrant tachycardia (AVRT) (see Chapter 14)
- Paced tachycardia: tracking at high rates or pacemaker-mediated tachycardia (see Chapter 28).
- **History:**
  - Patient's baseline clinical history and ECG can help suggest the cause of WCT:
    - If the patient has a history of coronary artery disease, myocardial infarction (MI), or cardiomyopathy, then the tachycardia is highly likely to be VT
    - A bundle branch block at baseline with the same QRS morphology as the WCT suggests SVT with aberrancy
    - A delta wave is highly suggestive of an antidromic AVRT or atrial fibrillation or AV nodal re-entrant tachycardia with pre-excitation
    - Other clues on the ECG include long QT, Brugada pattern, and epsilon waves (see Chapter 22).

- **Physical exam:**
  - Some patients, particularly those on antiarrhythmic drugs or with structurally normal hearts, can have relatively slow or well-tolerated VT. Hemodynamic stability itself, therefore, does not exclude VT
  - Evidence of AV dissociation, such as cannon A-waves, is indicative of VT.
- **ECG criteria:**
  - Distinguishing VT from other WCT is often difficult on the ECG
  - When in doubt, the rule is to assume VT unless proven otherwise
  - A few ECG findings are diagnostic of VT:
    - **AV dissociation:** P-waves march out independent of QRS complexes
    - **Fusion beats:** ventricles are depolarized simultaneously by the descending sinus beat and ectopic ventricular beat. QRS complex resembles a fusion of the sinus beat and VT
    - **Capture beats:** during VT, there can be intermittent QRS complexes that are identical (usually narrow) to normal sinus complexes. These are sinus beats conducted via the AV node at just the right time; seen particularly during slower VTs
  - Several published ECG criteria attempt to differentiate SVT with aberrancy from VT; Box 15.1 describes the Brugada criteria, the most commonly used. Most have sensitivities of 80–95% but specificities of 40–70%. VT is therefore difficult to rule out based solely on these criteria
  - Criteria to help distinguish VT from SVT are shown in Box 15.2.

Work-Up

- Once VT has been established and stabilized, the first step is to identify acutely reversible causes:
  - Ongoing cardiac ischemia/infarct
  - Electrolyte disturbances (hyperkalemia)
  - Drug toxicity (QT-prolonging drugs)
  - Hypoxia
  - Myocarditis
  - Heart failure.
- Next, any underlying structural heart disease should be identified, such as dilated, ischemic, hypertrophic or arrhythmogenic right ventricular cardiomyopathy or underlying scar.
- If no structural heart disease is identified and the QRS morphology is consistent with known patterns, then one of the idiopathic VT syndromes should be considered.
- With this in mind, it is important to remember that the vast majority of VT is associated with coronary disease, ischemic and nonischemic cardiomyopathies.

Box 15.1 Brugada criteria

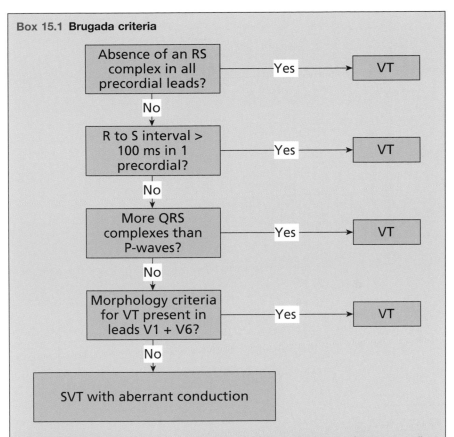

Although initially reported to have very high accuracy (high 90s), confirmatory studies have shown this set of criteria to be comparable to older algorithms.

- RS complex is seen in at least one precordial lead (V1–V6) in all SVT and 26% of VTs. So if there is no RS complex, then it is most likely VT. Consistently positive or negative QRS deflection across the precordium, called "concordance," also supports VT.

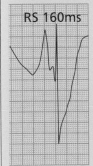

- Measuring the R–S interval – initial upstroke of the QRS to the nadir of the S-wave. In general, the wider the QRS complex, the more likely it is to be VT.
- AV dissociation is highly specific for VT; however, P-waves are usually difficult to make out during VT. Likewise more QRS complexes than P-waves is diagnostic, but difficult to determine.
- Morphology criteria (see below) are more challenging to memorize and interpret. In general, WCT that looks like typical right (RBBB) or left bundle branch block (LBBB) is more likely to represent aberrant conduction.

Box 15.2 Right and left bundle branch block patterns favoring VT and SVT

Favors VT

Favors SVT

RBBB pattern (more positive in V1)
V1: Monophasic R or QR or RS
V6: R-to-S ratio <1; QS or QR

V1: Triphasic rSR' (right "bunny ear" is bigger)
V6: R-to-S ratio >1; qRs pattern

LBBB pattern (more negative in V1)
V1: R > 40ms; nadir of S > 70ms; notched S
V6: QR or QS pattern

V1: No significant R-wave
V6: Monophasic R

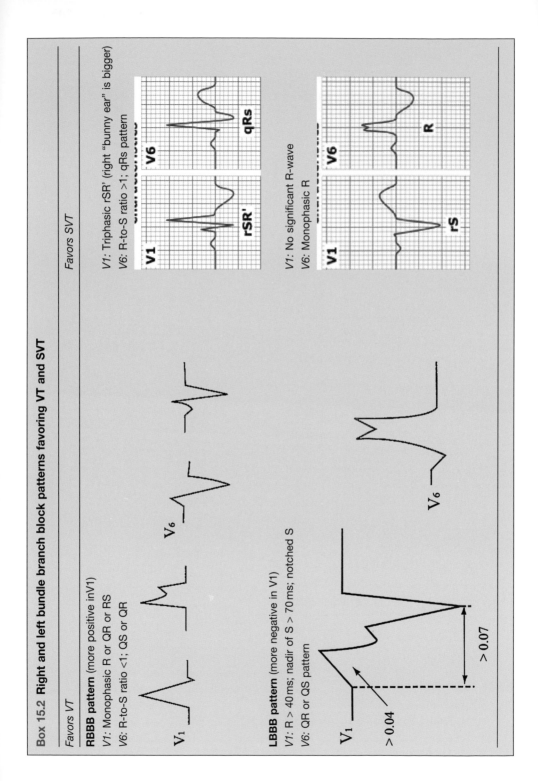

Acute Setting

- History: focus on signs of ischemia, heart failure, and myocarditis, such as chest pain or shortness of breath, illicit drug use, QT-prolonging medications, history of renal insufficiency (hyperkalemia)
- Baseline ECG: quickly identify signs of ischemia or infarction once VT has terminated. Also assess for a prolonged QT interval, Brugada pattern/epsilon waves/digoxin scooping (see Chapter 22)
- Cardiac enzymes: to rule out MI
- Electrolytes: particularly K^+, Ca^{2+}, and Mg^{2+}
- Toxicology screen: assess for cocaine or amphetamine use

Further Testing

- Echocardiogram: all patients should have an assessment of their left ventricular function, wall motion abnormalities, and right ventricular size and function.
- Coronary evaluation:
  - Consider stress testing in younger, low-risk patients
  - VT in older or at-risk patients may reflect underlying coronary artery disease and would benefit from coronary angiography directly.
- Cardiac MRI: consider in patients with structurally normal hearts to better evaluate for scar, myocarditis, RV size and function, as well as fatty infiltrates [seen in arrhythmogenic right ventricular cardiomyopahty (ARVC)].
- Electrophysiologic studies: consider in all patients with structurally normal hearts and no reversible cause of VT, especially if ECG suggests one of the VT syndromes discussed below.
- Signal-averaged ECG (SAECG):
  - Low diagnostic yield
  - May help reveal the late potentials seen in ARVC.

VT Syndromes

Patients with structurally normal hearts who have VT should be evaluated for one of several VT syndromes. Electrophysiologic studies can help diagnose the type of VT and curative ablation is sometimes possible.

Right or Left Ventricular Outflow Tract (RVOT, LVOT) Tachycardia

- A tachyarrhythmia originating in the outflow tracts
- Highly positive QRS complexes in the inferior leads during VT suggest outflow tract tachycardia
- LBBB with a relatively narrow (<140 ms) QRS indicates RVOT VT
- Generally benign, but often symptomatic
- Responds to beta-blockers and calcium channel blockers (CCBs)
- Ablation can be successful in >90% of cases

Idiopathic Left Ventricular Tachycardia
- Also called "fascicular VT" because of its origin in the left posterior fascicle
- ECG during tachycardia shows RBBB with left anterior hemiblock morphology (left axis deviation)
- Responds to verapamil and sometimes beta-blockers
- Other fascicular tachycardia may be from an anterior fascicular location
- Ablation successful in 75–80%

Arrhythmogenic Right Ventricular Cardiomyopathy (ARVC)
- Due to fibrofatty deposition in the right ventricle, can involve left side
- Although usually associated with RV enlargement or dysfunction, this is not always evident
- Diagnosis based on several criteria (Box 15.2)
- MRI not officially part of criteria, but fatty infiltrates in RV often seen
- Underlying RBBB with a VT that is of LBBB morphology is suggestive
- Implantable converter defibrillator (ICD) usually indicated if VT is evident
- Ablation success is less well studied

Long QT Syndrome (LQTS)
- Prolonged QTc interval, either congenital or secondary to several possible drugs, predisposes to Torsades de Pointes
- Schwartz criteria used in borderline cases (Box 15.2)
- Beta-blocker is indicated if no evidence of arrhythmia
- ICD is considered if ventricular arrhythmia is documented or if recurrent symptoms on beta-blocker
- No current role for catheter ablation
- Pacing may be necessary in the setting of bradycardia-related QT prolongation

Brugada Syndrome
- Genetic disease due to abnormal sodium channel function
- Diagnosis is based on ventricular arrhythmias or syncope in the setting of a typical ECG pattern (Box 15.3)
- ICD indicated if VT is evident
- No clear benefit of medications as first-line therapy; no current role for ablation

Other Syndromes
- Catecholaminergic polymorphic VT : rare, genetic VT associated with exercise, nl QT
- Idiopathic VF: genetic disease, VF in setting of normal heart
- Bundle branch re-entry: associated with dilated cardiomyopathy. Involves re-entry circuit usually antegrade down RBB and retrograde up LBB. Ablation of RBB is indicated with an ICD

Box 15.3 Diagnostic features of VT syndromes

Long QT syndrome (Schwartz criteria)		*ARVC*	*Brugada syndrome*
QTc		**Family history:**	Diagnosis based on symptoms
>480 ms	3 pts	Major: tissue diagnosis	in the setting of a typical ECG
460–480 ms	2 pts	Minor: clinical diagnosis or	pattern with RBBB
450–460 ms	1 pt	SCD < 35 years	
Torsades not associated with medication	2 pts	**ECG findings:** Major: QRS > 110 ms only in V1–V3 or epsilon waves	
T-wave alternans	1 pt		
Notched T-wave in 3 leads	1 pt		V2
Syncope		V1	
With stress	2 pts		Type 1: coved ST segment,
Without stress	1 pt		inverted T-wave
Family history		Minor: late potentials on	
Of LQTS	1 pt.	SAECG or T-wave	
Of SCD < 30 years	0.5 pt	inversion V2–V3 with no signs of RBBB	
Total		**Tissue characterization:**	V2
Low probability	0–1 pt	Major: fibrofatty infiltrate	
Moderate probability	2–3 pt	**Structural abnormalities:**	
High probability	≥4 pt	Major: severe RV dilation, dysfunction or aneurysm	Type 2: saddleback ST segment > 1 mm, positive or
		Minor: mild RV dilation, dysfunction or aneurysm	biphasic T-wave
		Arrhythmias: Minor: LBBB VT or frequent PVCs (>1000/24 h)	
			V2
		Diagnostic criteria: 2 major, 1 major + 2 minor Or 4 minor	
			Type 3: saddleback ST segment < 1 mm, positive T-wave

Treatment

EVIDENCE-BASED PRACTICE

Antiarrhythmics Versus Implantable Defibrillators (AVID)

Context: Until this trial, the benefits of secondary prevention with ICDs had not been demonstrated.

Goal: To compare antiarrhythmic therapy to ICD in patients with sustained or unstable VT or VF.

Methods: Multicenter, RCT. 1016 patients with prior MI, VT, or VF, randomized to ICD or antiarrhythmics, mostly amiodarone.

Results: There was a greater reduction in total mortality in patients randomized to ICD.

Take-home message: Patients with coronary disease and documented ventricular arrhythmia benefit from ICDs.

- **Unstable VT:**
  - For any unstable patients with hemodynamic compromise, treatment is rapid direct current cardioversion (DCC) and advanced cardiac life support (see Chapter 21).
- **Acute treatment of stable VT:**
  - If a reversible cause such as ischemia is identified, treatment of the underlying condition is necessary
  - In the immediately acute setting, amiodarone (150 mg bolus IV over 30 min, followed by 1 mg/min drip) is a good first-line agent
  - Lidocaine (1 mg/kg bolus, followed by 1 mg/min) is a good second-line agent, especially in the setting of ischemia
  - In a very stable patient, cautious use of beta-blockers may suppress VT
  - If polymorphic VT is noted, then empiric use of magnesium (2 g IV bolus) is indicated, especially if prolonged QT is seen
  - Calcium infusion (5 mL of 10% IV over 2 min) will stabilize the myocardium if hyperkalemia is suspected.
- **Secondary prevention of VT:**
  - Unless a reversible cause of VT is identified and treated, the primary intervention is implantation of an ICD to prevent sudden death from recurrent ventricular arrhythmias
  - Antiarrhythmic therapies alone have not performed as well as ICDs, and are used to suppress arrhythmias after ICD implant to prevent shocks
  - For the majority of VTs which are associated with structural heart disease, Class III agents are first-line therapies
  - Several VT syndromes with structurally normal hearts (see above), can be treated with beta-blockers or CCB.

- **PVCs and nonsustained VT:**
  - Although in theory, preventing ventricular ectopy with antiarrhythmics might be desired, Class Ic drug trials in patients without SVT have shown worsened arrhythmic death rates
  - More recent trials with Class III agents have shown reductions in arrhythmic death, but no reduction in overall death.
- **Primary prevention of sudden cardiac death:**
  - Thanks to the efficacy of ICDs, identifying patients who have never had SVT or VF, but are at high risk of sudden death from ventricular arrhythmias, has become necessary
  - EF is the single strongest predictor of ventricular arrhythmic death
  - For a detailed discussion of the role of ICDs in primary prevention of SCD, see Chapter 7.

EVIDENCE-BASED PRACTICE

Cardiac Arrhythmia Suppression Trial (CAST)
Context: Can suppression of ventricular ectopy reduce arrhythmic death?
Goal: To compare outcomes in patients randomized to Class Ic antiarrhythmic agents versus placebo.
Methods: RCT. 1727 patients post-MI, mild-to-moderate reduction in ejection fraction (EF) followed for an average of 10 months.
Results: Patients randomized to antiarrhythmics had less ectopy, but higher rates of arrhythmic death.
Take-home message: Class Ic treatment alone in patients without SVT worsens outcomes.

Recommended Reading

Clinical Trials and Meta-Analyses

Brugada P, Brugada J, Mont L, Smeets J, Andries EW. A new approach to the differential diagnosis of a regular tachycardia with a wide QRS complex. *Circulation* 1991;**83**:1649–1659.

The Antiarrhythmics versus Implantable Defibrillators (AVID) Investigators. A comparison of antiarrhythmic-drug therapy with implantable defibrillators in patients resuscitated from near-fatal ventricular arrhythmias. *N Engl J Med* 1997;**337**:1576–1583.

The Cardiac Arrhythmia Suppression Trial (CAST) Investigators. Preliminary report: effect of encainide and flecainide on mortality in a randomized trial of arrhythmia suppression after myocardial infarction. *N Engl J Med* 1989;**321**:406–412.

Guidelines

Zipes DP, Camm AJ, Borggrefe M et al. ACC/AHA/ESC 2006 guidelines for management of patients with ventricular arrhythmias and the prevention of sudden cardiac death – executive summary. *Eur Heart J* 2006;**27**:2099–2140.

16 Bradycardia

Jeffrey Hsing and Paul Wang
Department of Internal Medicine, Division of Cardiology, Stanford
University School of Medicine, Stanford, CA, USA

Normal Conduction System (Figure 16.1)

- Sinoatrial (SA) node: cells with automaticity initiate the sinus impulse and generates the electrical signal for atrial depolarization.
- Atrioventricular node: responsible for conduction of electrical signals from the atrium to the ventricle.
- His–Purkinje system: specialized, rapidly conducting tissue that carries the signal from the AV node and helps evenly depolarize the right and left ventricles.

Bradycardia, or a heart rate <60 bpm, can be caused by slowing of sinus node activity or abnormalities of atrioventricular (AV) conduction when a slowing or block occurs at any level of the normal conducting system.

- Since bradycardia can be transient, ECG monitoring is often necessary.
- Next step is to identify reversible causes of the bradycardia.
- Final step is to determine whether or not pacing or other interventions are indicated, which depends on the presence of symptoms and the degree and level of the block.

Definitions

- Sinus bradycardia: sinoatrial node impulses at <60 bpm
- Sinus pause: failure of impulse formation at the sinus node for a period that is longer than the normal P–P interval
- Sinus arrest: a prolonged sinus pause (>2–3 s). Also called sinus or atrial standstill
- Sick sinus syndrome: often used interchangeably with sinus node dysfunction, but in general is used in the setting of irreversible causes of sinus disease
- Tachy brady syndrome: coexistence of bradycardia due to sinus node dysfunction and atrial arrhythmias such as atrial fibrillation. The term implies

A Practical Approach to Cardiovascular Medicine, First Edition. Edited by Reza Ardehali,
Marco Perez, Paul Wang.
© 2011 Blackwell Publishing Ltd. Published 2011 by Blackwell Publishing Ltd.

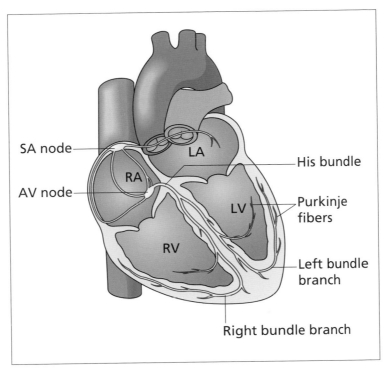

Figure 16.1 Normal conduction system

that tachycardia is difficult to rate control because of periods of bradycardia and may require pacing
- AV block or heart block: abnormalities of AV conduction.

Sinus Node Dysfunction

Bradycardia originating at the level of the sinus node can be due to a number of causes. Reversible causes must first be excluded with basic history and relevant testing. In the elderly particularly, sinus node dysfunction may be progressive.

Causes
- **Irreversible:**
  - Sinus node degeneration and/or fibrosis: most common cause of progressive conduction system disease that is usually seen with advancing age
  - Infiltrative disease: amyloidosis, tuberculosis, scleroderma, hemochromatosis, and tumors such as lymphoma. There are case reports of these reversing with treatment, but response is slow

- Trauma: can be seen after cardiac surgery or catheter ablation
- Congenital: rare genetic abnormalities such as *SCN5A* and *HCN4* mutations.
- **Reversible:**
  - Medications:
    - All nodal agents, such as beta-blockers, calcium channel blockers (CCBs), and digoxin; cimetidine, reserpine, lithium, some antiarrhythmic drugs (propafenone, amiodarone, sotalol)
    - Digoxin use should always be asked about and levels checked, especially in the setting of renal failure
  - Enhanced vagal tone: sinus impulse formation depends on a balance between vagal and sympathetic tone:
    - History of vigorous exercise often leads to elevation of baseline vagal tone
    - Carotid hypersensitivity may lead to transient sinus slowing
    - Transient vagal tone increase can be seen with vagal maneuvers: carotid massage, valsalva maneuver.
  - Inferior infarction: up to 5% of patients can have sinus node dysfunction, which is almost always reversible, but may require transient pacing
  - Epicardial disease: pericarditis or tumors in the epicardium
  - Inflammatory: rheumatic fever, Lyme disease, diphtheria, Chagas' disease
  - Other: hypothyroidism, hypothermia, hypoxia, muscular dystrophy, sleep apnea, hyperkalemia, elevated intracranial pressure.

Severity

Sinus node dysfunction due to any of the above causes can present with a spectrum of severity ranging from simple sinus bradycardia to prolonged sinus arrest. Treatment will depend on severity, progression, and symptoms (Box 16.1).

- **Sinus bradycardia:**
  - Manifest by a sinus rate of 60 bpm or less
  - Every P-wave is followed by a QRS complex and every QRS complex is preceded by a P-wave
  - Seen in up to one-third of healthy individuals under age 25 and in well-conditioned athletes
  - Treatment is generally indicated only if associated symptoms are due to the bradycardia.
- **Chronotropic incompetence:**
  - "Relative" sinus bradycardia, due to the inability to mount a sufficient sinus response in the setting of exercise or other hemodynamic changes
  - Suspect in elderly patients with exertional symptoms who have low heart rates at rest
  - Can be confirmed with exercise treadmill testing
  - Treatment is generally with a rate-adaptive pacemaker.

Box 16.1 Pacemaker indications

Sinus node dysfunction

Class I:
- Sinus node dysfunction with documented symptomatic bradycardia, including frequent sinus pauses that produce symptoms
- Symptomatic chronotropic incompetence

Class IIa:
- Sinus node dysfunction occurring spontaneously or as a result of necessary drug therapy with heart rate <40 bpm, when a clear association between significant symptoms consistent with bradycardia and the actual presence of bradycardia has not been documented

Class IIb:
- In minimally symptomatic patients, chronic heart rate <30 bpm while awake

Class III:
- Sinus node dysfunction in asymptomatic patients, including those in whom substantial sinus bradycardia (heart rate <40 bpm) is a consequence of long-term drug treatment
- Sinus node dysfunction in patients with symptoms suggestive of bradycardia that are clearly documented as not associated with a slow heart rate
- Sinus node dysfunction with symptomatic bradycardia due to nonessential drug therapy

Atrioventricular conduction abnormalities

Class I:
- Third-degree AV block associated with:
  - Symptomatic bradycardia
  - Asystole >3 s
  - Escape rate <40 bpm
  - Post AV junction ablation
  - Postoperative AV block not expected to resolve
  - Neuromuscular disease with AV block (Kearns–Sayre syndrome, Erb's dystrophy, myotonic muscular dystrophy)
- Second-degree AV block regardless of type or site of block, with associated symptomatic bradycardia

Class IIa:
- Asymptomatic third-degree AV block at any anatomic site with average awake ventricular rates >40 bpm
- Asymptomatic type II second-degree AV block
- Asymptomatic type I second-degree AV block at intra- or infra-His levels found incidentally at electrophysiologic study for other indications

(Continued)

Box 16.1 *(Continued)*

- First-degree AV block with symptoms suggestive of pacemaker syndrome and documented alleviation of symptoms with temporary AV pacing

Class IIb:
- Marked first-degree AV block (>0.30 s) in patients with LV dysfunction and symptoms of congestive heart failure in whom a shorter AV interval results in hemodynamic improvement, presumably by decreasing left atrial filling pressure

Class III:
- Asymptomatic first-degree AV block
- Asymptomatic type I second-degree AV block at the supra-His (AV node) level or not known to be intra- or infra-Hisian
- AV block expected to resolve and unlikely to recur (e.g. drug toxicity, Lyme disease)

- **Sinus pause and arrest**:
  - Transient prolongation of the sinus interval
  - Short pauses can be seen in healthy individuals
  - In general, patients with sinus pauses >3 s during waking hours are at increased risk for the development of symptoms and progression of disease, and should be considered for pacemaker implant.
- **Sinoatrial exit block:**
  - Failure of the sinus impulse to reach and depolarize the atrium
  - Can be classified in a manner similar to the types of AV nodal block (see below)
  - First-degree block will not be evident on ECG
  - Second-degree block, type I, will appear as gradual prolongation of the P–P interval followed by a "dropped" P-wave
  - Second-degree block, type II, will appear as an occasional doubling of the P–P interval
  - Third-degree block will appear as sinus arrest.

Atrioventricular Conduction Abnormalities

Bradycardia from atrioventricular conduction abnormalities can be due to nearly any of the causes of sinus node dysfunction (see above). In fact, many patients will present with both sinus and AV conduction abnormalities. Some notable differences are that AV conduction disease:

- Can be seen with anterior myocardial infarction (MI) (as opposed to inferior), and should be suspected when a new bundle branch block occurs.
- Is more common in certain types of surgeries involving the membranous septum, such as aortic valve replacement or myomectomy.

Treatment or intervention depends on symptoms, progression, and severity of AV conduction abnormalities.

Severity and Localization

Determining the severity and localization of AV conduction abnormalities is particularly important to determine the most appropriate therapeutic strategy. AV conduction abnormalities due to block below the level of the AV node is highly likely to progress with a slow escape rhythm and is an indication for pacemaker implantation, regardless of symptoms.

- **First-degree AV block**:
  - Defined on ECG by a P–R interval >0.2 s (Figure 16.2)
  - A narrow QRS and prolonged P–R interval is consistent with delay in the AV node
  - Treatment not indicated if asymptomatic.
- **Second-degree AV block: Mobitz type I (Wenckebach)**:
  - On ECG, there is progressive lengthening of the P–R interval and an eventual P-wave is not followed by a QRS complex (nonconducted, or dropped beat) (Figure 16.3)
  - Other ECG characteristics include a subtle, progressive shortening of the R–R interval, but this is not always present
  - R–R interval containing the nonconducted P-wave should be less than two P–P intervals
  - Final P–R interval before the dropped beat is usually markedly longer than the first P–R interval following the dropped beat
  - This infrequently progresses to complete heart block (CHB) and treatment is not indicated if asymptomatic.
- **Second-degree AV block: Mobitz type II**:
  - On ECG, an occasional, nonconducted P-wave is observed without a preceding change in the P–R interval (Figure 16.4)
  - In nearly all cases the QRS is wide, indicating distal conduction system disease
  - Infrequently the baseline QRS complex is narrow, suggesting the block is within the His bundle
  - These patients are at high risk of progression to CHB and pacemakers are usually indicated regardless of symptoms.

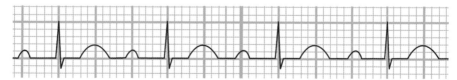

Figure 16.2 ECG of first-degree AV block

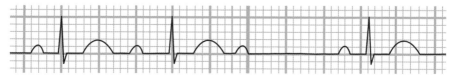

Figure 16.3 ECG of second-degree AV block: Mobitz type I

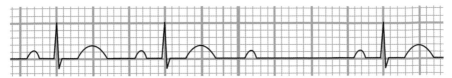

Figure 16.4 ECG of second-degree AV block: Mobitz type II

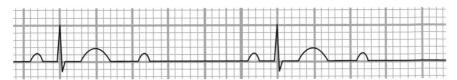

Figure 16.5 ECG of 2:1 AV block

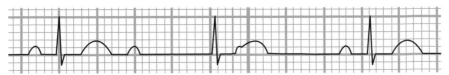

Figure 16.6 ECG of third-degree AV block

- **2:1 AV block**:
  - Every other P-wave is not conducted (Figure 16.5)
  - Presence of a narrow QRS indicates that the level of block is likely within the AV node
  - Alternately, if the QRS is wide, the level of the block may be below the His bundle.
- **Third-degree AV block (Figure 16.6)**:
  - CHB occurs when there is complete failure of conduction between the atria and the ventricles and can be due to block anywhere from the AV node to the His–Purkinje system
  - If the escape rhythm is a narrow QRS and occurs at a rate of 40–55 bpm, block is usually within the AV node
  - If the escape rhythm is a wide QRS and occurs at a rate of <40 bpm, the block is usually below the AV node
  - If atropine improves AV conduction, the site of block is likely to be at the AV node
  - If conduction worsens, then the site of block is more likely below the AV node
  - Conversely, vagal maneuvers worsen conduction if the block is at the AV node and improve AV conduction with infranodal block
  - Pacemaker implantation is indicated in most cases of complete AV block.

Treatment

- **Acute:**
  - For patients showing any signs of hemodynamic instability, the ACLS bradycardia guidelines should be followed (see Chapter 21)
  - In general, atropine (0.04 mg/kg IV bolus) is a first-line agent in the acute setting, but should be used with caution in patients with wide QRS complexes and AV block where infranodal disease is more likely and the degree of AV block can worsen
  - Isoproterenol (starting at 1 μg/min IV) can also be used with caution until temporary pacing is achieved
  - Temporary transcutaneous pacing is difficult to successfully achieve reliably and is usually quite uncomfortable for the patient, often requiring sedation
  - Temporary transvenous pacing is usually indicated in this setting and a catheter can be floated into the right ventricle at the bedside if necessary.
- **Permanent:**
  - As mentioned earlier, reversible causes of nodal disease should be excluded and treated before a more permanent form of pacing is sought
  - In general, symptomatic bradycardia is treated with a permanent pacemaker.

  The indications for pacemaker implantation are listed in Box 16.1.

CLINICAL PEARLS

- Always assess for digoxin use and toxicity, especially with new renal failure.
- New bundle branch block in the setting of an anterior MI is an indication for temporary pacing due to high risk of rapid progression to AV block.
- Evidence of progressive AV block in the setting of suspected endocarditis warrants further evaluation for abscess formation.
- Patients with high-degree AV block and wide QRS complexes should not be given atropine.
- Asymptomatic sinus bradycardia, particularly during sleep, does not usually require intervention.

Recommended Reading

Guidelines

ACC/AHA/HRS 2008 guidelines for device-based therapy of cardiac rhythm abnormalities. *Heart Rhythm* 2008;5(6):934–955.

17 Syncope

Farheen Shirazi and Karen Friday

Department of Internal Medicine, Division of Cardiology, Stanford University School of Medicine, Stanford, CA, USA

Syncope is defined as transient, self-limited loss of consciousness and postural tone followed by rapid and complete recovery. Although conditions such as seizure activity and stroke are not typically categorized as "syncope," they can present with transient loss of consciousness and must be included in the differential diagnosis.

Syncope is a common presenting complaint and accounts for up to 6% of all hospital admissions. While the majority of syncope is due to benign processes such as vasovagal syncope and orthostatic hypotension, it can be the initial presentation of more serious, life-threatening diseases that must be ruled out in high-risk individuals.

Differential Diagnosis

Keeping the differential diagnosis (Box 17.1) in mind is critical to the evaluation and subsequent management of patients with syncope.

Neurally-Mediated Syncope (~40%)
- Syncope caused by increased parasympathetic tone, decreased sympathetic tone, or a combination thereof is referred to as neutrally mediated.
- Increased parasympathetic tone leads to sinus and AV node suppression, manifested by sinus bradycardia and varying degrees of AV block.
- Decreased sympathetic tone leads to a vasodepressor response which is manifested by hypotension.
- Encompasses a range of syndromes with overlapping features and underlying etiologies:
  - **Neurocardiogenic syncope:**
    - Most frequent cause of syncope
    - Also known as the "common faint," reflex syncope, and vasovagal syncope

---

A Practical Approach to Cardiovascular Medicine, First Edition. Edited by Reza Ardehali, Marco Perez, Paul Wang.

Box 17.1 Common causes of syncope

Neurally-mediated syncope (40%)
Neurocardiogenic
Carotid sinus syncope
Situational syncope

Orthostatic hypotension (20%)
Autonomic dysfunction
Volume depletion
Postural orthostatic tachycardia syndrome
Drug-induced

Structural heart disease (10%)
Cardiomyopathy
Acute myocardial infarction or ischemia
Valvular disease
Hypertrophic cardiomyopathy
Congenital heart disease
Atrial myxoma
Aortic dissection
Pulmonary embolus

Primary cardiac arrhythmias (10%)
Conduction system disease
Ventricular tachycardia
Supraventricular tachycardia

Neurologic (5%)
Seizures
Stroke
Subclavian steal syndrome
Psychogenic

Idiopathic (15%)

- It is likely caused by reflex activation of vagal efferent pathways and sympathetic inhibition triggered by various neurologic inputs, including vagal afferents, pain pathways, and other central pathways.
- **Carotid sinus syncope:** a relatively common cause of syncope in the elderly which is due to oversensitivity of the baroreceptors found in the carotid sinus. These receptors normally respond to increases in BP by augmenting vagal efferents, leading to vasodilation.
- **Situational syncope:**
  - Some patients experience reproducible syncope in the setting of a wide range of very specific activities
  - Some of the more common situations include micturition, cough, postprandial and postexercise syncope
  - The mechanism is similar to that of neurocardiogenic syncope.

Orthostatic Hypotension (~20%)

- Maintenance of adequate vascular tone necessary for brain perfusion after an abrupt change in posture requires a complex set of autonomic responses.
- Common causes are:
  - **Autonomic dysfunction:**
    - Can be secondary to a number of associated conditions, such as diabetic neuropathy, or can be primary without a clear underlying etiology
    - Situational autonomic failure, as in postexercise or postprandial syncope, can also be present
  - **Volume depletion:** dehydration from either lack of fluid intake or excess loss (diarrhea, hemorrhage)
  - **Postural orthostatic tachycardia syndrome (POTS):**
    - Characterized by an exaggerated heart rate increase with a mild drop in BP following postural changes
    - Although a relatively common cause of dizziness in younger adults, it rarely causes syncope
  - **Drug-induced:** orthostatic hypotension can arise from medication or alcohol use.

Structural Heart Disease (~10%)

- Structural heart diseases lead to syncope either via associated ventricular arrhythmias or obstruction of flow.
- Conditions that must be considered:
  - **Cardiomyopathy:** patients with either ischemic or nonischemic cardiomyopathy, particularly those with ejection fraction (EF) <35%, are at high risk of ventricular arrhythmias
  - **Myocardial infarction or ischemia:** patients can manifest with ventricular arrhythmias due to ischemia or scar
  - **Valvular disease:** although any valvular disease can lead to syncope, critical aortic stenosis (AS) is the usual culprit
  - **Hypertrophic cardiomyopathy (HCM):** relatively rare condition, but must be suspected in young patients with exertional syncope. Syncope can be related to either obstruction or associated ventricular arrhythmias
  - **Congenital heart disease:** can be associated with both arrhythmias and obstructive disease
  - **Atrial myxoma:** although rare, these masses can grow large enough to cause valvular obstruction
  - **Aortic dissection:** a flap in the aortic lumen can lead to obstruction of aortic blood flow
  - **Pulmonary embolus:** large, bilateral emboli can obstruct pulmonary arterial blood flow.

Primary Arrhythmic Disease (~10%)

- Both brady- and tachy-arrhythmias can lead to syncope.
- Arrhythmic disease can initially be brief and self-limiting before it progresses to a more lethal form (see Chapter 17).

- Conditions that must be considered:
  - **Conduction-system disease:** any dysfunction from the level of the sinus node, through the AV node and down to the His–Purkinje system can cause significant bradycardia or asystole
  - **Ventricular tachycardia:**
    - There are several VT syndromes that occur in the absence of structural heart disease (see Chapter 15)
    - At high heart rates, diastolic filling time is compromised and cardiac output can drop precipitously
    - Ventricular fibrillation is often a terminal arrhythmia, but can also be self-limited
  - **Supraventricular tachycardia (SVT):** alone rarely causes syncope, unless there is associated volume depletion, a rapidly conducting accessory pathway, or structural heart disease (see Chapter 14).

Neurologic Conditions (~5%)
- Conditions that must be considered:
  - **Seizures:** primary, generalized seizure activity leads to loss of consciousness. However, it is important to remember that brain hypoperfusion can present with seizure-like activity. Cardiogenic disease, for example, can be missed if seizure-like activity was observed by the family during the syncopal event
  - **Stroke:** strokes and transient ischemic attacks rarely cause loss of consciousness. Very large, bilateral strokes or strokes involving the brain stem are the rare exceptions
  - **Subclavian steal syndrome:** shunting of blood from the vertebral arteries to the subclavian artery distal to a subclavian stenosis. Suspect in patients with peripheral vascular disease, upper extremity complaints or syncope following head turning
  - **Psychogenic:** suspect only after other causes have been ruled out with thorough evaluation.

Idiopathic (~15%)
- Despite thorough investigation, some patients who present with syncope remain undiagnosed.

Work-up

The work-up of syncope can be challenging because of the myriad tests available, many of which are not very sensitive or specific. A thorough patient history and exam often leads to the correct diagnosis and can help risk-stratify patients who may need additional, targeted testing.

History
- Allowing the patient to tell a detailed "story" of the syncopal episode is invaluable.

- Key components of the history that should be assessed in all patients:
  - Establish true loss of consciousness (LOC), approximate duration and number of episodes
  - Triggers: patients can usually point out events or unusual situations around the time of syncope
  - Postural changes: ask what position or changes in posture the syncope happened in
  - Prodrome: dizziness, nausea, palpitations, and diaphoresis can precede neurocardiogenic syncope, but these findings are nonspecific. AV block and ventricular tachycardias are usually more sudden in onset
  - Recovery: contrary to common belief, incontinence, confusion, and tongue biting are not specific for seizure disorders
  - Associated medical history: assess for pre-existing cardiovascular and neurologic disease
  - Family history: ask about cardiac disease and sudden cardiac death (SCD), including unexplained drownings and car accidents
  - Associated drug and medication use
  - Interview witnesses who observed event to assess duration and activity.

Physical Exam
- A thorough physical examination can provide clues to the etiology of syncope.
- Special attention should be given to the following physical findings:
  - Resting pulse: make note of irregularity, tachycardia, or bradycardia
  - Orthostatic hypotension: measure BP after lying supine for at least 5 min and standing for 1 min. Defined as:
    - Decrease in systolic BP (SBP) ≥20 mmHg regardless of symptoms
    - Decrease of SBP to <90 mmHg regardless of symptoms
    - A 10-point drop in diastolic BP with symptoms
  - Heart murmurs: assess for valvular disease, particularly AS, and HCM
  - Carotid sinus massage: moderate pressure over the carotid pulse for 5–10 s, continuous ECG monitoring, and frequent BP measurements. If carotid bruits or risk of stroke are present, avoid carotid sinus massage. Definitive hypersensitivity is defined as:
    - Syncope reproduced with asystole >3 s, or
    - Fall in systolic BP >50 mmHg.

Testing
The number of tests available to help elucidate the cause of syncope can be overwhelming. Given that syncope is a common presentation, tests must be ordered judiciously. The following is a guide to the options and recommendations on appropriate usage:
- ECG:
  - Everyone who presents with syncope should have an ECG performed (see Chapter 22 for a detailed description of findings)

- Special attention to be given to:
  - Rhythm
  - Presence of Q-waves (myocardial scar)
  - Prolonged QT interval
  - Conduction system abnormalities: marked sinus bradycardia or sinus pause >3 s; significantly prolonged PR interval or AV block; alternating left (LBBB) and right bundle branch block (RBBB); RBBB with left fascicular block
  - Pre-excitation (Wolf–Parkinson–White syndrome)
  - Brugada syndrome (RBBB with ST elevation V1–V3, epsilon waves, deeply inverted T-waves in V1–V3)
  - Marked LV hypertrophy (AS or HCM).
- **Echocardiogram:**
  - There should be a low threshold for cardiac echocardiography in anyone without a clear cause of syncope or those with suspected cardiac disease based on history, physical exam, and ECG
  - Echo is used to assess for structural heart disease, most commonly left ventricular dysfunction and valvular disease in the elderly, and HCM in the younger populations.
- **Exercise testing:**
  - Should be performed in patients with a history of or at risk for coronary artery disease
  - Although primarily used to assess for ischemia, rhythm disturbances or autonomic failure may become manifest
  - Echo should be performed first to rule out obstructive disease.
- **Ambulatory monitoring:**
  - Arrhythmias responsible for syncope can be intermittent and transient, with no clues on baseline studies
  - Unless an alternative cause of syncope has been identified, extra care should be taken in ruling out arrhythmias with ambulatory monitoring
  - Holter monitor:
    - Continuous 24–72-h monitoring
    - Only useful if syncope or associated symptoms are frequent
  - Loop/event monitoring:
    - Usually the preferred method of monitoring after initial presentation with syncope
    - Monitoring period is typically 21–30 days
    - Monitors are triggered automatically by heart rate or manually by the patient
  - Implantable loop recorder:
    - Implanted substernally
    - Patient or heart-rate triggered
    - Batteries on current devices can last approximately 2 years
    - Useful if syncope is very infrequent and cause remains a mystery.

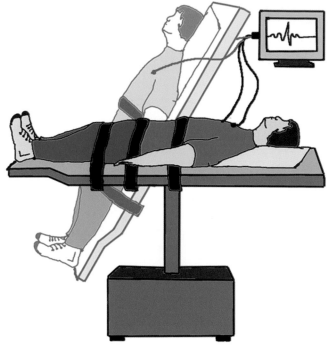

Figure 17.1 Tilt table testing

- **Upright tilt table testing** (Figure 17.1):
  - Given the limited specificity, sensitivity, and reproducibility of tilt table testing, its appropriate use in the setting of syncope remains controversial
  - Although many (about 40%) patients exhibit excessive hemodynamic or chronotropic changes during testing, it is often difficult to correlate these findings with clinical symptoms
  - Testing may be useful in:
    - Recurrent syncope or presyncope without evidence of structural or arrhythmic heart disease
    - Proving susceptibility of patient to neurally-mediated syncope
    - Patients involved in high-risk environmental/occupational conditions
    - Evaluating jerking motions to help differentiate neurocardiogenic syncope from primary seizure disorders.
  - Testing procedures vary by institution, but generally involve:
    - A special tilt table able to safely and rapidly position patients
    - Continuous ECG monitoring
    - Tilting the patient 60–80° for 25–40 min
    - If no initial response is seen, isoproterenol infusion or sublingual nitroglycerin are often used to increase positivity during the last 15–20 min of the study
    - Test is considered positive only if syncope occurs

- Possible responses (Figure 17.2):
  - Cardioinhibitory: HR falls to <40 bpm for 10 s, or asystole >3 s
  - Vasodepressor: BP falls without cardioinhibition
  - Mixed: BP falls with minimal cardioinhibition (drop in HR, but >40 bpm or asystole <3 s)
  - POTS: excessive heart rate rise (>130 bpm) before syncope
  - Chronotropic incompetence: heart rate rises <10% of baseline.
- **Electrophysiology study (EPS):**
  - Can be useful in a very select group of patients to establish conduction system disease or arrhythmia inducibility (see Chapter 29); however, findings can also be difficult to correlate with clinical symptoms
  - In the past, this test was often performed in patients with systolic dysfunction to evaluate for implantable cardioverter defibrillator (ICD) implantation; however, randomized trials have established the benefit of defibrillators in patients with severely reduced EF for primary prevention regardless of EPS
  - In addition, patients who meet other clinical criteria for pacemaker implantation (see Chapter 16) can also bypass the EPS
  - Test should be considered in syncopal patients with:
    - Suspected conduction system disease (bifascicular block, borderline sinus node dysfunction)
    - Strong family history of SCD
    - Nonsustained VT in the setting of mild-to-moderately reduced systolic function (EF 35–50%)
    - Presence of pre-excitation (Wolf–Parkinson–White syndrome)
  - Assesses the following:
    - Sinus node function (sinus node recovery time, sinoatrial conduction time)
    - AV nodal function (AV conduction and refractoriness)
    - Infranodal conduction system disease (prolonged HV interval)
    - Induction of ventricular or supraventricular tachycardia
  - If significant conduction system disease is identified, then a pacemaker is indicated (see Chapter 29)
  - If ventricular tachycardia is induced, then a defibrillator may be warranted
  - Induction of SVT with associated symptoms would prompt treatment with either medication or ablation, especially in the setting of an accessory pathway.
- **Head CT/brain MRI:**
  - Frequently obtained, often in the acute setting
  - If the patient is alert and a thorough neurologic examination is normal, then the yield is low.
- **EEG:**
  - Useful in distinguishing seizure-like activity during syncope from epilepsy

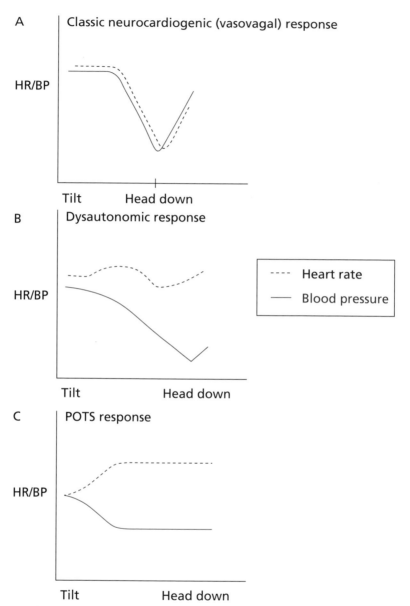

Figure 17.2 Heart rate and BP responses to tilt table testing (reproduced from Grubb BP. Neurocardiogenic syncope. In: Grubb BP, Olshansky B, eds. *Syncope: Mechanisms and Management*. Oxford: Blackwell Publishing Ltd, 1997, with permission)

- A single study has poor sensitivity and often must be repeated if the suspicion for epilepsy is high.
- **Carotid ultrasound:**
  - Often routinely ordered in the elderly population
  - Yield is low unless there is a history of peripheral vascular disease or presence of carotid bruits
  - Of note, for carotid disease to cause syncope, the patient must have significant bilateral disease.

Criteria for Hospital Admission

Patients at high risk of sudden death or injury from recurrent syncope should be hospitalized for further evaluation. These primarily include older patients and those suspected of having cardiovascular disease. Repeat hospitalization for recurrent syncope is of limited value.

The main indications for hospitalization include:
- Risk factors or history of coronary disease
- Signs or symptoms suspicious of structural or arrhythmic heart disease, including:
  - Heart failure
  - Abnormal ECG
  - Sudden syncopal event, without prodrome
- Exertional syncope
- Significant associated injury
- Family history of SCD.

Treatment

Once the diagnosis has been established, treatment of the underlying problem is recommended. The choice of therapy, however, can be challenging in many cases where, despite thorough investigation, the underlying cause is not clear. In this section, treatment for neutrally-mediated syncope and orthostatic hypotension is addressed. Refer to the relevant chapters for recommendations on treatment of other cardiovascular conditions.

Neurally-Mediated Syncope
The mainstays of treatment are reassurance and patient education. Vasovagal syncope is relatively common and if infrequent, does not necessitate intervention beyond patient education.
- **Education:**
  - Patients should avoid known triggers and assume a supine position when prodromal symptoms begin
  - Learning counterpressure maneuvers, such as fist clenching, leg pumping, leg crossing, and arm tensing, can delay syncope, particularly during long periods of standing
  - Moderate exercise may also have a beneficial effect.

- **Beta-blockers:**
  - Randomized trials have failed to show consistent benefit and may be harmful in younger populations.
- **Midodrine:**
  - Small trials and observational studies have shown varying degrees of benefit
  - Starting dose is 2.5 mg tid, which can be titrated to 10 mg tid
  - Avoid usage in patients with coronary disease, heart failure, or supine hypertension
  - Often prescribed in patients with recurrent syncope despite lifestyle changes.
- **Other drugs:**
  - Small randomized trials have shown reduction of syncope and/or improvement in tilt-table syncope with selective serotonin reuptake inhibitors, but their clinical use in syncope is not well established
  - Fludrocortisone for neurally-mediated syncope is not as well studied as it is for orthostatic hypotension.
- **Pacemakers:**
  - Four randomized trials, each with no >100 patients, have been performed with conflicting results. Two double-blinded trials were ended prematurely because of pacemaker complication rates without demonstrable benefit in syncope recurrence
  - Although bradycardia can be a major contributor to syncope, pacemakers do not prevent vasodilatory responses
  - A pacemaker may be considered for recurrent symptoms if significant bradycardia associated with syncope has been documented either spontaneously or with tilt-table testing.

Orthostatic Hypotension

Identification of the underlying cause of orthostasis will guide treatment. Acute volume depletion should be treated with replacement of fluid loss. Alcohol use and suspicious medications should be discontinued, particularly antihypertensive medications, antidepressants, diuretics, and antianginal medications. Additional treatments include:

- **Education:**
  - Rising slowly, raising the head of the bed 10–20°, using elastic stockings, increased exercise, smaller meals with less carbohydrates, leg tensing by crossing legs while standing, and avoiding alcohol are simple measures that can be recommended to all patients.
- **Salt and water intake:**
  - Autonomic disorders may be associated with increased salt and water excretion
  - High sodium diets and salt tablets along with increased water intake can also be advised.

- **Fludrocortisone:**
  - This mineralocorticoid is the first-line agent for most patients and is usually well tolerated
  - Starting dose is 0.1 mg/day with a max 1.0 mg/day
  - Patients must be monitored for supine hypertension, hypokalemia, and edema.
- **Midodrine:**
  - This alpha-1-adrenergic agonist is often added to fludrocortisones as a second-line agent
  - Starting dose is 2.5 mg tid which can be titrated to 10 mg tid
  - Avoid usage in patients with coronary disease, heart failure, or supine hypertension.
- **Other drugs:**
  - Since fludrocortisones and midodrine are not well tolerated or ineffective in many patients, a number of other medications have been studied, including caffeine, erythropoietin, pyridostigmine, NSAIDs, desmopressin, yohimbine and metoclopramide, with varying degrees of success, and their use is not well established.
  - Beta-blockers: no longer recommended in the treatment of orthostatic hypotension given their side effects and relative ineffectiveness.

CLINICAL PEARLS

- History and physical examination provide a diagnosis in the majority of cases.
- Seizure-like activity can be seen with any disorder causing brain hypoperfusion.
- Unless there is a clear etiology for syncope, most patients should have an ECG and echo performed early in the evaluation.
- Further testing should be targeted, otherwise, work-up can become costly and be of low yield.

Recommended Reading

Clinical Trials and Meta-Analyses

Connolly SJ, Sheldon R, Roberts RS, Gent M. The North American Vasovagal Pacemaker Study (VPS). A randomized trial of permanent cardiac pacing for the prevention of vasovagal syncope. *J Am Coll Cardiol* 1999;**33**:16–20.

Connolly SJ, Sheldon R, Thorpe KE et al. Pacemaker therapy for prevention of syncope in patients with recurrent severe vasovagal syncope. Second Vasovagal Pacemaker Study (VPS II): a randomized trial. *JAMA* 2003;**289**:2224–2229.

Ward CR, Gray JC, Gilroy JJ, Kenny RA. Midodrine: a role in the management of neurocardiogenic syncope: *Heart* 1998;**79**:45–49.

Guidelines

Brignole M, Albone P, Benditt DG et al. Guidelines of management (diagnosis and treatment) of syncope – update 2004. *Europace* 2004;**6**:467–537.

Epstein AE, DiMarco JP, Ellenbogen KA et al. ACC/AHA/HRS 2008 Guidelines for Device-Based Therapy of Cardiac Rhythm Abnormalities: a report of the American College of Cardiology/American Heart Association Task Force on Practice Guidelines. *J Am Coll Cardiol* 2008;**51**:e1–62.

Review Articles

Kapoor WN. Syncope. *N Engl J Med* 2000;**343**:1856–1862.

VI Cardiovacular Disease in Special Populations

18 Congenital Heart Disease

Patrick Yue

Department of Internal Medicine, Division of Cardiology, Stanford University School of Medicine, Stanford, CA, USA

Fundamental Underlying Principle

A patient's long-term prognosis is largely determined by the amount of systemic blood flow delivered to the pulmonary vasculature. Increased pulmonary flow increases the risk of irreversible pulmonary vascular obstructive disease (also known as Eisenmenger's syndrome). Accordingly, repairing a lesion *before* the onset of Eisenmenger's is critical.

Common Congenital Lesions

Atrial Septal Defects
- **Four types:**
  - Secundum (75% of all ASDs): located in the region of the fossa ovalis (i.e. the center of the atrial septum)
  - Primum (15%): located in the inferior septum
  - Sinus venosus (10%): located in the superior septum
  - Coronary sinus (<1%): "unroofed" coronary sinus = communication between the left and right atrium (LA and RA).
- **Associations:**
  - Secundum defects are classically associated with mitral valve prolapse
  - Primum defects:
    - Often coexist with superior ventricular septal defects (VSDs) to form an atrioventricular septal defect
    - Another commonly noted association is with a cleft anterior mitral leaflet and consequent mitral regurgitation
  - Sinus venosus defects are frequently (up to 85%) associated with partial anomalous pulmonary venous return (PAPVR) from the right upper (or

A Practical Approach to Cardiovascular Medicine, First Edition. Edited by Reza Ardehali, Marco Perez, Paul Wang.
© 2011 Blackwell Publishing Ltd. Published 2011 by Blackwell Publishing Ltd.

less frequently, lower) pulmonary vein (PV) to the RA or inferior vena cava (IVC)
- Atrial septal defects (ASDs) in general are thought in some circles to be related to migraine headaches, though this association is controversial.
- **Epidemiology:** 1 per 1500 live births (second to bicuspid aortic valve as most common adult congenital lesion).
- **Exam findings:**
  - Unless severe, subtle at best. The ASD itself does not produce a murmur
  - Wide, fixed splitting of S2 as inspiration-associated venous return is diverted to LA
  - Soft systolic ejection murmur in the second left intercostal space due to increased pulmonary artery (PA) flow.
- **Natural history:**
  - Progression to Eisenmenger's relatively rare (<5%) due to low pressure differential between LA and RA
  - Larger ASDs (>1.5 cm) result in chronic volume overload → remodeling of the RA, LA, and right ventricle (RV) → tricuspid regurgitation (TR), RV failure, and atrial arrhythmias, by the fourth or fifth decade of life
  - Death is most frequently caused by either heart failure or thromboembolic stroke.
- **Echo:**
  - Best view: apical four-chamber
  - Sinus venosus defects are notoriously difficult to detect on transthoracic echocardiography (TTE), and may require transesophageal echocardiography (TEE) or CT/MRI to visualize them
  - Even if a sinus venosus defect is seen on echo, CT/MRI may be necessary to identify an associated PAPVR.

Ventricular Septal Defects
- **Types:**
  - No complete consensus
  - At Stanford, VSDs are typically categorized into four groups:
    - Membranous (75–80%): located basally in the membranous septum just inferior to the aortic valve
    - Muscular (5–20%): situated in the apical trabeculum. ≥2 muscular VSDs frequently coexist in the same patient (i.e. "Swiss Cheese" VSD)
    - Inlet (5–10%): due to proximity, inlet VSDs are sometimes lumped with membranous VSDs. However, inlet VSDs are located posterior/inferior to membranous VSDs, close to the septal leaflet of the tricuspid valve
    - Outlet [also known as supracristal, doubly committed; 5–7%; more frequent in Asians (25–30%)]: located in the fibrous continuity between the pulmonic and aortic valves (i.e. between the two outflow tracts).
- **Associations:**
  - Chromosomal syndromes (e.g. trisomy 13, 18, and 21); only 5% of VSDs are associated with these disorders.

- **Epidemiology:**
  - 2–6 per 1000 live births, making them more common than ASDs in children
  - However, given the significant attrition rate (see below), the prevalence drops with age.
- **Exam findings:**
  - Holosystolic murmur at lower left sternal border ± palpable thrill
  - Smaller VSDs produce louder, higher-pitched murmurs
  - Lateral displacement of the apical impulse and mid-diastolic rumble due to volume overload.
- **Natural history:**
  - 25–40% close spontaneously before age 10 (esp. if in muscular septum).
  - 60–75% remain open into adulthood
  - Chronic left-to-right shunting, with high pressure gradient, leads to eventual progression to Eisenmenger's if the defect is large enough
  - If so, patients survive only 30–50 years.
- **Echo:**
  - Usually easy to identify on TTE
  - However, more basal VSDs (inlet and outlet) can be elusive, and sometimes require TEE and/or CT/MRI
  - By VSD type, the best echocardiographic windows are:
    – Membranous: parasternal long axis, apical four- and five-chamber
    – Muscular: apical four- chamber
    – Inlet: parasternal short axis at the level of the AV valves, apical four-chamber
    – Outlet: basal parasternal short axis.

Patent Ductus Arteriosus

In adults, the ligamentum arteriosum is what remains of the left sixth primitive aortic arch, which in fetal life is commonly referred to as the ductus arteriosus. The ductus, which connects the left main pulmonary artery with the descending aorta just distal to the left subclavian take-off, remains patent throughout gestation, but closes during or shortly after birth. When this does not occur, the result is a patent ductus arteriosus (PDA).

- **Associations:**
  - Assumed to be present in preterm infants
  - Increased prevalence in individuals with chromosomal abnormalities
  - Classically associated with maternal rubella.
- **Epidemiology:** 1–20 per 10 000 live births (variation may be due to the inclusion and/or exclusion of preterm neonates in various clinical studies).
- **Exam findings:**
  - Widened pulse pressure
  - Continuous "machinery" murmur loudest around S2 in the left second intercostal space.

- **Natural history:** Variable depending on size.
  - Small PDAs are generally inconsequential (albeit with increased endocarditis/endarteritis risk)
  - Moderately-sized PDAs develop volume overload, with LA/LV enlargement and atrial fibrillation. Additionally, the PDA itself can develop calcification, dilatation, and/or rupture
  - Large PDAs with increased left-to-right shunting can progress toward Eisenmenger's.
- **Echo:**
  - Best visualized in the basal parasternal short axis
    - Suprasternal approach also possible.

Pulmonic Stenosis

- **Types:**
  - Most are valvular (80–90%)
  - Remainder are either supra- or sub-valvular.
- Associations:
  - Williams syndrome
  - Noonan syndrome.
- **Epidemiology:** 1 in 1500 live births, though the incidence is suspected to be greater.
- **Exam findings:**
  - Wide split S2 (wider than any other lesion)
  - Systolic ejection murmur along the left sternal border that increases with inspiration
  - Systolic ejection click.
- **Natural history:** dependent on the pressure gradient across the pulmonic outflow tract:
  - If the mean gradient is <50 mmHg, no significant sequelae will develop
  - More severe cases progress to RV hypertrophy and failure.
    - **Echo:** best view is the basal parasternal short axis.

Tetralogy of Fallot (TOF)

Involves:

- Pulmonic stenosis (PS)/atresia
- Overriding aorta
- VSD
- RV hypertrophy.

Conceptually an interesting lesion as it involves a VSD (typically an acyanotic condition), yet produces a cyanotic phenotype.

- **Associations:**
  - Sometimes clumped with other lesions to form such entities as the pentalogies of Fallot (TOF plus ASD) and Cantrell (TOF plus aortic coarctation)

- Coronary anomalies [particularly an anomalous origin of the left anterior descending artery (LAD) from the right coronary artery (RCA)].
- **Epidemiology:** 3–6 per 10000 live births (most common cyanotic lesion).
- **Exam findings:**
  - Cyanotic.
  - RV heave
  - Palpable thrill is often appreciated along the left sternal border
  - Single S2 due to obliteration of the pulmonic valve
  - Overriding aorta (which is frequently dilated) results in a systolic ejection click
  - Systolic ejection murmur along the left sternal border, which is caused by flow across the obstructed right ventricular outflow tract (RVOT).
- **Natural history:**
  - Uncorrected: death by 30–40 years; usually RV failure
  - Surgical repair (VSD closure, relief of RVOT obstruction) in infancy markedly improves survival, though patients are often left without a pulmonic valve
  - Progressive pulmonary regurgitation (PR) leads to RV dilatation and failure over time
  - Pulmonic valve replacement is thus often necessary.
- **Echo:**
  - Parasternal long axis: sufficient to visualize the VSD, the overriding aorta, and the right ventricular hypertrophy (RVH)
  - Basal parasternal short axis: for RVOT obstruction.
    - Given associations, a complete study should evaluate for ASDs, other AV shunts, and aortic coarctation.

Transposition of Great Arteries

- **Types:**
  - **D-transposition** (D-TGA; or complete TGA): aorta arises from the morphologic right ventricle, and the pulmonary artery arises from the morphologic LV. Accordingly, the systemic and pulmonary circuits are uncoupled, an arrangement which, unless mitigated by an AV shunt, is incompatible with life
  - **L-transposition** (L-TGA; or congenitally corrected TGA): the RA enters the morphologic LV, which empties into the pulmonary artery, and the left atrium enters the morphologic RV, which empties into the aorta. Thus a normal circulation exists (two wrongs make a right), but the ventricles are mismatched, leading to downstream sequelae (see below).
- **Associations:**
  - D-TGA: by necessity, associated with a shunt, usually an ASD, PDA, or VSD
  - L-TGA: VSDs (70%; typically perimembranous) and subvalvular PS (40%).

- **Epidemiology:**
  - D-TGA:
    - Relatively common cause of newborn cyanosis
    - Adults with this condition have typically undergone some form of corrective surgery
  - L-TGA: comparatively rare, probably because of underdiagnosis.
- **Exam findings:**
  - Single, loud S2 (anterior aorta = loud A2; posterior PA = soft P2)
  - Holosystolic murmur arising from systemic AV valvular regurgitation (location dependent on ventricular situs).
- **Natural history:**
  - L-TGA: asymptomatic until early adulthood:
    - Gradual dilatation/failure of systemic (i.e. morphologic) RV associated with systemic AV valvular regurgitation
    - Survival to 40–50 s.
    - Mode of exodus pump failure and/or arrhythmias
  - D-TGA: prognosis dependent on the type of repair performed (see below):
    - Post-Mustard patients are functionally identical to L-TGA with similar risk of systemic ventricular failure
    - Post-Jatene patients: prognosis undefined, as first patients are only now reaching adulthood
    - Common sequelae to both: atrial arrhythmias, coronary stenoses, baffle leaks/obstructions/infections.
- **Echo:** because of the juxtaposition of the PA and aorta (and at times, the LV and RV), TGAs are among the most difficult congenital lesions to properly visualize. Echocardiographic hallmarks:
  - Parasternal long axis (as well as the apical three- and five-chamber): the systemic and pulmonic outflow tracts run parallel with each other, i.e. the PA and the aorta can be visualized longitudinally with the same cut
  - Parasternal short axis: aortic root anterior to PA (use "Mercedes" sign of aortic valve to confirm aorta's identity)
  - Configuration of the ventricles is variable:
    - D-TGA: morphologic RV and LV are in "proper" locations (post-Mustard patients will have morphologic RV dilatation/dysfunction)
    - L-TGA: morphologic RV dilatation/dysfunction, but this ventricle will be located on the left.

Patients Who Most Benefit from Surgical Repair

The morbidity and natural history of many, if not most, congenital lesions often dictate that a corrective procedure, whether curative or merely palliative, be strongly considered. If intervention is to be entertained, however, two questions must be addressed:

- **For acyanotic lesions with left-to-right shunt, what is the shunt fraction?**
  - Applies not only to "conventional" left-to-right shunts (i.e. ASDs, VSDs, and PDAs), but also to surgically palliated cyanotic lesions with residual L-R shunting
  - Shunt fraction, or the ratio of pulmonary and systemic blood flows (Qp/Qs), can generally be determined by Doppler echocardiography or MRI, though occasionally it is necessary to use invasive means (i.e. cardiac catheterization) to do so
  - Commonly accepted threshold for intervention is ≥1.5, though this has not been formally validated.
- **Is there evidence of pulmonary vascular obstructive disease?**
  - Threshold for pulmonary hypertension at risk for pulmonary veno-occlusive disease (PVOD) is generally considered to be a mean pulmonary pressure ≥2/3 the mean systemic arterial pressure [analogously, the pulmonary vascular resistance (PVR) and systemic vascular resistance (SVR) should also obey the same ratio]
  - If a patient exceeds this level, invasive catheterization with a nitrous oxide challenge should be performed to determine the reversibility of the increased pulmonary resistance
  - If the PVR cannot be brought down below 2/3 the SVR, the disease is deemed irreversible (i.e. Eisenmenger's physiology) and intervention is therefore contraindicated.

Eisenmenger's Syndrome

Eisenmenger's syndrome represents a special case in that:
- No efficacious medical therapies exist
- Survival, as compared to patients with primary pulmonary hypertension, is significantly longer
- Patients are exquisitely sensitive to hemodynamic shifts.

Thus, the predominant mode of treatment for these individuals should be one of nonintervention and prevention.

Considerations specific to Eisenmenger's patients are:
- **Hemodynamics:**
  - Balance between right-to-left and left-to-right shunting is precarious in these patients. Therefore, alteration of this balance should not be disturbed
  - Avoid:
    - Factors with direct influence on vascular tone (e.g. vasodilator drugs, hot tub use)
    - Factors that decrease cardiac output (e.g. phlebotomy, hemorrhage, dehydration).
- **Hypoxemia:**
  - As with all patients with pulmonary hypertension, oxygenation (and those factors that tend to decrease it) should be properly addressed

- If necessary, supplemental oxygen is often useful, if only for symptomatic relief of dyspnea.
- **Hemoptysis:**
  - Due to pulmonary infarction, hemorrhage, embolism
  - Frequently devastating because of the potential hemodynamic consequences (see above).
- **Erythrocytosis:**
  - Never phlebotomize except as a last resort (Hct >65%)
  - If considered, concomitant fluid replacement should also be entertained to maintain hemodynamic homeostasis.
- **Surgery:**
  - Should be avoided unless absolutely necessary
  - Sources of risk:
    - Hemodynamic effects of anesthetic agents
    - Frequent intra- and post-operative fluid shifts
    - Iatrogenic embolic phenomena.
- **Pregnancy:**
  - Associated with roughly 40–50% maternal mortality
  - *Strictly* contraindicated.

Imaging a Patient with Suspected Congenital Heart Disease

One of the more intimidating "on call nightmares" for the cardiologist is a request to perform an echocardiogram on a patient with previously uncharacterized congenital disease.

Tips to provide a framework that may make this endeavor easier:
- **Adult patient:**
  - There are only so many lesions that allow for survival to adulthood
  - Truly complex (mostly cyanotic) lesions are typically "weeded out"
  - Postoperative patients have a stereotypical postsurgical configuration with relatively little variation.
- **Sort out the RV from the LV:**
  - Do not assume that the ventricle on the right is the RV, and the ventricle on the left is the LV, especially if TGA is suspected
  - Conventional cues (e.g. chamber shape, wall thickness, trabeculation pattern, moderator band) may be unreliable
  - Compare the septal insertions of the AV valves:
    - Apical insertion = morphologic RV
    - Basal insertion = morphologic LV.
- **Image from the bottom up:**
  - Parasternal view is frequently limited by acoustic shadowing of RV from sternum
  - Subcostal and apical views often better

- Somewhat dictated by tradition (pediatric echoes are subcostal due to smaller intercostals spaces and rib shadowing).
- **If you do not know what something is, track it:**
  - Often useful to sweep through the field with the ultrasound probe to identify structures contiguous with the unknown chamber
  - Use color Doppler to determine direction of flow
  - If flow is visualized, measure the pressure gradient to determine whether the chamber belongs to the systemic or pulmonary circuit.
- **If you find something, do not stop:**
  - Never assume a lesion is isolated
  - Many associations (e.g. primum ASD with cleft mitral valve) exist
  - Ultimately, patient's anatomy should match the clinical picture (an ASD should not be the only finding in a 20-year-old cyanotic patient).

Most Commonly Encountered Surgical Corrections

Blalock–Taussig (1945), Potts (1946), and Waterston (1962) Shunts

- Indicated for complex cyanotic heart disease
- Palliative in nature and have largely been replaced by more definitive corrective surgeries (see below)
- All involve creation of anastomosis between the systemic and pulmonary circulations:
  - Blalock–Taussig: subclavian artery to pulmonary artery
  - Waterston: ascending aorta to right PA
  - Potts: descending aorta to left PA
  - Modified Blalock-Taussig (1962):
    - Subclavian artery to pulmonary artery via Gore-Tex graft
    - Performed if patient too sick for more involved procedure.
- These procedures have been largely abandoned:
  - Systemic load to the pulmonary vasculature, which if left uncorrected, leads to Eisenmenger's
  - Chronic LV volume overload due to now left-to-right shunt.

Glenn (1958)

- As with the above, also indicated for various complex cyanotic lesions.
- Involves anastomosis between systemic *vein* and pulmonary circulation (as opposed to the above, which connect systemic *artery* and pulmonary circulation).
- Thus pulmonary pressures are preserved, preventing development of Eisenmenger's.
- Classic Glenn: end-to-side anastomosis between superior vena cava (SVC) and distal right PA.
- Bidirectional Glenn (current configuration): same as Classic except the right PA is not isolated from the main PA, allowing systemic venous return to both lungs.

- Current indication: bridge procedure in young (<1–5 years) patients pending more definitive repair, especially if PA pressures too high to tolerate full Fontan circuit (see below).

Fontan (1971)
- Current gold standard for lesions with a single ventricle (e.g. hypoplastic left heart, tricuspid atresia, double inlet ventricle, etc.).
- Fontan principle: an RV is dispensable to deliver venous return to the lungs, provided there is:
  - Low enough pulmonary vascular resistance, and
  - Adequate systemic cardiac output.
- Aim: to reconnect (by whatever means) all systemic return to the pulmonary arteries.
- Most up-to-date configuration:
  - Bidirectional Glenn to account for SVC inflow
  - Connection between the IVC and the PA, using either an extracardiac conduit or a tunnel incorporating a baffle against the lateral right atrial wall.

Mustard Atrial Switch (1958)
- Initially indicated for patients with complete D-type TGA.
- A bypass conduit, or "baffle," is constructed within the atria to redirect incoming flow from the IVC and pulmonary veins to the correct chamber.
- Unfortunately, it leaves the patient with an anatomy functionally identical to a congenitally corrected transposition.
- Post-Mustard patient is thus consigned to the natural history of an L-TGA and its attendant sequelae.
- Accordingly, the Mustard has largely been abandoned.

Jatene Arterial Switch (1976)
- Gold standard procedure for D-TGA.
- Has essentially replaced the Mustard procedure as it restores normal connectivity of systemic pulmonary circuit without ventricular mismatch.
- PA and ascending aorta are transected then switched.
- Coronaries are then reimplanted in the neo-aorta.

Percutaneous Repair
- Gaining acceptance.
- Repair of choice for PDA (closure device implantation) and PS (balloon valvuloplasty).
- ASD/VSDs:
  - Closure devices also available
  - However due to anatomic variation/limitations, only secundum ASDs and muscular VSDs are eligible.

Complications Relevant to Adults

- **Arrhythmias:**
  - Most frequent reason for ER visits in adults with CHD, and are notoriously difficult to treat
  - Both brady- and tachy-arrhythmias (atrial fibrillation and flutter most common) are known to affect patients with congenital heart disease
  - Underlying factors:
    - Late consequence of operative repair
    - Progressive atrial and/or ventricular remodeling
    - Associated primary dysrhythmia (e.g. congenital heart block, WPW)
    - Occult hemodynamic derangement, be it obstruction or leakage
  - Treatment:
    - Bradyarrhythmias: pacemaker if high grade (Mobitz II or greater) block present
    - Tachyarrhythmias: prompt rhythm control (i.e. chemical ± electrical cardioversion) often essential.
- **Hyperviscosity:**
  - Erythrocytosis alone does not connote hyperviscosity
  - Symptoms: often nonspecific (excess bleeding, headache, fatigue, visual disturbances)
  - Treatment: therapeutic phlebotomy:
    - Used only if symptomatic and Hct >65.
    - Concomitant IV hydration should take place
    - Complications: iron-deficiency anemia due to rebound erythropoesis; air embolism (*air filters for IV lines!*)
- **Protein-losing enteropathy:**
  - 4–13% of post-Fontan patients
  - Results from chronically increased systemic venous pressures leading to lymphatic congestion and subsequent loss of protein (e.g. albumin, immunoglobulins) into the intestine
  - Present with generalized edema, ascites, and/or diarrhea
  - Poor prognosis (50% 5-year survival)
  - No definitive treatment modalities (save cardiac transplantation) currently exist.

CLINICAL PEARLS

- Endocarditis prophylaxis should be administered to *all* patients with congenital heart disease, except:
  - Isolated secundum ASD
  - Corrected ASD, VSD, PDA (>6 months after correction).
- ECG findings in ASD:

(Continued)

- Secundum ASD: *right* axis deviation and an incomplete right bundle branch block (RBBB)
- Primum ASD: *left* axis deviation (due to left ventricular hypertrophy secondary to cleft mitral valve/mitral regurgitation) and an incomplete RBBB.
- Ebstein's anomaly:
  - Inferior displacement of tricuspid valve leading to a small, frequently vestigial RV and decreased forward flow
  - Infrequent (5.2 per 100 000 live births) but overrepresented in board exams
  - Physical exam: loud, wide split S1, due to delayed closure of the grossly enlarged anterior leaflet of the tricuspid valve; peripheral cyanosis with central sparing; a systolic ejection click; a wide split S2; murmur of tricuspid regurgitation
  - Chest X-ray: "box-like" or "wall-to-wall" heart due to right atrial enlargement, generalized cardiomegaly, and underdevelopment of the pulmonary trunk
  - ECG: gigantic ("Himalayan") P-waves due to size of the RA and atrialized RV; right axis deviation; RBBB
  - Associated lesions: secundum ASD or PFO (80%); accessory pathway (20–25%); classic historical association: mother with lithium exposure.

Recommended Reading

Guidelines

Warnes CA, Williams RG, Bashore TM et al. ACC/AHA 2008 Guidelines for the Management of Adults with Congenital Heart Disease: a report of the American College of Cardiology/ American Heart Association Task Force on Practice Guidelines (writing committee to develop guidelines on the management of adults with congenital heart disease). *Circulation* 2008;**118**:e714–833.

Review Articles

Brickner ME, Hillis LD, Lange RA. Congenital heart disease in adults. First of two parts. *N Engl J Med* 2000;**342**:256–263.

Brickner ME, Hillis LD, Lange RA. Congenital heart disease in adults. Second of two parts. *N Engl J Med* 2000;**342**:334–342.

Mavroudis C, Backer CL, Deal BJ. Venous shunts and the Fontan circulation in adult congenital heart disease. In: Gatzoulis MA, Webb GD, Daubeney PEF, eds. *Diagnosis and Management of Adult Congenital Heart Disease*. Edinburgh: Churchill Livingstone, 2003.

Warnes CA. Adult congenital heart disease. In: Murphy JG, Lloyd MA, eds. *Mayo Clinic Cardiology: Concise Textbook, 3rd edn*. Rochester, MN: Mayo Clinic Scientific Press, 2007.

Webb GD, Smallhorn JF, Therrien J, Redington AN. Congenital heart disease. In: Libby P, Bonow RO, Mann DL, Zipes DP, eds. *Braunwald's Heart Disease: A Textbook of Cardiovascular Medicine*, 8th edn. Philadelphia: Saunders Elsevier, 2007.

19 Cardiology Consultation and Management of Perioperative Complications

Azar Mehdizadeh and Stanley G. Rockson
Department of Internal Medicine, Division of Cardiology, Stanford University School of Medicine, Stanford, CA, USA

Preoperative Cardiac Evaluation

Cardiac complications can lead to significant mortality and morbidity in patients who require noncardiac surgeries. Therefore, a thorough cardiac evaluation is an essential component of perioperative assessment. It is imperative that clinicians tailor their evaluations to specific patient- and procedure-related features. Of course, this approach is only feasible in elective, nonemergent circumstances. In all such cases, a through evaluation is warranted. Preoperative evaluation begins with a thorough history, a complete physical examination, and a 12-lead electrocardiogram (ECG).

History
- History should focus on a patient's:
  - Symptoms (e.g. chest pain, dyspnea on exertion)
  - Past cardiac history [e.g. myocardial infarction (MI), congestive heart failure, arrhythmia]
  - Cardiac functional status (e.g. sedentary vs. active).
- Baseline exercise capacity plays a major role in assessing a patient's risk profile.
- Activity scale [in metabolic equivalents (METs)] to determine a patient's baseline functional status:
  - 1 – taking care of one's self, e.g. eating, dressing
  - 4 – walking up a flight of stairs or a hill
  - 4–10 – heavy work around the house, e.g. scrubbing or moving furniture
  - >10 – strenuous sports, e.g. basketball, football

A Practical Approach to Cardiovascular Medicine, First Edition. Edited by Reza Ardehali, Marco Perez, Paul Wang.
© 2011 Blackwell Publishing Ltd. Published 2011 by Blackwell Publishing Ltd.

Physical Exam

- A detailed cardiovascular examination is an invaluable tool in identifying cardiac pathology such as heart failure or valvular disease.
- Clinicians must carefully assess the vital signs, volume status, pericardial palpation and auscultation, and vascular system, including the carotids and peripheral vessels.

ECG

- Abnormal ECG findings, such as pathologic Q-waves or significant ST segment deviations, are associated with an increased risk of preoperative cardiac complications.
- ACC/AHA guidelines recommend an ECG in patients with a recent episode of chest pain or an ischemic equivalent in patients undergoing an intermediate- or high-risk surgical procedure, and consider an ECG reasonable in asymptomatic patients with diabetes.

Risk Stratification of Cardiac Events

Three elements need to be assessed as part of the preoperative evaluation to determine the risk of cardiac events.

- **Patient-specific risk profile:**
  - Box 19.1 lists the clinical predictors, as defined by the ACC/AHA guidelines, that are associated with increased perioperative cardiac events (including MI, heart failure and death)
  - Major predictors require further evaluation and management, and may result in a delay or cancellation of non-emergent surgeries.
- **Surgery-specific risk profile:**
  - Type of surgery is another major factor that determines a patient's risk of adverse cardiac events
  - Box 19.2 summarizes the risk profile of various surgeries and procedures

---

Box 19.1 Clinical predictors of increased preoperative cardiovascular risk

Major predictors

Acute MI (within 7 days)

Recent MI (within 8–30 days)

Unstable angina

Decompensated heart failure

High-grade atrioventricular block

Symptomatic ventricular arrhythmias in patients who have underlying heart disease

Supraventricular arrhythmias with a poorly controlled ventricular rate

Severe heart valve disease

Box 19.1 *(Continued)*

Intermediate predictors

Mild angina

Previous myocardial infarction as determined from the history or the presence of pathologic Q-waves

Compensated heart failure or a prior history of heart failure

Diabetes mellitus

Renal failure with serum creatinine >2

Minor predictors

Advanced age

Abnormal ECG (left ventricular hypertrophy, left bundle branch block, ST-T abnormalities)

Rhythm other than sinus rhythm (e.g. atrial fibrillation)

Low functional capacity

History of stroke

Uncontrolled hypertension

Box 19.2 Cardiac risk stratification for specific noncardiac surgical procedures

High

Emergent surgery

Aortic and other major vascular surgery

Peripheral vascular surgery

Prolonged surgery associated with large fluid shifts or blood loss

Intermediate

Carotid endarterectomy

Head and neck surgery

Intraperitoneal and intrathoracic surgery

Orthopedic surgery

Prostate surgery

Low

Endoscopic procedures

Superficial procedures

Cataract surgery

Breast surgery

- Reported cardiac risk for high-, intermediate- and low-risk surgery groups are >5%, <5%, and <1%, respectively.
- **Functional status:**
  - As discussed above, baseline exercise capacity plays a major role in determining a patient's risk profile
  - Lack of ischemic symptoms in a patient with a sedentary lifestyle is not reassuring and may lower a clinician's threshold for further evaluation
  - See activity scale above.

Stepwise Approach to Perioperative Cardiac Evaluation

Part 1: Risk Stratification

The ACC/AHA guidelines provide a stepwise guide to assessing the need for investigation.

- Noninvasive stress testing is generally utilized to further evaluate those patients with clinical risk factors who will undergo noncardiac surgeries.
- It is important to keep in mind that, as with any other test, noninvasive stress testing should be performed in patients in whom an abnormal result will lead to an intervention that can improve the outcome or change the management strategy.
- Based on current guidelines, patients with active cardiac conditions such as unstable angina, severe valvular disease, or decompensated heart failure, need to be evaluated and treated prior to noncardiac surgeries.
- It is reasonable to perform noninvasive stress testing in patients with three or more clinical risk factors, if the outcome of the test will be used to potentially change the patient's management.
- Poor functional status (4 METs) lowers the threshold for noninvasive stress testing in patients with fewer risk factors.
- Exercise ECG testing is preferred in most ambulatory patients since it can assess a patient's functional status and detect coronary ischemia.
- In patients with an abnormal baseline ECG, stress cardiac imaging is recommended.
- If patients are unable to exercise, pharmacologic stress testing should be considered.

Part 2: Risk Modification

Currently the two treatment options available for preoperative cardiac mortality are medical therapy and revascularization. Assessment of the need for medical or interventional therapy is discussed below.

Medical Therapy

Beta-Blockers
- Perioperative use of beta-blockers is controversial in the absence of conclusive data.

- Previously, numerous randomized controlled trials showed promising benefits from the use of beta-blockers in high-risk patients undergoing high-risk noncardiac surgeries.
- However, the cardioprotective effect of beta-blockers that previously had been attributed to heart rate control has become more questionable in light of more recent data.

EVIDENCE-BASED PRACTICE

Effect of atenolol on mortality and cardiovascular morbidity after noncardiac surgery

Context: Effect of beta-blocker therapy on perioperative cardiovascular mortality.

Goal: To compare the effect of atenolol with that of a placebo on overall survival and cardiovascular morbidity/mortality in patients with CAD risks undergoing non cardiac surgery.

Methods: RCT, double-blind, placebo-controlled. 200 patients assigned to atenolol versus placebo.

Results: Reduction in death from cardiac causes in the atenolol group at 6 months, 1 year, and 2 years postoperatively but not during hospitalization.

Take-home message: Perioperative use of beta-blockers may have a protective effect.

EVIDENCE-BASED PRACTICE

Meta-analysis of the effect of heart rate achieved by perioperative beta-adrenergic blockade on cardiovascular outcomes

Context: Assessment of the cardioprotective properties of beta blockers

Goal: To investigate the association between the heart rate achieved with perioperative beta-blockade and the incidence of perioperative cardiac complications.

Methods: Meta-analysis of eight randomized trials

Results: Perioperative use of beta-blockers is not associated with a reduction in the incidence of cardiac complications.

Take-home message: That heart rate control with beta-adrenergic blockers is cardioprotective is not confirmed.

- Based on current available evidence, the ACC/AHA guidelines recommend beta-blockers in two groups:
  - Patients who are taking beta-blockers for angina, symptomatic arrhythmia, or hypertension
  - Patients scheduled for vascular surgery and with ischemic findings on preoperative testing.

- It is reasonable to use cardioselective beta-blockers and titrate the dose to attain the target resting heart rate of <65/min.
- Beta-blockers are probably also beneficial in patients with more than one clinical risk factor undergoing intermediate risk surgeries.
- However, it is uncertain if low-risk patients who have one or no risk factors would benefit from beta-blockade.

Statins
- Evidence suggests that perioperative use of statins may lower the rate of adverse cardiac events.
- However, most data are derived from observational studies and the time-to-initiation of statin therapy and optimal duration of therapy remain poorly characterized.
- Current guidelines recommend:
  - Continuing statin for patients currently taking this medication
  - Considering statin therapy in patients with at least one clinical risk factor undergoing noncardiac surgery.

Alpha-2 Agonists
- A few studies, including a prospective and meta-analysis, have looked at the effects of alpha-2 agonists on postoperative mortality and cardiac adverse events with promising results.
- Current guidelines recommend that clinicians can consider using alpha-2 agonists (clonidine) to control hypertension in patients with known coronary artery disease (CAD) and at least one clinical risk factor.

Revised Cardiac Risk Score (Risk Indices)
Various multivariable analyses have identified combinations of factors that could help to estimate the risk of cardiac complications. These factors are mainly derived from clinical and laboratory data. The revised cardiac risk index (RCRI) is one of the best validated risk prediction indices; it is simple to use and has excellent predictive value.

The RCRI is based on six predictors, each of which is given a score of 1:
- Ischemic heart disease
- Congestive heart failure
- Cerebrovascular accident
- Diabetes mellitus
- Creatinine >2
- High-risk surgery

Preoperative evaluation strategies can be based on the RCRI score.

Table 19.1 summarizes this strategy by combining a patient's risk score, noninvasive functional study results, and use of beta-blockers.

Table 19.1 Role of RCRI score in adverse event rate prediction and perioperative assessment

RCRI	RCRI score	Adverse cardiac event rate (%)	Recommendations	
			Beta-blocker	Non-invasive test
Ischemic heart disease				
CHF	0	0.4–0.5	No	No
CVA	1	0.9–1.3	Uncertain	No
DM	2	4–6.6	Yes	No
Cr >2	>3	9–11	Yes	Yes
High risk surgery				

EVIDENCE-BASED PRACTICE

Derivation and prospective validation of a simple index for prediction of cardiac risk of major non cardiac surgery

Context: Establishing a reference index for prediction of cardiac risk of major noncardiac surgery.

Goal: To derive and validate a simple index for the prediction of the risk of cardiac complications in major elective noncardiac surgeries.

Methods: Prospective cohort study of 4325 patients undergoing noncardiac surgery. RCRI was used to evaluate the major cardiac complications.

Results: Diagnostic performance of the RCRI was superior to other risk-prediction indices.

Take-home message: RCRI has a better predictive value of cardiac risk for patients undergoing noncardiac surgery.

Revascularization

Studies have shown that coronary artery bypass graft (CABG) or percutaneous coronary intervention (PCI) several months to years prior to a surgery may offer a degree of protection from adverse cardiac events. However, revascularization immediately before a surgery may actually lead to an increase in perioperative cardiovascular mortality and morbidity. The optimal time interval for cardioprotection following a revascularization strategy has not been defined – some reports that protection from revascularization may not be evident in surgeries done within 2 months after revascularization.

- ACC/AHA guidelines recommend coronary revascularization before noncardiac surgery in patients with high-risk unstable angina or acute MI and patients with stable CAD but significant left main coronary artery disease or three-vessel disease (especially when the left ventricular ejection fraction is <50%).
- No conclusive evidence to support revascularization in high-risk patients with abnormal noninvasive functional studies.
- Routine, prophylactic coronary revascularization is not recommended in patients with stable CAD.

EVIDENCE-BASED PRACTICE

Coronary artery revascularization before elective major vascular surgery
Context: Role of prophylactic revascularization in vascular surgery patients.
Goal: To evaluate whether prophylactic revascularization prior to vascular surgery reduces mortality in patients with stable CAD.
Methods: Randomized study. 510 patients assigned to revascularization strategy or not with most patients at intermediate risk with an RCRI >2.
Results: There was no difference between the two groups in long-term all-cause mortality at ~3 years, perioperative mortality or MI.
Take-home message: Prophylactic coronary artery revascularization in vascular surgery patients does not appear to have a protective effect.

CLINICAL PEARLS

- Adverse cardiac events are a major cause of perioperative mortality.
- Careful preoperative cardiac evaluation can identify those patients at higher risk.
- Thorough perioperative cardiac evaluation starts with a comprehensive history and physical exam.
- Patient's risk profile, surgery risk profile, and functional status are the three major elements of risk stratifying patients undergoing noncardiac surgeries.
- RCRI score is one of the best validated risk prediction indices that can estimate adverse cardiac events.
- ACC/AHA guidelines provide a framework for risk stratification and risk modification of patients undergoing noncardiac surgeries based on the current evidence.
- Noninvasive stress testing should be used in high-risk patients with multiple risk factors if the results will change their management.
- Perioperative use of beta-blockers remains controversial in light of new data.
- High-risk patients may benefit from cardioprotective properties of beta-blockers; however, this benefit has not been definitively shown in intermediate-/low-risk patients.
- Coronary revascularization (CABG or PCI) immediately prior to a noncardiac surgery has not been shown to improve mortality in patients with stable CAD.

Recommended Reading

Clinical Trials and Meta-Analyses

Fleischmann KE, Beckman JA, Buller CE et al. 2009 ACCF/AHA focused update on perioperative beta blockade. *J Am Coll Cardiol* 2009;**54**:2102–2128.

Ford MK, Beattie WS, Wijeysundera DN. Systematic review: prediction of perioperative cardiac complications and mortality by the revised cardiac risk index. *Ann Intern Med.* 2010;**152**:26–35.

Monaco M, Stassano P, Di Tommaso L et al. Systematic strategy of prophylactic coronary angiography improves long-term outcome after major vascular surgery in medium- to high-risk patients: a prospective, randomized study. *J Am Coll Cardiol* 2009;**54**:989–696.
Poldermans D, Hoeks SE, Feringa HH. Pre-operative risk assessment and risk reduction before surgery. *J Am Coll Cardiol* 2008;**51**:1913–1924.

Guidelines

Fleisher LA, Beckman JA, Brown KA et al. ACC/AHA 2007 Guidelines on perioperative cardiovascular evaluation and care for noncardiac surgery: a report of the American College of Cardiology/American Heart Association Task Force on Practice Guidelines (Writing Committee to Revise the 2002 Guidelines on Perioperative Cardiovascular Evaluation for Noncardiac Surgery): developed in collaboration with the American Society of Echocardiography, American Society of Nuclear Cardiology, Heart Rhythm Society, Society of Cardiovascular Anesthesiologists, Society for Cardiovascular Angiography and Interventions, Society for Vascular Medicine and Biology, and Society for Vascular Surgery. *Circulatio.* 2007;**116**:e418–499.

Review Articles

Fleisher LA, Eagle KA. Lowering Cardiac Risk in Noncardiac Surgery. *N Engl J Med* 2001;**345**:1677–1682.
Sun JZ, Maguire D. How to prevent perioperative myocardial injury: the conundrum continues. *Am Heart J.* 2007;**154**:1021–1028.

20 Management of Pre- and Post-Cardiac Surgery Patients

Mohammad Haghdoost[1] and Ramin Beygui[2]

[1]Department of General Surgery
[2]Department of Internal Medicine, Division of Cardiology, Stanford University School of Medicine, Stanford, CA, USA

Preoperative Assessment for Cardiac Surgery

- **History:** important points to clarify are:
  - Bleeding history
  - Antiplatelet and anticoagulant treatment
  - GI bleeding
  - Peripheral vascular disease
  - Any vascular reconstruction, vein stripping
  - Diabetes
  - Neurologic diseases
  - Urologic symptoms
  - Active infection
  - Smoking
  - Alcohol abuse
  - Medications and allergies.
- **Physical examination:** particular attention should be paid to:
  - Heart and lung exam
  - Vascular examination
  - Differential arm BP
  - Varicose veins
  - Skin infection
  - Presence of scars
  - Presence of dental caries.
- **Laboratory tests:** CBC, PT, PTT, platelet count, electrolytes, BUN, creatinine, blood sugar, LFTs, urinalysis, CXR PA and lateral, and ECG.

A Practical Approach to Cardiovascular Medicine, First Edition. Edited by Reza Ardehali, Marco Perez, Paul Wang.
© 2011 Blackwell Publishing Ltd. Published 2011 by Blackwell Publishing Ltd.

Preoperative Anticoagulation

- Stop Aspirin (ASA), cyclo-oxygenase inhibitor, 3–7 days preop (although, some surgeons recommend continuation of ASA until the time of surgery)
- Stop clopidogrel, ADP-mediated aggregation inhibitor, 5–7 days preop
- Stop abciximab, IIb/IIIa receptor inhibitor, 12–24 h preop
- Stop epitifibatide, IIb/IIIa receptor inhibitor, 2–4 h preop
- Stop tirobfibon, IIb/IIIa receptor inhibitor, 2–4 h preop
- Stop warfarin, 4 days preop and start heparin when INR becomes subtherapeutic
- If the patient has a compelling reason for being on warfarin (i.e. mechanical valve), admission to hospital and heparin therapy until the day of surgery is indicated
- If the patient is on warfarin and going for an urgent surgery, 5 mg of vitamin K IV significantly reduces INR within 12–24 h; however, fresh frozen plasma may be used for more emergent situation

Postoperative Assessment

- All cardiac surgery patients should be admitted to ICU.
- Communicate intraoperative course with anesthesiologist and surgeon.
- Find the relevant past medical and surgical history and comorbidities.
- Perform a thorough physical exam (heart, lung, peripheral perfusion, lines, tubes, pacemaker wires, and underlying rhythm)

Orders and Assessment
- **Neurology:**
  - Pain and anxiety control can be a challenge, particularly during first few days postoperatively. In general, benzodiazepines with short half-life are superior to the long-acting ones
  - Propofol and midazolam may be used while the patient is intubated
  - Morphine, as infusion or patient-controlled anesthesia (PCA), is a good choice of pain control
  - Ketoralac 15–30 mg IV q6h PRN may be administered for breakthrough pain and discontinue after 48 h (should be used cautiously in renal failure and watch for raising creatinine level)
  - Fentanyl 25 µg IV PRN may be given for shivering (mepridine 25 mg IV PRN for shivering should be use cautiously as accumulation of normeperidine in renal failure has deleterious effects).
- **Cardiovascular:**
  - Expected hemodynamic values:
    - Mean arterial pressure (MAP): 60–90 mmHg
    - Systolic BP (SBP): 90–140 mmHg
    - Right atrial pressure (RAP): 5–15 mmHg
    - Cardiac index (CI): 2.2–4.4 L/min/m^2

Box 20.1 Vasoactive medications

	Principal use	Other considerations
Inotropes		
Dopamine	General circulatory support	Vasopressor effects
Epinephrine	Inotrope and chronotrope	increasing with dose
Dobutamine	Inotrope and chronotrope	Alpha-adrenergic effect
Digoxin	Inotrope, AV node block	increasing with dose
Milrinone	Low CI with pulmonary and	Peripheral vasodilator
	systemic hypertension (HTN)	Toxicity, low K+, renal
		elimination
		Preferred vasodilator for
		diastolic heart failure
Vasopressors		
Dopamine	Shock with low SVR	See above
Norepinephrine	Shock with low SVR, CI <4 L/	Moderate inotrope
Phenylephrine	min/m2	Some reflex slowing of pulse
Epinephrine	Hyperdynamic shock with CI	rate
Vasopressin	4 L/min/m2	Use only for inotropic effects
	Shock with low SVR and low	H2O retention (?)
	CI	
	Hyperdynamic shock with low	
	SVR	
Vasodilators		
Nitroglycerin	HTN, fluid overload, high PVR	Inhibits hypoxemia,
Sodium nitroprusside	HTN, high SVR (HTN crisis)	pulmonary vasoconstriction
Nicardipine	HTN, cerebral vasospasm	Cyanide toxicity, renal
Milrinone	Low CI with pulmonary and	elimination
	systemic HTN	Reflex tachycardia
		Preferred vasodilator for
		diastolic heart failure

- Pulmonary artery wedge pressure (PAWP): 10–15 mmHg
- Systemic vascular resistance (SVR): 1400–2800 dyn/s/cm^5
- Commonly used vasoactive medications (Box 20.1) in ICU and indications:
  - Metoprolol 25 mg PO/NG tube q12h (to start after discontinuation of inotropic agents), then hold for HR <60 or SBP <100. Use of beta-blockers while the patient is on inotropic agents is counterproductive and should be avoided.
  - Dopamine 3–5 µg/kg/min infusion to keep CI >2.2, SBP >100
  - Dobutamine 3–5 µg/kg/min infusion to keep CI >2.2
  - Epinephrine 2–50 ng/kg/min infusion to keep CI >2.2, SBP >100
  - Norepinephrine to keep SBP >100

- Phenylephrine to keep SBP >100
- Nitroprosside (reduces afterload) to keep SBP <130
- Nitroglycerin (reduces preload and coronary artery spasm) to keep SBP <130
- Milrinone at $0.375–0.75\,\mu g/kg/min$ is helpful in patients with low CI and pulmonary hypertension with adequate or high systemic arterial pressure. May also be preferred to dobutamine because of its lack of effect on myocardial O_2 consumption

- **Pulmonary:**
  - Assessment includes physical exam, chest X-ray, and ABG
  - Chest X-ray on arrival and daily while in ICU to assess placement of endotracheal tube (2–3 cm above carina), nasogastric tube, widening of mediastinum, pneumothorax, hemothorax, pacemaker, central-line
  - ABG on arrival to ICU, then q4h and prior to weaning and prior to extubation
  - Connect chest tube to $20\,cmH_2O$ suction, record hourly output. If chest tube output >100 mL/h check PT/PTT, platelet count, and fibrinogen level and act accordingly.
  - Common ventilator settings:
    - Synchronized intermittent mandatory ventilation (SIMV)
    - FIO_2: 100% on arrival to ICU, wean to 40% within 24 h
    - Rate: 12–18/min
    - Tidal volume: 6–10 mL/kg
    - Positive end-expiratory pressure (PEEP): $5\,cmH_2O$
    - Pressure support: $10\,cmH_2O$
    - Wean ventilator and plan to extubate within 24 h to eliminate risk of ventilator-associated pneumonia (VAP).

- **Gastrointestinal:**
  - Proton pump inhibitors or H_2 blockers reduce risk of stress gastric ulcer and should be given perioperatively. Also daily laxative may be helpful by avoiding straining and valsalva maneuver.

- **Renal:**
  - Frequent urine output and electrolyte monitoring are extremely important and replacement should be done.
  - Cardiac surgery patients very often develop edema and third space fluid retention. Start furosemide, postoperative day 2–3 with KCl supplement and continue for 5–7 days, until the peripheral edema improves.

- **Hematology:**
  - For long-term anticoagulation, see Chapter 10
  - Give ASA 325 mg PO/NG tube daily (or 81 mg daily in some patients concurrently with clopidrogel or warfarin), starting 6 h after arrival and hold for platelet count <75 000 or chest tube drainage >75 mL/h
  - Heparin infusion:
    - Should be given on postoperative day 3, for atrial fibrillation, prosthetic heart valves, deep vein thrombosis, or pulmonary emboli

– Check platelets and hemoglobin level while on heparin to assess for heparin-induced thrombocytopenia and/or bleeding.

- **Infectious disease:**
  - Prophylaxis perioperative antibiotic is a standard of care practice for cardiac surgery patients
  - Cefazolin 1 g IV q8h for 48h only or vancomycin 1 g IV q12h two doses if allergic to cefazolin are recommended.
- **Endocrine:**
  - **Diabetes:**
    – Goal of glycemic control is blood glucose <150 mg/dL
    – Insulin infusion is used for the first 24 h if patient is diabetic or glucose >150 mg/dL and may be switched to insulin sliding scale sub-Q afterwards
    – Significance of tight glycemic control post cardiac surgery remains controversial
  - **Adrenal dysfunction:**
    – Subclinical adrenal insufficiency is present in 20% of elderly population and can be unmasked by stress of surgery
    – Cortisol level should be high at postsurgical stress status
    – Suspect for any patient with prolonged, unexplained vasodilatory shock and check cortisol level. If it is low or normal may check using Cosyntropin test and consider giving dexamethasone or hydrocortisone tapering stress doses
    – Any patient taking exogenous steroid within 6 months of surgery may receive stress-dose steroid perioperatively.

Postoperative Complications

Low Cardiac Output
- Bradycardia:
  - If HR <60, increase atrial pacing to 90–110
- Low preload:
  - CVP <10 mmHg, PAWP <12–15 mmHg
  - Give 500 mL colloid bolus or consider transfusion if Hct <25%
- Increased afterload:
  - Normal systemic afterload 800–1400 dyn/s/cm^5
  - Sodium nitroproside 1–10 µg/min:
    – Short half-life
    – Arterial vasodilator
    – Cyanide toxicity after several days
  - Cyanide toxicity:
    – Elevated mixed venous O_2, metabolic acidosis, convulsion, disorientation, muscle spasms, anorexia
    – Give IV infusion of 25% sodium thiosulphate 150 mg/kg over 15 min

- Milrinone at 0.375–0.75 µg/kg/min is helpful in patients with low CI and pulmonary hypertension with adequate or high systemic arterial pressure

Contractility and Myocardial Dysfunction
- Give inotropic drugs (dopamine, dobutamine, epinephrine, milrinone)
  - Start at low dose, titrate to the desired effect, and then wean gradually
- Consider phosphodiesterase inhibitors (milrinone) for patients with right ventricular failure and those with low cardiac output, high pulmonary artery (PA) pressure, and high pulmonary vascular resistance (PVR).

Tamponade
- Signs:
  - Low cardiac output
  - Low urine output
  - Central venous pressure (CVP) higher than mean PA pressure
  - Fast increase in left and right atrial pressure tends to equalize
  - Abrupt reduction of chest tube output
  - Beck's triad (high CVP with distended neck veins, hypotension, muffled heart sounds) is difficult to assess in post open-heart surgery patients
- Chest X-ray: progressive widening of mediastinum shadow
- Bedside echocardiogram shows poor right ventricular filling due to free-wall compression
- Treatment:
  - Vigorous stripping of mediastinal chest tube
  - Inotropes and volume expander
  - Taking patient to the OR for exploration and evacuation of clots emergently.

Arrhythmia
- Common complication after cardiac surgery
- Prevention for all types of arrhythmias include: beta-blocker, avoiding hypothermia (T <35°C), hypoxia and acidosis, and replacement of K^+, Ca^{2+} and Mg^{2+}
- **Atrial fibrillation:**
  - Up to one-third of post-cardiac surgery patients
  - Hemodynamically unstable:
    – Synchronized electrical cardioversion, starting from 100 J, may increase up to 300 J
  - Hemodynamically stable:
    – Start with rate control agents such as beta-blockers, amiodarone, or digoxin
    – Correct arrhythmia with antiarrhythmic agents, such as amiodarone and procainamide; for details, see Chapter 13

- **Atrial flutter:**
  - Hemodynamically unstable:
    - Cardioversion starting from 100 J and may increase up to 300 J
  - Hemodynamically stable:
    - Rapid atrial pacing
    - See management of atrial fibrillation above
- **Ventricular arrhythmia:**
  - Premature ventricular complex (PVC):
    - Unifocal PVC – possibly due to misplaced PA catheter and endocardial stimulation: check electrolytes and replace; give a bolus dose of lidocaine followed by infusion; if no response, relocate PA catheter
    - Multifocal PVC – most likely due to electrolyte imbalance: check electrolytes and replace; give a bolus dose of lidocaine followed by infusion
  - Ventricular tachycardia and fibrillation:
    - Immediate cardioversion
    - Amiodarone bolus of 150 mg or lidocaine bolus 100 mg followed by infusion

Hemorrhage
- Postoperative bleeding is either coagulapathic, surgical, or both
- **Surgical postoperative bleeding:**
  - Indications for re-exploration per chest tube output are:
    - >400 mL/h for 1 h
    - >300 mL/h for 2–3 h
    - >200 mL/h for 4 h
- **Coagulopathic postoperative bleeding:**
  - Hemodynamically stable patient should be reassessed and the coagulopathy should be corrected:
    - Prolonged ACT: indication for administration of protamin to reverse the effect of heparin
    - Prolonged PT/PTT: need for fresh frozen plasma (FFP)
    - Hypofibrinogenemia: give cryoprecipitate.
    - Thrombocytopenia: (platelets <50 000/mm^3) is treated with pooled platelet transfusion. If on ASA preoperatively, transfuse platelets regardless of platelet count
    - Hct, in general, should be maintained >24% postoperatively. However, consider transfusion of packed red blood cell (PRBC) at higher Hct for elderly patients and those with ECG changes, low BP, or significant tachycardia.

Renal Failure
- Oliguria (urine <30 mL/h or <0.5 mL/kg/h) requires renal perfusion assessment.
- Keep SBP >100 mmHg, CI >2.2 L/min/m^2

- Rule out bladder obstruction
- Start furosemide 20 mg IV and increase by 20 mg increments until good urine output is achieved
- Start ethacrynic acid 50 mg, metolazone 2.5–20 mg, or torsemide if no response to furosemide.

Neurologic Complications
- **Cerebrovascular accident (CVA):**
  - Incidence of 2–4% after cardiac surgery and is associated with higher mortality rate
  - Needs thorough neurologic exam and CT scan of head and neurology consult
  - Supportive measures:
    - Avoiding hypoglycemia and hypoxia
    - Maintain a higher SBP (>150 mmHg) for better cerebral perfusion using volume expanders or inotropes
  - Usage of anticoagulation is controversial and should be balanced between risk of postoperative bleeding and chance of recurrent CVA
- **Peripheral nerve injury:**
  - Quite common and resolves within a few months after surgery
  - Nerve injuries include:
    - Brachial plexus injury
    - Ulnar nerve stretch injury
    - Unilateral vocal cord paralysis
    - Phrenic nerve damage
    - Saphenous nerve neuropathy and femoral nerve damage
  - Treatment with physiotherapy and relevant neurologic consultation
- **Neuropsychiatry changes:**
  - Precipitating factors for postoperative psychosis include: high age, alcohol withdrawal, withdrawal from selective serotonin reuptake inhibitors (SSRI; such as flextime, setraline), preoperative psychiatric illness, hypoxia, electrolyte imbalance, sleep deprivation, narcotic and benzodiazepine use, and ICU environment
  - Treatment includes:
    - Reorientation to time, date, and place
    - Discontinuing contributing medication
    - Correction of hypoxia and electrolyte imbalance
- **Seizure:**
  - Causes include: hypoxia, air embolization during surgery, CVA, severe hyperglycemia, hypoglycemia, hypomagnesemia, hypocalcemia, hyponatremia, low levels of anticonvulsants in patients with epilepsy, lidocaine toxicity, and chronic meperidine use
  - Treatment:
    - Secure airway and oxygenation
    - Lorazepam 2–4 mg IV

- Phenytoin 15 mg/kg IV loading dose and continue to reach the therapeutic level
- If convulsion persists (or status epilepticus unresponsive to treatment), consider general anesthesia with neuromuscular blockade.

Gastrointestinal Complications

- **Cholecystitis:** consider nonsurgical management
- **Bowel perforation:** incidence of GI bleeding and duodenal perforation has reduced significantly due to the use of H_2 blockers and proton pump inhibitors
- **Bowel ischemia:**
  - Infrequent complication but catastrophic
  - Risk factors: long duration of bypass, use of pressor support, use of intra-aortic balloon pump (IABP), atrial fibrillation, peripheral vascular disease, and heparin-induced thrombocytopenia
  - Early surgical intervention within 6 h is associated with 48% mortality rate
  - Late surgical intervention after 6 h is associated with 99% mortality rate
- **Pancreatitis:**
  - Usually diagnosed with elevated serum amylase and lipase
  - Treatment:
    - Bowel rest
    - Supportive care.

Infection

- Incidence is 10–20% and may be related to surgical wound, lung, urinary tract, invasive lines and devices and gastrointestinal tract.
- **Deep wound infection with mediastinitis:**
  - Incidence of 1–2% with mortality rate of 10%
  - Common organisms: *Staphylococcus epidermidis*, MRSA, Corynebacterium and enteric Gram-negative bacilli
  - Predisposing factors: obesity, diabetes, chronic obstructive pulmonary disease (COPD), renal dysfunction, low serum albumin, use of both internal mammary arteries, prolonged cardiopulmonary bypass time, and decreased cardiac output following surgery
  - Treatment:
    - Broad-spectrum IV antibiotics
    - Surgical exploration and extensive debridement
    - Possible removal of sternum with primary or secondary closure with muscle or an omental flap
- **Superficial wound infection:**
  - Same organisms and predisposing factors as deep wound infection
  - Treatment:
    - Broad-spectrum IV antibiotics
    - Opening the wound and culture

- Local wound care
- Antibiotic adjustment per culture
- **Pneumonia:**
  - Incidence of VAP increases 1%/day
  - Diagnosis:
    - Chest X-ray: progressive infiltrate
    - Raised WBC
    - Fever
    - Sputum Gram stain: >25 neutrophils/low power field suggest infection
    - Sputum culture of 10^5–10^6 colony per milliliter is indicative of infection
  - Treatment: first-line of empiric antibiotic should cover Gram-negative organisms and this can be further refined per culture and sensitivity results
- **Urinary tract infection (UTI):**
  - Confirm diagnosis with urine analysis and urine culture
  - Start IV or PO antibiotic empirically and change antibiotic per culture result if needed.

Complications of Specific Operations
- **Graft occlusion:**
  - 5–10% incidence postoperatively
  - Signs:
    - Sudden hypotension
    - Ventricular arrhythmias
    - ECG changes (ST segment elevation)
  - Diagnosis: emergent cardiac catheterization
  - Treatment: immediate reoperation or percutaneous coronary intervention if feasible
- **Mammary artery spasm:**
  - Presentation and diagnosis are the same as for graft occlusion
  - Treatment:
    - Nifedipine SL followed by nipride and nitroglycerin infusion
    - Refractory spasm with hemodynamic instability warrants replacement of mammary artery with vein graft.

EVIDENCE-BASED PRACTICE

Interventions to reduce adverse outcomes after CABG surgery

Context: Cardioprotective strategies implemented to prevent ischemic events in patients at risk for cardiovascular disease have decreased morbidity and prolonged survival.

(Continued)

Goal: To identify the interventions with most benefit in minimizing ischemic events and survival following CABG surgery.

Method: Therapeutic interventions available to minimize ischemic events in the post-CABG patient were analyzed using ACC/AHA Classifications and Level of Evidence criteria. Number-needed-to-treat (NNT) analyses were performed to determine the effectiveness of each intervention compared to the number of patients needed to be treated before a benefit was apparent.

Results: Strongest evidence and recommendation to improve quality of life and prolong survival after CABG surgery are:
- **Antiplatelets:** Class I recommendation and Level A evidence.
- **ACE inhibitors:** Class I recommendation and Level A evidence.
- **Statins:** Class I recommendation and Level A evidence.
- **Beta blockers:** Class I recommendation and Level B evidence.

Take home message: All CABG patients should receive ASA, statin, beta-blocker, and ACE inhibitor upon discharge.

CLINICAL PEARLS

- Venous graft occlusion occurs in 8–12% of patients before they leave hospital, and by 1 year post-CABG, 15–30% of vein grafts have become occluded. The overall occlusion rate by 10 years is 40–50%.
- Internal mammary artery grafts have a much better patency rate than vein grafts: 95%, 88%, and 83% at 1, 5, and 10 years, respectively.
- Baroreceptor dysfunction may occur after carotid endarterectomy, resulting in tachycardia, abrupt elevation of BP, and variable sensitivity to antihypertensive vasodilator medications.
- Factors that have been shown to increase the risk of post-CABG MI include emergency operation, an aortic cross-clamp time >100 min, MI during the week preceding CABG, and history of previous revascularization (percutaneous or surgical).
- ECG is the most reliable tool for diagnosing perioperative MI. The single most important criterion on the ECG is the presence of new and persistent Q waves once the early postoperative rewarming period is completed.
- Ventricular aneurysms must be resected in patients with heart failure, recurrent ventricular arrhythmias, angina, and peripheral emboli.
- Patients with hypertrophic obstructive cardiomyopathy who undergo myectomy are at high risk for developing left bundle branch block, whereas those undergoing alcohol ablation are at high risk for developing right bundle branch block.

Recommended Reading

Guidelines

Bonow RO, Blase A, Carabello BA et al. 2008 Focused update incorporated into the ACC/ AHA 2006 Guidelines for the Management of Patients With Valvular Heart Disease. *Circulation* 2008;**118**:e523–e661.

Review Articles

Arora R, Sowers JR, Saunders E, Probstfield J, Lazar HL. Cardioprotective strategies to improve long-term outcomes following coronary artery bypass surgery. *J Card Surg* 2006;**21**:198–204.

Bojar MB. *Manual of Perioperative Care in Adult Cardiac Surgery*, 4th edn. Oxford: Blackwell, 2005.

Charlson ME, Isom OW. Care after coronary-artery bypass surgery. *N Engl J Med* 2003;**348**(15):1456–1463.

Clary BM, Milano CA. *The Handbook of Surgical Intensive Care*, 5th edn. St Louis: Mosby, 2000.

Cohn LH. *Cardiac Surgery in the Adult*, 3rd edn. New York: McGraw Hill, 2008.

McKhann GM, Grega MA, Borowicz LM Jr et al. Encephalopathy and stroke after coronary artery bypass grafting: incidence, consequences, and prediction. *Arch Neurol* 2002;**59**:1422–1428.

Specialized Testing and Therapeutics

21 | Adult Advanced Cardiac Life Support

Anurag Gupta and Amin Al-Ahmad

Department of Internal Medicine, Division of Cardiology, Stanford University School of Medicine, Stanford, CA, USA

Overview of Sudden Cardiac Arrest and Resuscitation

Guidelines Source

- The most current guidelines were developed during the 2005 International Consensus Conference on Cardiopulmonary Resuscitation and Emergency Cardiovascular Care Science with Treatment Recommendations, hosted by the American Heart Association (AHA). The guidelines form the basis for the information presented in this chapter.
- Given the challenges of performing large clinical resuscitation trials in human subjects adequately powered to demonstrate improved neurologically intact survival to hospital discharge, such studies are limited. The guidelines thus largely reflect evidence gathered from nonrandomized or retrospective studies, clinical trials using intermediate outcomes, animal models, extrapolations, and/or expert consensus.

Epidemiology

- Sudden cardiac arrest (SCA) is a common cause of death in the United States; though estimates vary, approximately 300000–350000 adults, and potentially as high as 450000 adults, succumb to sudden cardiac death (SCD) in the United States annually.
- SCA accounts for >50% of deaths due to cardiovascular disease and thus represents the most common lethal manifestation of heart disease.
- Notwithstanding, at least 50% of SCD occurs in individuals as their first clinical manifestation of heart disease, or in those who were deemed to be at low risk for SCA.
- Among the initial rhythm disturbances documented in nontraumatic cardiac arrests in adults, *ventricular* arrhythmias are common, with estimates varying widely though generally reported to be between 20% and 40%.

A Practical Approach to Cardiovascular Medicine, First Edition. Edited by Reza Ardehali, Marco Perez, Paul Wang.

© 2011 Blackwell Publishing Ltd. Published 2011 by Blackwell Publishing Ltd.

- Despite advances in resuscitation, survival following SCA remains low. Though estimates vary widely depending upon the populations studied, recent prospective studies suggest that adult survival to hospital discharge is 18% following inhospital SCA and 5% following out-of-hospital SCA.

Elements of Successful Resuscitation

- The AHA "Chain of Survival" offers a paradigm for optimizing resuscitation outcomes and includes:
  - Early recognition and activation of emergency medical services
  - Early bystander cardiopulmonary resuscitation (CPR)
  - Early defibrillation
  - Early advanced life support.
- Early CPR and defibrillation are key and complementary elements of successful resuscitation:
- For witnessed ventricular fibrillation (VF) SCA, survival decreases 7–10% for every minute from collapse to defibrillation without CPR as opposed to 3–4%/min from collapse to defibrillation if bystander CPR is provided.
- Consequently, the expansion of automated external defibrillators (AEDs) into the community and education of individuals in their use (e.g. via public access defibrillation and first-responder AED programs) have led to improvements in resuscitation outcomes.
- The addition of advanced life support capabilities, such as endotracheal intubation, IV line insertion, and IV medication administration, though considered important elements of resuscitation, has not consistently shown significant improvements in survival to hospital discharge following SCA; they are generally considered as adjunctive therapies.

Notable Guideline Modifications

The guidelines are elaborated below. The notable revisions in the most recent 2005 adult guidelines for trained rescuers compared to 2000 include:

- *Simplified* CPR instructions and/or algorithms. Studies examining the treatment of individuals with SCA continue to demonstrate that providers, including well-trained hospital staff, deliver too few compressions, inadequate compression force, and/or excess ventilation.
- Increased emphasis on providing *chest compressions* during CPR.
- Use of therapeutic *hypothermia* in some victims of SCA, as improved neurologic outcomes have been documented in clinical trials. Mechanisms may include reduction in cerebral oxygen requirements and amelioration of deleterious biochemical processes.

Basic and Advanced Management of Adult Cardiac Arrest

Complete evaluation and management strategies are provided in the Adult BLS healthcare provider algorithm and ACLS pulseless arrest algorithm [2005 American Heart Association Guidelines for Cardiopulmonary Resuscitation and Emergency Cardiovascular Care. *Circulation* 2005;**112** (Suppl IV):1–211)].

Additional points include:
- **Positioning**: place the patient on a hard surface in the supine position.
- **Airway instructions**:
  - Healthcare providers should open the airway using the head tilt–chin lift maneuver unless cervical spine injury is suspected, in which case the jaw thrust maneuver without head extension is preferred, if feasible
  - If an advanced airway is inserted, proper placement should be confirmed.
- **Rescue breath instructions**:
  - Give breaths *over 1 s* with sufficient volume to achieve visible chest rise for all forms of ventilation during CPR.
  - *Excess ventilation is detrimental* as it, in part, increases intrathoracic pressure and decreases venous return to the heart, overall reducing cardiac output, coronary and cerebral perfusion, and survival.
- **Chest compression instructions**:
  - Push with sufficient force and speed (*"push hard, push fast"*) with *minimized interruptions* to compressions.
  - More specifically, compress the center of the chest (at the lower half of the sternum at the nipple level), with the goal of depressing the chest by approximately 1.5–2″ using the heel of one hand with the other hand on top, to achieve approximately *100 chest compressions*/min while still achieving complete chest recoil (with approximately equal compression and relaxation times).
- **Compression-to-ventilation ratios**:
  - Use a single compression-to-ventilation ratio of *30:2 for single rescuers.*
  - Once an advanced airway is in place (e.g. endotracheal tube, esophogeal–tracheal combitube, or laryngeal mask airway), the compressing rescuer should then provide 100 chest compressions/min *continuously*, without pauses for ventilation, while the rescuer delivering ventilation should provide 8–10 breaths/min (with care to avoid excess ventilation).
  - If spontaneous circulation is present and ventilation alone is required, 10–12 breaths/min should be provided.
  - *Alternate rescuers*: approximately every 2 min to prevent fatigue and to maintain the quality of chest compressions.
  - Chest compressions may be more important than ventilations during the initial minute(s) of SCA due to VF, because oxygen delivery to the tissues may initially be more dependent upon blood flow than relatively preserved initial arterial oxygen saturation. Notwithstanding, combining some ventilation with minimally interrupted compressions is recommended and may be optimal, particularly for asphyxial arrest and prolonged arrest.
  - The minute ventilation required during CPR is less than under normal circumstances as this can match the diminished systemic and lung perfusion. 100% inspired oxygen should be administered initially when available to enhance arterial oxygen content.

- **Defibrillation**:
  - Defibrillation refers to high-energy unsynchronized shock that depolarizes myocardial cells, extinguishes activation wavefronts, and terminates VF. It is indicated for VF, pulseless ventricular tachycardia (VT), or polymorphic VT.
    - There is no evidence to support shock delivery for asystole.
    - **Synchronized cardioversion**, in which shock delivery is timed to the QRS complex, should be used for unstable tachyarrhythmias with pulses, including monomorphic VT.
    - Critical role of rapid defibrillation is based in part on two well-demonstrated principles:
      Presentation with a shockable rhythm (VF or pulseless VT) is common and compared to other initial rhythm disturbances in SCA confers the highest probability of successful resuscitation in adults.
      Time to treatment is the most critical variable in determining the success of resuscitation.
  - **Technique:**
    - Place electrode pads or paddles on the patient's bare chest. Transthoracic impedance is reduced with conductive materials and is accomplished by use of self-adhesive pads (preferred), gel pads, or electrode paste with paddles.
    - Electrode pads or paddles should be placed in the sternal–apical (anterolateral) position; i.e. the sternal chest pad is placed in the right superior–anterior (infraclavicular) chest and the apical chest pad is placed in the inferior lateral chest (lateral to the left breast). Other acceptable positions include placement of pads on the left and right lateral chest wall (biaxillary) or in the standard apical position and right or left upper back position.
    - If an implantable medical device is present, place the pads at least 1″ away from the devices. Interrogate permanent pacemakers and internal cardioverter–defibrillators following resuscitation episodes incorporating these devices.
    - **Monophasic waveforms:** reasonable to deliver 360 J for the initial and subsequent defibrillation.
    - **Biphasic waveforms:** device-specific energy levels, generally *120–200 J* for initial shock followed by escalating energy delivery if needed, should be employed; 200 J may be used as a default dose if the optimal doses are not known and/or labeled.
  - **Coordinating CPR with defibrillation:** as noted, concurrent early defibrillation and CPR are critical for successful resuscitation outcomes. However, the critical importance of chest compressions in effecting successful defibrillation and/or overall resuscitation outcomes are emphasized in the guidelines, as reflected in the following considerations. It should be stressed though that for inhospital settings with continuous monitoring, the doctor may elect to modify this sequence:

– Consideration of emergency medical services (EMS) providing about five cycles of CPR (approximately 2 min) prior to defibrillation in cases of unwitnessed, out-of-hospital arrest, when the response time is >c. 4 min. Immediate defibrillation for VF of short duration, such as witnessed cardiac arrest with prompt availability of AED or in-hospital settings, remains preferable.

– Consideration of rescuers providing about five cycles of CPR (approximately 2 min) – between rhythm checks for pulseless electrical activity (PEA) and immediately after defibrillation for VF/pulseless VT arrest, prior to reassessing the rhythm or pulse.

– Consideration of immediately resuming CPR after 1 shock for VF/pulseless VT instead of three stacked shocks. This reflects high first-shock efficacy of defibrillation, and if unsuccessful, the importance of chest compressions in restoring the myocardial substrate for effective subsequent defibrillation attempts or in restoring a perfusing rhythm if PEA or asystole is induced.

- **Underlying etiology**:
  - In all cases of SCA, potentially reversible underlying and/or complicating etiologies must be considered and possibly treated during CPR.
  - When compared to a shockable rhythm (namely VF or pulseless VT), survival rates for PEA and asystole are far inferior. As defibrillation is not thought to be appropriate nor effective for PEA or asystole, identification and treatment of the underlying and/or complicating causes is particularly critical and is often necessary to effect a successful resuscitation.
  - Directed interventions can be considered on a case-by-case basis, such as but not limited to:
    – Fibrinolysis for acute thrombosis
    – IV magnesium for suspected torsades de pointes
    – IV fluids in cases of hypovolemia
    – sodium bicarbonate in cases such as tricyclic antidepressant overdose, hyperkalemia, or pre-existing metabolic acidosis
    – acute therapies for severe hyperkalemia, such as calcium chloride, sodium bicarbonate, insulin with glucose, and/or nebulized albuterol.
  - Of note, there is neither a clear role nor recommendation for attempting pacing with asystolic cardiac arrest. The indications for pacing in symptomatic bradycardia are covered below.
- **Adjunctive pharmacologic therapy**:
  - Establishing IV access and/or administering pharmacologic therapy should serve as an *adjunctive* therapy that does not interfere with CPR and defibrillation:
    – Though drug administration is incorporated in resuscitation algorithms and may have important salutary effects in certain individuals, controlled trial data are lacking that demonstrate improved intact

survival to hospital discharge by administering any drug at any stage of arrest.

– See ACC/AHA algorithms for specific drug recommendations.

- **Access:**
  - **Peripheral** venous access and infusion is generally adequate during resuscitation and does not require interruption of CPR. Given an approximately 1–2 min delay to reach central circulation, peripherally administered drugs should be given as bolus injection followed by a 20 mL bolus of IV fluid with the extremity elevated.
  - **Central** venous access may be indicated if feasible, and if resuscitation is not achieved despite initial efforts, including defibrillation and peripheral drug administration. Intraosseous (IO) cannulation is an alternative mode of central drug administration.
  - **Endotracheal** drug administration is an option if IV or IO access is not available, though the latter modes are preferred given more effective and predictable drug delivery. If endotracheal delivery is used, consider administering approximately *2–2.5 times* the recommended IV dose of the drug, diluting the drug in 5–10 mL of water or normal saline, and directly injecting into the endotracheal tube.

Management of Symptomatic Bradycardia and Tachycardia

Complete evaluation and management strategies are provided in the ACLS bradycardia and tachycardia algorithms [2005 American Heart Association Guidelines for Cardiopulmonary Resuscitation and Emergency Cardiovascular Care. *Circulation* 2005;**112** (Suppl IV):1–211)].

Additional points include:

- **General points:**
  - Assess the impact of the rhythm disturbance on the patient's clinical condition, specifically assessing the *adequacy of organ perfusion*:
    - Symptoms and signs of diminished perfusion include, but are not limited to, decreased level of consciousness, acutely altered mental status, seizure, syncope, chest pain, congestive heart failure, hypotension, and other manifestations of shock.
  - Tailor treatment decisions to the rhythm disturbance *and* its clinical impact on the patient, not solely to the rhythm disturbance. If a patient is deemed *unstable,* prepare for immediate *pacing* if the patient is bradycardic, or synchronized *cardioversion* if the patient is tachycardic; if synchronization is not possible, deliver a high-energy unsynchronized shock.
  - When evaluating a patient with clinically significant bradycardia or tachycardia, prompt attention should be paid to establishing *airway and breathing support*, establishing *IV access*, and assessing potential underlying *etiologies*.
  - If feasible, obtain a *12-lead ECG* to confirm the rhythm diagnosis.

- **Symptomatic bradycardia**:
  - **Pacing:** prepare to initiate pacing immediately in symptomatic/unstable patients, particularly in patients who are *severely symptomatic* and/or are suspected to have *AV block at or below the His level* (e.g. if presenting with Mobitz type 2 second-degree AV block or third-degree AV block, especially when associated with wide QRS >120 ms).
    - It may be reasonable to begin with *transcutaneous* pacing, though reliable capture is extremely *difficult* and it may further be associated with significant patient discomfort requiring sedation and analgesia.
    - If transcutaneous pacing is attempted, effective mechanical capture must be verified (e.g. by assessment of pulse or continuous arterial pressure monitoring if available) as the pacing stimulus artifact may obscure and/or be misinterpreted as electrical capture.
    - Immediate capacity for transvenous pacing and/or expert consultation is thus recommended.
  - **Atropine:** generally the first-line drug for acute symptomatic bradycardia, as it may be effective in cases of sinus bradycardia and/or AV block at the level of the AV node.
    - In cases of Mobitz type 2 second-degree AV block due to block at or below the level of His, administration of atropine may exacerbate AV block.
    - Administering doses less than the recommended 0.5 mg IV may result in paradoxical bradycardia.
  - **Other drugs:** such as epinephrine, dopamine, and glucagon (for bradycardia associated with excess beta-blockers or calcium channel blockers), may be considered as alternative temporizing agents.
- **Symptomatic tachycardia**:
  - Irrespective of the arrhythmia origin, if a symptomatic/unstable tachyarrhythmia with pulses is present, prompt cardioversion should be delivered.
  - Characterization of the arrhythmia and its origin aids in the optimal acute as well as long-term management, including pharmacologic therapy.
  - Accurate arrhythmia diagnosis requires careful analysis, including characterization of the atrial and ventricular relationships, axis, morphology, mode of arrhythmia initiation and termination, and/or arrhythmia response to perturbations. However, assessment of *QRS duration* and its *regularity* during arrhythmia may provide rapid clues regarding the origin of the arrhythmia and forms the basis for urgent treatment algorithms.
  - **Narrow-QRS-complex (<120 ms) tachycardias** generally result from supraventricular tachycardias (SVTs) with activation of the ventricle over the His–Purkinje system leading to a narrow-QRS-complex. The differential diagnosis includes:
    - Sinus tachycardia
    - Atrial fibrillation (AF)
    - Atrial flutter

  - AV nodal reentry tachycardia
  - Accessory pathway-mediated tachycardia (with antegrade conduction over the AV node)
  - Atrial tachycardia
  - Multifocal atrial tachycardia
  - Junctional tachycardia
  - Some forms of VT (uncommon).
- **Wide-QRS-complex (>120 ms) tachycardias** often represent:
  - VT
  - Though the differential diagnosis further includes SVT (as above) with aberrant conduction and/or pre-existing bundle branch block, and pre-excited tachycardia (with antegrade conduction over the accessory pathway).
- **Shock therapy:** the recommended initial energy via synchronized cardioversion (if feasible) is suggested below, though optimal values are not well established and alternate doses are reasonable; subsequent doses may be escalated.
  - **Monophasic waveform:** for AF administer 100–200 J initially; for atrial flutter and other SVTs administer 50–100 J initially; for monomorphic VT with pulses administer 100 J initially.
  - **Biphasic waveform:** for AF administer 100–120 J initially, though optimal doses for AF and other tachyarrhythmias are less well established.
  - For arrhythmias due to increased automaticity as opposed to re-entry, such as atrial tachycardia, multifocal atrial tachycardia, and junctional tachycardia, cardioversion is generally not effective.

Ethical Considerations

- Efforts should be made to obtain information regarding advanced directives and living wills and/or to discuss care with surrogate decision-makers, when feasible.
- Nonetheless, recognizing that decisions regarding resuscitation are made emergently, often without clear knowledge of a patient's advanced directives, and with difficultly in predicting the subsequent outcome, resuscitation efforts should generally be initiated promptly to all patients.
- Exceptions may include presence of:
  - Legally valid instructions not to intervene [such as a valid Do Not Attempt Resuscitation (DNAR) order, interpretable advanced directives, or valid surrogate directives]
  - Signs of irreversible death such as rigor mortis (principle of futility)
  - An expectation that such efforts will not restore effective circulation due to deterioration of vital functions despite maximal medical therapy, such as in cases of progressive shock (principle of futility)
  - Risk of physical injury to the rescuer (such as in some cases of out-of-hospital arrest).

- Guidelines for terminating resuscitation efforts are likewise limited and largely dependent upon individual patient characteristics, including consideration of time to CPR and/or defibrillation, comorbid disease(s), prearrest status, initial arrest rhythm, and continual reassessment of response to resuscitation interventions.
- Providing emotional support to family members is a critical element of resuscitation. Consideration should be made to inviting select family member(s) to be present during resuscitation, given data suggesting that this may be desirable in some instances, though attitudes and opinions regarding this topic vary widely.
- Issues regarding organ and tissue donation should be considered in cases of failed resuscitation.

Recommended Reading

Clinical Trials and Meta-Analyses

Abella BS, Alvarado JP, Mykleburst H et al. Quality of cardiopulmonary resuscitation during in-hospital cardiac arrest. *JAMA* 2005;**293**:305–310.

Hallstrom AP, Ornato JP, Weisfeldt M et al. The Public Access Defibrillation Trial Investigators. Public-access defibrillation and survival after out-of-hospital cardiac arrest. *N Engl J Med* 2004;**351**:637–646.

Hypothermia After Cardiac Arrest Study Group. Mild hypothermia to improve neurological outcome after cardiac arrest. *N Engl J Med* 2002;**346**:549–556.

Nadkarni VM, Larkin GL, Peberdy MA et al. First documented rhythm and clinical outcome from in-hospital cardiac arrest among children and adults. *JAMA* 2006;**295**:50–57.

Stiell IG, Wells GA, Field B et al. Advanced cardiac life support in out-of-hospital cardiac arrest. *N Engl J Med* 2004;**351**:647–656.

Guidelines

2005 American Heart Association Guidelines for Cardiopulmonary Resuscitation and Emergency Cardiovascular Care. *Circulation* 2005;**112** (Suppl IV):1–211.

Review Articles

Cooper JA, Cooper JD, Cooper JM. Cardiopulmonary resuscitation: history, current practice, and future direction. *Circulation* 2006;**11**:2839–2849.

Myerburg RJ, Kessler KM, Castellanos A. Sudden cardiac death: epidemiology, transient risk, and intervention assessment. *Ann Intern Med* 1993;**119**:1187–1197.

22 ECG Interpretation

Marco Perez and Victor F. Froelicher

Department of Internal Medicine, Division of Cardiology, Stanford
University School of Medicine, Stanford, CA, USA

The 12-lead ECG remains the most commonly used test in patients suspected
of having cardiovascular disease. It supplies a wealth of information regarding the health of the conduction system, presence of structural abnormalities,
such as hypertrophy, and signs of injury. The trick to reading a 12-lead ECG
is being methodical in approach and learning to recognize certain patterns.
This chapter will assume prior knowledge about basic ECG function and will
concentrate on a practical approach to reading the ECG.

Checklist

- Rate
- Rhythm
- Axis
- Intervals: PR, QRS, QT
- Hypertrophy: LV, RV, LA, RA
- R-wave progression
- Ischemia and injury: Q-waves, ST- and T-wave patterns
- PR depression
- Voltages: calibration, low voltage, and electrical alternans
- Lead reversal
- Clinical syndromes

Rate
The normal adult heart rate (HR) is 60–100 bpm.
- If a slow HR is seen, SA or AV nodal disease should be assessed (see
  Chapter 18).
- A fast HR should flag a check for a tachyarrhythmia (see Chapters 15–17)
  before calling the rhythm sinus tachycardia.

A Practical Approach to Cardiovascular Medicine, First Edition. Edited by Reza Ardehali,
Marco Perez, Paul Wang.
© 2011 Blackwell Publishing Ltd. Published 2011 by Blackwell Publishing Ltd.

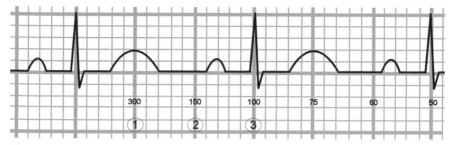

Figure 22.1 Example ECG

Count the number of "large boxes" to quickly estimate heart rate. Memorize the HRs at each of the large boxes. In Figure 22.1, three large boxes translates to 100 bpm. If the distance is somewhere between two large boxes, make an approximate estimate, e.g. four and a half large boxes would work out to be about half way between 75 and 60, or approximately 68.

Rhythm

Sinus rhythm is determined when every P-wave is followed by a QRS complex, every QRS complex is preceded by a P-wave, and the P-wave is upright in II and biphasic in V1. If these criteria are not met, an attempt to identify the rhythm should be made:

Ask:

- Fast or slow
- Narrow or wide
- Regular or irregular
- Where are the Ps?

Figure 22.2 is not a comprehensive algorithm, but will identify the majority of arrhythmias.

If no clear pattern is present, remember to check for frequent premature atrial contraction (PACs) and premature ventricular contractions (PVCs).

Axis

The normal QRS axis is between −30 and +90. If leads I and aVF are predominantly positive then the axis is between 0 and +90 (Figure 22.3). If lead I is positive and aVF is negative, lead II will help determine normal versus left axis deviation (Figure 22.3). A negative lead I and positive lead aVF means there is right axis deviation.

Intervals (Figure 22.4)

- **PR:**
  - 0.12–0.20 s
  - Measured from beginning of p to beginning of QRS
  - Quick read: less than one "big box"

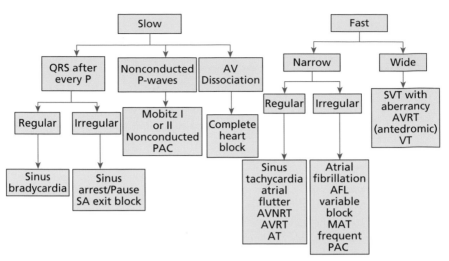

Figure 22.2 Algorithm for arrhythmia identification

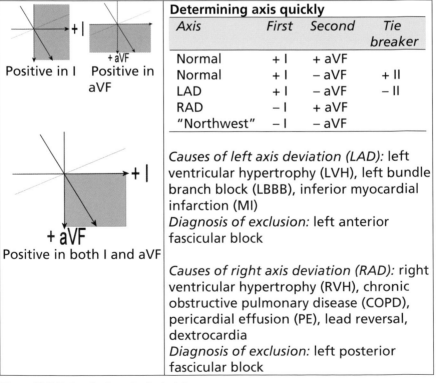

Figure 22.3 Determination of axis deviation

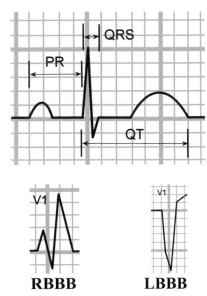

Figure 22.4 Intervals and bundle branch blocks

- **QRS:**
  - Normal: <0.10; prolonged: >0.12
  - Measured from beginning of QRS to end of QRS
  - Quick read: less than half of one "big box"
- **QT:**
  - 0.35–0.43 s
  - Measured from beginning of QRS to end of T-wave
  - Correct for HR: QTc = QT/(sqrt R–R)
  - Quick read: less than half the R–R interval

Bundle Branch Blocks

In a prolonged QRS, identify the morphology (Figure 22.4):
- Quick read: right bundle branch block (RBBB) looks like an "M" in V1
- Quick read: left bundle branch block (LBBB) looks like a "V" or "W" in V1

Hypertrophy

Left Ventricle

There are several criteria that can be used, each with varying sensitivities and specificities. The best strategy is to choose a couple that can be remembered. A few are described below.
- **Cornell criteria:** R in aVL + S in V3 >28 mm in males or >20 mm in females
- **Precordial lead criteria:** S in V1 + R in V5 or V6 >35
- **Limb lead criteria**: R in aVL ≥12

- **Estes criteria:** point system, cumbersome. Just remember discordant ST abnormalities, large left atrium, and left axis deviation associated with LVH are often seen

Right Ventricle
Any of the following:
- R >S in V1
- R in V1 ≥ 7 mm
- rSR' in V1 with R' > 10

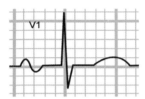

Left Atrium
- Wide P (>0.12 s) in II *or*
- Neg. P in V1 > 1s × 1 mm

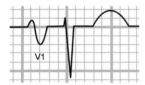

Right Atrium
- Tall P (>2.5 mm) in II or
- Pos. P in V1 > 1.5 mm

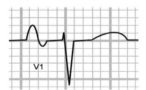

R-Wave Progression
- Abnormal R-wave progression should be a flag that something is abnormal.
- Normally the R-wave starts off small in V1 and gradually enlarges towards V6.
- The transition where the R-wave is bigger than the S-wave is usually V2–V4.

- Late transition: LVH, COPD, anterior MI, LBBB, cardiomyopathy
- Early transition: RVH, posterior MI, RBBB, Wolff–Parkinson–White (WPW), precordial lead reversal
- Reverse R-wave progression: dextrocardia, significant anterior injury.

Ischemia and Injury: Q-Waves, ST- and T-Wave Patterns

The leads can be grouped together according to anatomic distribution (Figure 22.5). Q-waves and ST elevations can then be localized based on this distribution. Note that ST depressions and TWI can*not* be localized in this manner.

- **Pathologic Q-waves:**
  - Any Q-wave in V1–V3
  - Q >1 mm deep *and* >0.03 s in other leads
  - Must be present in two contiguous leads
- **Significant ST elevation** (Figure 22.6):
  - Must be >2 mm in V1–V3
  - STE >1 mm in other leads
  - Must be present in two contiguous leads
- **Ischemic ST depressions:**
  - Horizontal or down sloping
  - At least 1 mm deep
  - Must be present in two contiguous leads
- **Ischemic T-waves:**
  - Deeply inverted
  - Biphasic (positive then negative).

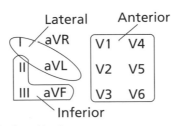

Figure 22.5 Anatomic distribution of leads

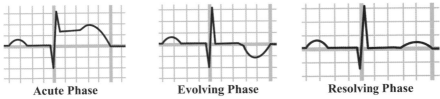

Acute Phase   **Evolving Phase**   **Resolving Phase**

Figure 22.6 Evolution of an ST elevation myocardial infarction

PR Depression

PR depression is due to abnormal atrial repolarization seen in acute pericarditis. PR elevation of 1 mm is seen in aVR, while PR depression and ST elevation are seen in all other leads. If PR depression is seen, look for low voltages or electrical alternans as further clues of coexistent PE. PR depression is easily missed.

Voltages

- **Calibration**:
  - Make sure the voltage calibration bracket covers two "large boxes"
  - If the voltages are abnormally high or low, some ECG machines may adjust the voltages to keep the tracings from overlapping.
- **Low voltages**:
  - QRS <5 mm in all limb leads and <10 mm in all precordial leads
  - Diagnosis: PE, COPD, obesity, infiltrative cardiomyopathy, extensive MI, myxedema
- **Electrical alternans** (Figure 22.7):
  - Alteration in amplitude from beat to beat, usually seen in QRS but can be noted of P- and T-waves
  - Diagnosis: PE, deep respiration, heart failure, rheumatic heart disease, coronary artery disease (CAD).

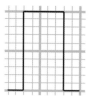

Lead Reversal

- **Limb leads**:
  - Most common lead reversal is that of the left and right arms (Figure 22.8) This results in a negative P-wave, QRS and T-wave in I and aVL

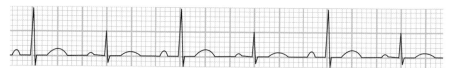

Figure 22.7 Electrical alternans

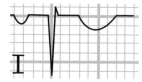

Figure 22.8 Left and right arm lead reversal

- Rule out dextrocardia if this is seen (see below)
- Other abnormally inverted limb leads, especially in lead III, are clues to alternative types of lead reversals.
- **Precordial leads:**
  - Next most common lead reversal is that of any two precordial leads
  - This appears as a disruption in the normal R-wave progression, with a sudden change in R-wave amplitude, followed by a return to normal progression (Figure 22.9).

Important Clinical ECG Patters

Patterns to look out for in the appropriate clinical scenarios are listed below, and characteristic ECG patterns are shown in Figure 22.10.

- **Hyperkalemia:**
  - Mild (5.5–6.5): peaked T-waves (limb leads >6mm, precordial leads >10mm), short QT
  - Moderate (6.5–7.5): AV block, QRS widening
  - Severe (>7.5): P-wave flattening, bundle branch block, ST elevation, VT/VF, asystole.
- **Hypokalemia:** QT prolongation, U-waves, ST depressions, AV block.

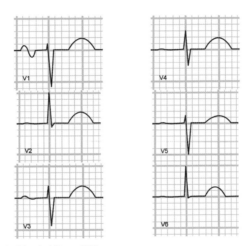

Figure 22.9 Reversal of leads V2 and V5

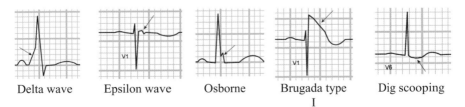

Delta wave   Epsilon wave   Osborne   Brugada type   Dig scooping
I

Figure 22.10 Characteristic ECG patterns

- **Digoxin effect:** scooping of ST, abnormal TW, short QT, U-wave, prolonged PR.
- **Digoxin toxicity:** any arrhythmia, atrial fibrillation or tachycardia with AV block, junctional/idioventricular.
- **Hypercalcemia:** short QT, PR prolongation.
- **Hypocalcemia:** prolonged QT, TW abnormalities.
- **Dextrocardia:** inverted lead I (negative P, QRS and T-waves) *and* reverse R-wave peak (RWP).
- **Chronic obstructive pulmonary disease:** RVH, right axis deviation, right atrial enlargement, late RWP, low voltages.
- **Pericardial effusion:** S1Q3T3 (large S in I, deep Q in III, inverted T in III), RBBB, inverted TW V1–V3.
- **Hypertrophic obstructive cardiomyopathy:**
  - Large amplitude QRS, large Q-waves throughout, large R-wave in V1
  - Left axis deviation, secondary ST/TW changes, left atrial enlargement
- **Wolff–Parkinson–White:** all of:
  - Delta wave
  - Short PR
  - Prolonged QRS.
- **Myxedema:** low voltages, sinus bradycardia, flat TW, prolonged PR, electrical alternans.
- **CNS disorder:** deep TW inversions in precordium, prolonged QT, prominent U.
- **Brugada:** prolongation of the QRS complex with a RBBB morphology and a persistent ST elevation in leads V1–V3. The morphology differs between the three subtypes.
- **Arrhythmogenic right ventricular dysplasia:** QRS may be prolonged with incomplete RBBB. TWI in V1 arrhythmogenic right ventricular dysplasia V3. Epsilon wave.
- **Hypothermia:** marked bradycardia, prolongation of PR, QRS, QT, Osborne waves, AF.

Lead Placement

Precordial Leads (Figure 22.11)
- V1: fourth intercostal space, right of the sternum.
- V2: fourth intercostal space, left of the sternum
- V3: directly between leads V2 and V4
- V4: fifth intercostal space at midclavicular line
- V5: level with V4 at left anterior axillary line
- V6: level with V5 at left midaxillary line

The four limb leads account for the six standard ECG limb vectors. The electrodes should be placed just above the wrists and ankles, although they can extend up to the shoulder or hips, respectively.

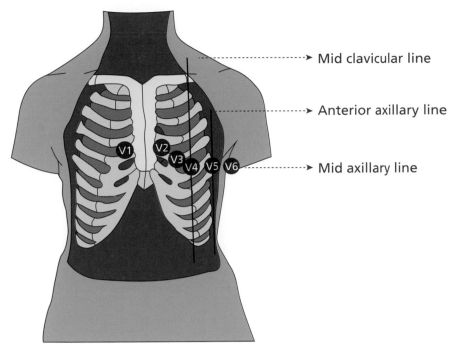

Figure 22.11 Lead placement

CLINICAL PEARLS

- In RBBB: Q-waves and axis can still be interpreted, and LVH criteria followed; standard criteria for RVH cannot be followed.
- In LBBB: Q-waves, axis, and LVH cannot be interpreted or standard injury criteria used; discordant ST elevations >5 mm or concordant ST depressions >2 mm suggest acute MI.
- Left anterior fascicle block (LAFB): unexplained left axis deviation + small Q-waves in I, aVL, and small R in III.
- Left posterior fascicle block: unexplained right axis deviation + small Q-waves in II, III, aVF, and small R in I. Rare compared to LAFB and often occurs with RBBB.
- Patients with inferior or posterior MI should have right precordial leads assessed. Right-sided V4 ST elevation >1 mm suggests RV infarct.
- Posterior infarcts: suspect when inferior infarct is seen. R > 0.04 ms and R > S in V1.
- Post-syncope: make sure you assess for Wolff–Parkinson–White, long QT, Brugada, complete heart block, Mobitz II and hypertrophic obstructive cardiomyopathy pattern.

Recommended Reading

Review Articles

Goldberger A. *Clinical Electrocardiography: A Simplified Approach*. St Louis: Mosby, 1999.

O'Keefe J, Hammill S, Freed M, Pogwizd S. *The Complete Guide to ECGs: A Comprehensive Study Guide to Improve ECG Interpretation Skills*. Royal Oak: Physician's Press, 2002.

23 Transthoracic and Transesophageal Echocardiography

Shahriar Heidary and Ingela Schnittger

Department of Internal Medicine, Division of Cardiology, Stanford University School of Medicine, Stanford, CA, USA

In transthoracic echocardiography (TTE), multiple ultrasound beams are transmitted from a transducer and bounce off various internal structures. The reflected signals are then integrated to produce real-time imaging based on the relationship:

- $c = \lambda \times f$
- c is speed of sound in body tissue (1540 m/s)
- λ is wavelength
- f is usually 2.5–4.0 MHz (up to 7.0 MHz for TEE)

Higher frequency means shorter wavelength, so there is better resolution but at the expense of less tissue penetration. In the obese patient, imaging should be tried at a lower frequency to get better penetration and possibly better images.

Imaging Views (Figure 23.1)
- Parasternal long axis (pLAX)
- Parasternal short axis (pSAX): rotate transducer 90° from pLAX; sweep from base to apex) (Figure 23.2)
- RV inflow (from pLAX tilt inferomedially and slightly clockwise)
- Apical four-chamber (angle anteriorly and get apical five-chamber view)
- Apical two-chamber (rotate counter-clockwise 60° from apical four-chamber view)
- Apical three-chamber (rotate counter-clockwise another 60° from apical two-chamber view)
- Subcostal [interrogate inferior vena cava (IVC) and descending aorta as well]
- Suprasternal (head extended, tilted; place transducer marker at 1 o'clock)

A Practical Approach to Cardiovascular Medicine, First Edition. Edited by Reza Ardehali, Marco Perez, Paul Wang.

© 2011 Blackwell Publishing Ltd. Published 2011 by Blackwell Publishing Ltd.

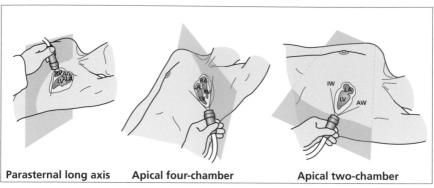

Parasternal long axis   **Apical four-chamber**   **Apical two-chamber**

Figure 23.1 Standard imaging planes. AW, anterior wall; IW, inferior wall

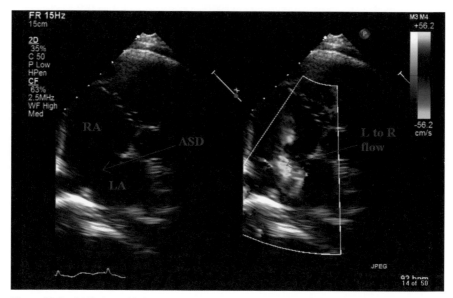

Figure 23.2 pSAX view with large secundum atrial septal defect (ASD) with left to right flow

Start imaging at a depth of 24 cm to get overall impression of cardiac and extracardiac structures (e.g. pleural effusion). Then readjust depth to make the heart larger. Use the zoom function freely, especially over valves.

Doppler Echocardiography

- Doppler is the best modality to evaluate blood flow direction, turbulence, and velocity.
- Color Doppler should be performed around each valve, the interatrial septum, interventricular septum (when needed), and ascending and descending aorta.
- Convention is BART: **B**lue **A**way = blood flow away from transducer; **R**ed **T**owards = blood flow towards transducer.

Box 23.1 Common Doppler-derived pressure gradients

Location	Clinical utility
Right ventricular (RV) inflow view	Across tricuspid valve (TV) = gradient between right atrium (RA) and RV. Right atrial pressure (RAP) + gradient = right ventricular systolic pressure (RVSP) or pulmonary artery systolic pressure (PASP) if no pulmonic stenosis
Apical five-chamber view	Get peak and mean gradients across aortic valve for aortic stenosis assessment
Suprasternal	Can see increased gradient (a step up) across an aortic coarctation Should be done in all patients but especially those with bicuspid AV or other congenital anomalies
Mitral inflow	Use pulse wave Doppler with sample volume of 1–2 mm between the tips of the mitral valve during diastole for peak inflow velocities Diastolic parameters obtained here Use continuous-wave Doppler for mean gradient for mitral stenosis
Subcostal	Get spectral Doppler across interatrial septum if atrial septal defect (ASD) RAP + gradient = left atrial pressure (LAP)

- Pressure gradients (Box 23.1) can be accurately estimated with the simplified Bernoulli equation:

Pressure = $4V^2$ (where V is the peak instantaneous velocity)

M-Mode
- "Ice-pick" view of heart
- Provides the highest temporal resolution; subtle motion of structures can be seen

Utility in Diagnosis of Disease
- Evaluation of cardiac structure/function for:
  - Shortness of breath, dyspnea on exertion, angina, coronary artery disease, myocardial infarction, syncope, transient ischemic attack, congenital disease (shunts), atrial fibrillation, diabetes mellitus, hypertension, edema, palpitations, fatigue, anemia, chronic obstructive pulmonary disease (COPD), chemotherapy
- Evaluation of hypotension, hemodynamic instability, pulmonary embolism, shock
- Evaluation of murmur, mitral valve prolapse, native and prosthetic valvular function

- Evaluation of intracardiac mass (cardiac source emboli), pericardial disease (constriction, pericarditis, tamponade)
- Evaluation of aortic disease (dissection, coarctation)
- Evaluation of heart failure, pulmonary hypertension, diastolic function, hypertension, ischemic and nonischemic cardiomyopathies (hypertrophic cardiomyopahty, amyloidosis, arrhythmogenic right ventricular dysplasia), dyssynchrony, LVAD, intracardiac devices

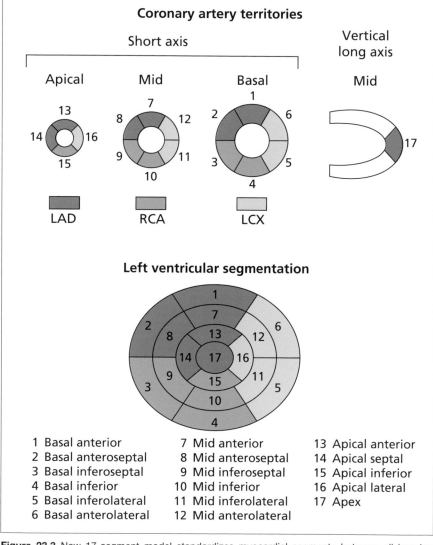

Figure 23.3 New 17-segment model standardizes myocardial segments between all imaging modalities, knowing that there is anatomic variability to coronary distribution

Coronary Artery Disease (Figure 23.3)

- Normal segment has thickening of 40–50% in systole (score = 1)
- Hypokinesis <30% thickening during systole (score = 2)
- Akinesis <10% (score = 3)
- Dyskinesis is systolic outward movement of a segment (score = 4)
- Aneurysm is a thinned segment; bowing out in systole and diastole (score = 5)
  - Wall motion score index (WMSI) = $\dfrac{\text{Sum of wall motion scores}}{\text{Number of segments visualized}}$
  - WMSI >1.7 associated with a perfusion defect of >20%
- Remember to always assess for LV thrombus (Figure 23.4), especially after an extensive MI.

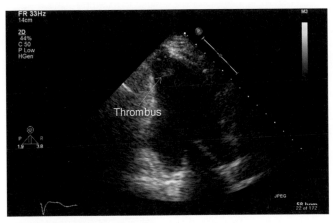

Figure 23.4 Round LV thrombus at the apex

Diastolic Dysfunction

See Box 23.2 and Figure 23.5.

Box 23.2 **Summary of diastolic dysfunction**		
Grade	Description	Findings
1	Impaired relaxation	E/A < 0.75; E' < 8 cm/s; DT > 240 ms; IVRT > 90 ms PVS > PVD Vp < 50 cm/s
2	Pseudonormalization (impaired relaxation with increased filling pressures)	E/A 1–1.5; E' < 8 cm/s DT 160–200 ms; IVRT < 90 ms PVS < PVD Vp < 50 cm/s
		(Continued)

Grade	Description	Findings
3	Restrictive physiology: reversible with Valsalva or reducing filling pressures	E/A > 1.5; E' < 8cm/s DT < 160ms; IVRT < 70ms PVS < PVD Valsalva (ΔE/A > 0.5) Vp < 50cm/s
4	Restrictive physiology: irreversible with Valsalva or reducing filling pressures	E/A > 1.5; E' < 8cm/s; DT < 160ms; IVRT < 70ms PVS < PVD Valsalva (ΔE/A < 0.5) Vp < 50cm/s

E, early diastolic filling wave; E', early diastolic mitral annular velocity (lateral); A, late diastolic filling wave from atrial contraction; DT, deceleration time; IVRT, isovolumic relaxation time; PVS, pulmonary venous systolic flow; PVD, premature ventricular depolarization

CLINICAL PEARLS

- RV inflow view gives one of the only pictures of the inferior leaflet of the tricuspid valve.
- Most common cause of dilated coronary sinus is persistent left superior vena cava (SVC).
- In evaluating bicuspid AV, note opening pattern: football = bicuspid; triangle = tricuspid.
- Four pulmonary veins seen in the "crab" view: short axis of aortic arch with posterior angulation.
- In aortic stenosis, the Doppler maximal instantaneous gradient is always higher than the peak-to-peak gradient at cath. It is better to use mean gradient when the two techniques are compared.
- Consider a bubble study to evaluate for shunt with right-sided enlargement without identifiable cause.
- If congestive heart failure, but E' >8cm/s, then consider constriction.
- For tamponade, best views are often subcostal but could be apical.
- Remember to reduce sweep speed from 50mm/s to 25mm/s for assessing respiratory variation of mitral and tricuspid inflows.
- In obese patients or those with COPD, subcostal as well as subcostal short axis views can be helpful.

- With pulmonary hypertension, classic signs of tamponade may not be seen.
- E' of medial annulus (≥10cm/s) is less than the E' of the lateral annulus (≥15cm/s).
- Tachycardia or primary atrioventricular block can cause fusion of E- and A-waves.
- Mitral valve deceleration time (DT) can be short in the young and the healthy.
- E/E' of lateral annulus ≥15 is associated with a pulmonary capillary wedge pressure (PCWP) ≥20mmHg; E/E' of lateral annulus ≤10 is associated with a PCWP ≤15mmHg.
- Pericardiocentesis to drain a hemorrhaging pericardial effusion caused by a Type A dissection can worsen the clinical situation. Need to go to surgery.

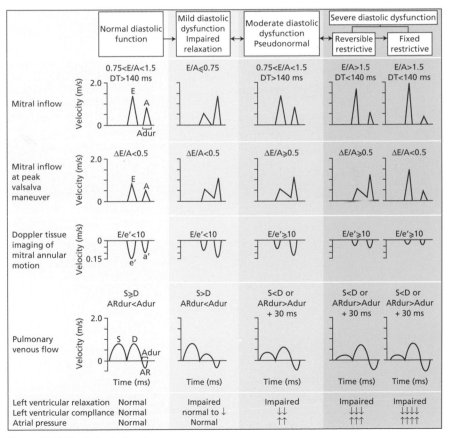

Figure 23.5 Diastolic dysfunction

Transesophageal Echocardiocardiography

Common Clinical Uses

- Evaluation of suspected aortic dissection or transsection:
  - Advantages over CT and MRI are portability and usability in unstable patients
  - Can also evaluate for AR, pulmonary embolism, and dissection into a coronary, resulting in segmental wall motion abnormalities (Figure 23.6).
- Diagnosis and management of endocarditis:
  - Useful in diagnosis in cases of moderate-to-high pretest likelihood
  - Useful in diagnosis with persistent fever and intracardiac device
  - Useful in diagnosis for suspected prosthetic valve endocarditis
  - Useful in management of endocarditis for suspected complications: aortic root/paravalvular abscess, perforation of leaflet, fistula.
- Used to guide invasive procedures:
  - Patent foramen ovale (PFO)/ASD closure (Figure 23.7)
  - Balloon mitral valvuloplasty

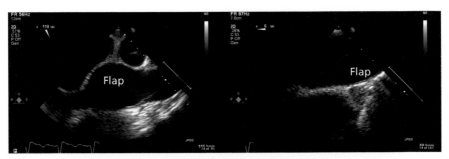

Figure 23.6 Intimal flap in the ascending aorta extending into the aortic arch

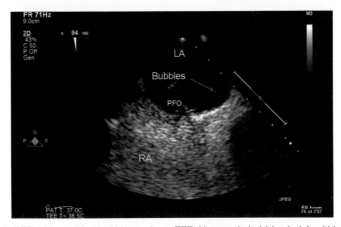

Figure 23.7 PFO with positive bubble study on TEE. Note early bubbles in LA within 1 beat

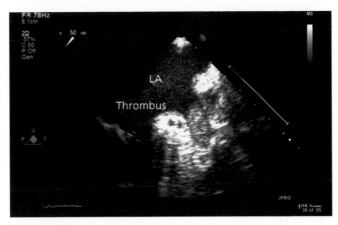

Figure 23.8 TEE with large thrombus in the left atrial appendage

- Alcohol septal ablation for hypertrophic cardiomyopathy (HCM)
- Guidance for transseptal punctures.
- Evaluate valvular regurgitation and its mechanism; particularly useful in cases when planning valve repair.
- Evaluation of patient with atrial fibrillation or atrial flutter prior to cardioversion or in patients with suspected cardiac source of embolization (Figure 23.8).
- Evaluation of structure/function: poor TTE windows (obese, critically ill, and ventilated), congenital heart disease.

CLINICAL PEARLS

- Deep transgastric view is often best for evaluating the gradient across AV or left ventricular outflow tract (LVOT).
- Use m-mode through a structure to help decide if it is an artifact or real.
- In general, turning the TEE probe to the right (clockwise) brings out right-sided heart structures (RA, SVC, IVC).
- In general, turning the TEE probe to the left (counterclockwise) brings out left-sided heart structures (AV, MV).
- Buckling of the TEE probe tip in the esophagus presents as resistance when trying to withdraw the probe. Solution is to advance into the stomach, straighten probe, and then withdraw, avoiding potential complications.
- Right pulmonary veins: start at 45° and turn right (clockwise).
- Left pulmonary veins: start at 110° and turn left (counterclockwise).
- Suspect methemoglobinemia if cyanosis after excessive topical anesthetic, especially benzocaine.
- Treatment for methemoglobinemia is methylene blue 1 mg/kg over 5 min.

Recommended Reading

Guidelines

American College of Cardiology/American Heart Association Task Force on Practice Guidelines; Society of Cardiovascular Anesthesiologists; Society for Cardiovascular Angiography and Interventions; Society of Thoracic Surgeons; Bonow RO, Carabello BA, Kanu C et al. ACC/AHA 2006 Guidelines for the Management of Patients With Valvular Heart Disease: A Report of the American College of Cardiology/American Heart Association Task Force on Practice Guidelines (Writing Committee to Revise the 1998 Guidelines for the Management of Patients With Valvular Heart Disease): Developed in Collaboration With the Society of Cardiovascular Anesthesiologists: Endorsed by the Society for Cardiovascular Angiography and Interventions and the Society of Thoracic Surgeons. *Circulation* 2006;**114**:e84–231.

Cerqueira MD, Weissman NJ, Dilsizian V et al. Standardized Myocardial Segmentation and Nomenclature for Tomographic Imaging of the Heart: A Statement for Healthcare Professionals From the Cardiac Imaging Committee of the Council on Clinical Cardiology of the American Heart Association. *Circulation* 2002;**105**:539–542.

Douglas PS, Khandheria B, Stainback RF et al. ACCF/ASE/ACEP/ASNC/SCAI/SCCT/ SCMR 2007 Appropriateness Criteria for Transthoracic and Transesophageal Echocardiography: A Report of the American College of Cardiology Foundation Quality Strategic Directions Committee Appropriateness Criteria Working Group, American Society of Echocardiography, American College of Emergency Physicians, American Society of Nuclear Cardiology, Society for Cardiovascular Angiography and Interventions, Society of Cardiovascular Computed Tomography, and the Society for Cardiovascular Magnetic Resonance Endorsed by the American College of Chest Physicians and the Society of Critical Care Medicine. *J Am Coll Cardiol* 2007;**50**:187–204.

Nagueh SF, Appleton CP, Gillebert TC et al. Recommendations for the evaluation of left ventricular diastolic function by echocardiography. *J Am Soc Echocardiogr* 2009;**22**: 107–133.

Review Articles

Redfield MM, Jacobsen SJ, Burnett JC Jr, Mahoney DW, Bailey KR, Rodeheffer RJ. Burden of systolic and diastolic ventricular dysfunction in the community: appreciating the scope of the heart failure epidemic. *JAMA* 2003;**289**:194–202.

Nagueh SF, Sun H, Kopelen HA, Middleton KJ, Khoury DS. Hemodynamic determinants of the mitral annulus diastolic velocities by tissue Doppler. *J Am Coll Cardiol* 2001;**37**: 278–285.

Oh JK, Seward JB, Tajik AJ. *The Echo Manual*, 3rd edn. Philadelphia: Lippincott, Williams & Wilkins, 2006.

24 Noninvasive Stress Testing

Arvindh Kanagasundram and Victor F. Froelicher

Department of Internal Medicine, Division of Cardiology, Stanford
University School of Medicine, Stanford, CA, USA

Estimating Pretest Probability

- Initial step in the diagnosis of coronary artery disease (CAD) should include an estimate of pretest probability that can guide the need for further diagnostic tests.
- Combined with the sensitivity and specificity of a particular test, this pretest probability can then give the post-test probability of having CAD.
- Patients with a low pretest probability of CAD will have a significantly higher rate of false-positive results, and this should be considered prior to ordering noninvasive tests in this group of patients.
- Pretest probability of CAD can be estimated using either the Diamond-Forrester estimates or the Morise score (Table 24.1).

Exercise Testing

Patients who meet the criteria for exercise testing should be referred for a treadmill or bicycle stress test (Box 24.1, Figure 24.1).

Exercise testing provides more information than pharmacologic stress testing for the following reasons:

- Able to gain insight into the actual functional ability of a patient and the level of exertion at which symptoms are elicited.
- Information about patient's symptoms.
- Maximal exercise capacity is the most powerful predictor of prognosis and hemodynamic responses, such as heart rate and BP, are ischemia-independent predictors for prognosis:
  - Worse cardiovascular outcomes are associated with the following:
    - Exercise capacity <5 metabolic equivalents (METs) for those <65 years of age

A Practical Approach to Cardiovascular Medicine, First Edition. Edited by Reza Ardehali, Marco Perez, Paul Wang.
© 2011 Blackwell Publishing Ltd. Published 2011 by Blackwell Publishing Ltd.

Table 24.1 Pretest probability of coronary disease

Variable			Score
Age	Men	Women	
	< 40	< 50	3
	40–54	50–64	6
	> 55	> 65	9
Estrogen-positive (women only)			–3
Estrogen-negative (women Only)			3
Nonanginal symptoms			1
Atypical anginal symptoms			3
Typical anginal symptoms			5
Diabetes			2
Hyperlipidemia			1
Smoking history			1
Hypertension			1
Family history of CAD			1
Obesity			1
Total:			
Low probability			0–8
Intermediate probability			9–15
High probability			≥16

Box 24.1 Exercise protocols

Protocol	Description
Ramp	Approach to exercise testing that has supplanted earlier protocols
	Work increases constantly and continuously and allows individualization of protocol
	A given test duration can be targeted
	Optimized patient performance and estimation of oxygen uptake
Bruce	Earliest adopted protocol limited by technology available when developed
Cornell	Developed for use with rate-related change in exercise induced ST-segment depression
	Could prove to be useful when heart rate-related changes are studied
Naughton	Early protocol with constant speed and 1-min changes in grade

- – Exercise-induced angina as the reason for stopping
- – Low peak systolic pressure, or a fall in systolic pressure during exercise
- – Poor heart rate recovery after maximal exercise
- • Exercise testing requires an incremental protocol, which progresses from low to higher workload, until a target endpoint is reached:

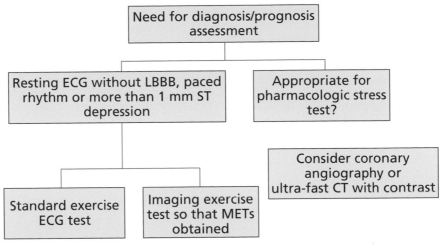

Figure 24.1 Choice of testing modality

Box 24.2 Contraindications to exercise testing

Absolute	Relative
Acute myocardial infarction (within 2 days)	Left main coronary stenosis
High-risk unstable angina	Moderate stenotic valvular lesion
Uncontrolled cardiac arrhythmias	Electrolyte abnormalities
Symptomatic severe aortic stenosis	Severe arterial hypertension
Uncontrolled symptomatic heart failure	Tachyarrhythmias or bradyarrhythmias
Acute pulmonary embolus or infarction	Hypertrophic cardiomyopathy and
Acute aortic dissection	other forms of outflow tract obstruction
	Mental or physical impairment leading
	to inability to exercise adequately
	High-degree AV block

- Target endpoint is usually maximal effort or signs and symptoms that preclude further exercise
- Note that protocols are usually chosen to match individual's functional capacity.

Though noninvasive, exercise testing is not without risks. Rare cases of myocardial infarction, serious arrhythmias, and deaths have been reported.

Contraindications to stress testing are listed in Box 24.2.

Exercise ECG (see Table 24.2)
- Patient selection:
- Patients who are able to exercise (free from orthopedic or neurologic limitations)

Table 24.2 Sensitivity and specificity of noninvasive tests for the detection of coronary artery disease

Diagnostic test	Sensitivity (Range)	Specificity (Range)	Studies	Patients
Planar thallium imaging	0.79 (0.70–0.94)	0.73 (0.43–0.97)	6	510
Single-photon emission CT	0.88 (0.73–0.98)	0.77 (0.53–0.96)	8	628
Echocardiography	0.76 (0.40–1.00)	0.88 (0.80–0.95)	10	1174
Positron emission tomography	0.91 (0.69–1.00)	0.82 (0.73–0.88)	3	206
Exercise electrocardiography	0.68	0.77	132	24 074

- Patients without the following ECG changes that can affect interpretation:
  - Pre-excitation syndrome (Wolff–Parkinson–White)
  - Paced rhythm
  - >1 mm ST depressions at rest
  - Left bundle branch block (LBBB)
- Interpretation of standard exercise test results:
  - **Electrographic:**
    - Maximal ST depression or elevation
    - Slope of ST depression (flat or downsloping is abnormal)
    - Leads showing ST depression (V4–5–6 most clinically significant, does not localize subendocardial ischemia)
    - Leads showing ST elevation (which localizes transmural ischemia)
    - Whether depression occurs during exercise and/or recovery (exercise-only depression is most sensitive, while recovery depression is more specific, particularly at 2–3 min recovery)
    - Exercise-induced ventricular arrhythmias
  - **Hemodynamic:**
    - Maximum exercise heart rate
    - Maximum exercise systolic BP (SBP)
    - Maximum exercise double product (HR × BP)
    - Maximal MET level achieved
    - Exertional hypotension
    - Chronotropic incompetence
    - Heart rate recovery
  - **Symptomatic:**
    - Whether exercise-induced angina occurred or was the reason for stopping
    - Other exercise-limiting symptoms, particularly specifying whether it was fatigue or shortness of breath
    - Time to onset of angina
  - **Prognostic markers:**
    - **Maximum exercise capacity:**
      Influenced by cardiac function as well as age, general physical conditioning, comorbidities and psychologic states, such as depression

Markers include: maximum MET level achieved; maximum heart rate, SBP (should rise >40 mmHg and not drop during exercise), and double product (should exceed 25 000)
- **Exercise-induced ischemia:**
Markers include: exercise-induced ST elevation or depression; exercise-induced angina
- **Chronotropic incompetence:**
Failure to achieve 80–85% of the age-predicted maximum exercise heart rate or a low chronotropic index (heart rate adjusted to MET level)
Failure of the heart rate to drop >20 bpm by the second minute of recovery after exercise
- **Ectopy:**
Premature ventricular contractions (PVCs) particularly during recovery have been found to be associated with an adverse prognosis.
- **Duke treadmill score:**
  - Treadmill score = METs: $5 \times$ (amount of ST – segment deviation in mm) – $4 \times$ exercise angina index (0 if there is no exercise angina; 1 if exercise angina occurred, and 2 if angina was the reason the patient stopped exercising)
  - Low risk: score ≥+5
  Average annual cardiovascular mortality rate of 0.5%
  - High risk: score ≤–11
  Average annual cardiovascular mortality rate ≥5%
  - In patients who are classified as low risk on the basis of clinical and exercise testing, there is no evidence that invasive interventions could alter outcomes.
  - Patients with intermediate-risk treadmill scores, however, might benefit from further imaging or intervention to determine if the ST response was a false positive.

EVIDENCE-BASED PRACTICE

Exercise treadmill score for predicting prognosis in coronary artery disease
Context: Use of treadmill exercise score to stratify prognosis in patients with suspected coronary artery disease
Goal: To determine the prognostic value of treadmill exercise testing
Methods: 2842 patients with chest pain who had both treadmill testing and cardiac catheterization were evaluated. The population was randomly divided into two equal-sized groups and the Cox regression model was used in one to form a treadmill score that was then validated in the other group.

(Continued)

> **Results:** Final treadmill score (Duke treadmill score) added independent prognostic information and was useful for stratifying prognosis in patients with suspected CAD.
>
> **Take-home message:** Treadmill score has prognostic value in patients with suspected CAD and is useful for clinical decision-making

Stress Echocardiography (see Table 24.2)

- Can be used to demonstrate the presence of coronary disease by showing inducible wall motion abnormalities (see Chapter 23).
- Of significant additive clinical value compared with standard exercise testing for detecting and localizing inducible myocardial ischemia.
- Multiple echo views are obtained at rest and stress and these are compared side-by-side in a continuous loop format.
- Wall motion abnormality is defined as a reduction in either amplitude or speed of thickening:
  - In segments with resting wall motion abnormalities, ischemia is noted by deterioration of the abnormality or a biphasic response with initial improvement and then deterioration.
- **Exercise echo:**
  - Typically performed with concurrent ECG monitoring with the same exercise protocols used for exercise ECG testing
  - Recommended as initial stress in patients who can exercise, but who have baseline ECG abnormalities
  - Predictive value of exercise echocardiography is enhanced by combining echocardiographic findings with exercise test data.
- **Pharmacologic stress echo:**
  - Can be performed with either adrenergic-stimulating (dobutamine or arbutamine) or vasodilating (dipyridamole or adenosine) agents
  - Pharmacologic stress might best be accomplished using adrenergic stimulants since these enhance myocardial performance which can be directly evaluated by echocardiography. Comparative studies have suggested a higher sensitivity using this modality.
- **IV contrast enhancement:**
  - Predictive value can be enhanced with contrast echocardiography
  - Information about myocardial perfusion is also obtained with this technique.
- **Diagnostic and prognostic value:**
  - Accuracy of dobutamine echocardiography is dependent on:
    - Degree of stenosis
    - Amount of myocardium at risk
    - Degree of deterioration of wall motion.
  - Prognosis varies with specific findings on stress echocardiography:
    - Number of abnormal territories at peak stress

- Abnormal left ventricular end-systolic volume response
- Whether wall motion abnormality occurs only during stress or is also present during rest.

EVIDENCE-BASED PRACTICE

Prediction of mortality by exercise echocardiography: a strategy for combination with the Duke treadmill score

Context: Predicting mortality from abnormal exercise echocardiography.

Goal: To study prediction of mortality with stress echocardiography and formulate a strategy for combination with standard exercise testing.

Methods: Clinical, exercise testing, and echocardiographic data were collected in 5375 patients undergoing exercise echocardiography.

Results: Over the first 6 years of follow-up, those with normal exercise echocardiograms had a mortality of 1%/year. Exercise echocardiography was able to further substratify patients with intermediate-risk Duke scores into groups with yearly mortality of 2–7%.

Take-home message: Normal exercise echo confers a low risk of death; whole positive results are an independent predictor of mortality.

EVIDENCE-BASED PRACTICE

A clinical and echocardiographic score for assigning risk of a major event after cobutamine echocardiograms

Context: Use of clinical and stress echocardiographic findings to predict prognostic score.

Goal: To develop a risk score combining both clinical and dobutamine echocardiographic features.

Methods: Data from a series of 1456 patients were used to develop a multivariate model for prediction of events. The model was then internally validated in the remaining dobutamine echo patients in the same series and externally validated in 1733 patients in an independent series.

Results: The following score was used to predict risk score:

$$\text{Risk score} = (\text{age} \times 0.02) + [(\text{heart failure history} + \text{rate-pressure product} < 15\,000) \times 0.4] + [(\text{ischemia} + \text{scar}) \times 0.6] \text{ (each variable as 1 if present and 0 if absent)}$$

- <1.2: low risk; >97% 5-year event-free survival
- 1.2–2.6: intermediate risk; 75–97% 5-year event-free survival
- >2.6: high risk; <75% 5-year event free survival

Take-home message: The devised risk score can be used to quantify risk of events after a dobutamine echocardiogram.

Echocardiography versus Myocardial Perfusion Imaging
- Choice should be based on both local availability and expertise.
- Advantages of stress echocardiography over stress myocardial perfusion imaging include:
  - Information regarding left ventricular mass and valvular function
  - Lower cost and shorter time commitment
  - Avoidance of radiation exposure

Radionuclide Imaging (see Table 24.2)
- Most commonly performed in the setting of known or suspected coronary artery disease.
- In contrast to 2D echocardiography, SPECT and PET provide true tomographic imaging, where all segments of the myocardium are visualized.
- Symptom-limited exercise is the preferred form if patient is able to fit the criteria stated above.
- Similar to stress echocardiography pharmacologic stress agents can be classified as either vasodilators or adrenergic stimulating agents.
- **Choice of agent:**
  - Adenosine and dipyradamole are the major vasodilators used. These agents cause vasodilation and resulting steal with differences in stenosed and normal vascular territories
  - Major adrenergic agent used is dobutamine which results in increased oxygen demand
  - Vasodilators are the first choice for pharmacologic stress. However, contraindications to vasodilators include:
    - Significant hypotension
    - Bronchospastic airway disease
    - Sick sinus syndrome and high-degree AV block.
- **Interpretation:**
  - In a stenotic artery there is blunted coronary flow reserve during vasodilator-induced hyperemia. The resulting regional differences in tracer uptake are then detected by imaging
  - Development of ST depressions during pharmacologic stress testing is less common compared with treadmill exercise testing, but has been shown to have a high positive predictive value
  - 17–20 segmental model is usually used in which visual estimates of perfusion defects are graded within each segment. Summing of the individual segmental scores to achieve global perfusion scores has been extensively studied and correlated with prognosis.
- **Diagnostic and prognostic value:**
  - As with the other modalities of stress testing, maximal exercise capacity, exercise-induced ischemia, and chronotropic incompetence are important prognostic signs
  - High-risk features on myocardial perfusion imaging include:
    - Ischemia involving >20% of the left ventricle

- Defects in more than one vascular supply region
- Reversible ischemia in multiple segments
- Stress-induced left ventricular cavity dilatation
- Stress-induced ventricular dyssynergy
- Increased lung uptake which is a marker for increased pulmonary capillary wedge pressure.

EVIDENCE-BASED PRACTICE

Incremental prognostic value of myocardial perfusion SPECT for the prediction of cardiac death

Context: Value of nuclear testing in predicting mortality

Goal: To define the incremental prognostic value of stress SPECT for the prediction of cardiac death.

Methods: 5183 patients with known or suspected CAD who underwent SPECT imaging with exercise or pharmacologic stress were followed up for the occurrence of cardiac death or MI. Visual interpretation was performed with short-axis and vertical long-axis myocardial tomograms divided into 20 segments. The sum of the differences between each of the 20 segments on the rest and stress images was defined as the summed difference score. Summed stress scores <4 were considered normal; 4–8, mildly abnormal; 9–13 moderately abnormal; and >13 severely abnormal.

Results: The annual rates of cardiac death in patients with mildly abnormal, moderately abnormal, or severely abnormal perfusion defects were 2.7%, 2.9%, and 4.2%, respectively. Patients with a normal scan had <0.5% risk for cardiac death per year.

Take-home message: Myocardial perfusion SPECT is valuable in predicting incremental prognostic information about cardiac-related mortality.

CLINICAL PEARLS

- Only ST elevation localizes territory of ischemia. ST depression is caused by generalized subendocardial ischemia and does not localize. ST elevation is arrythmogenic while ST depression is not.
- Chest discomfort during dipyridamole or adenosine infusion is a side effect of these drugs and unrelated to ischemia.
- Exercise testing in patients with hypertrophic cardiomyopathy and aortic stenosis provides valuable information about their physical limitations. However, arrhythmias, angina, and hypotension may occur and the test must be stopped immediately.
- In the event of a severe side effect with dipyridamole, it can be reversed by aminophylline.

(Continued)

- Principal factor affecting specificity of SPECT imaging is soft tissue attenuation (breast tissue artifacts in women and diaphragmatic attenuation in men). This attenuation occurs at a lower frequency with use of higher energy ^{99m}Tc agents and can be lessened by the body position during imaging.

Recommended Reading

Clinical Trials and Meta-Analyses

Hachamovitch R, Berman DS, Shaw LJ et al. Incremental prognostic value of myocardial perfusion single photon emission computed tomography for the prediction of cardiac death: Differential stratification for risk of cardiac death and myocardial infarction. *Circulation* 1998;**97**:535–543.

Mark DB, Hlatky MA, Harrell FE, Lee KL, Califf RM, Pryor DB. Exercise treadmill score for predicting prognosis in coronary artery disease. *Ann Intern Med* 1987;**106**:793–800.

Marwick TH, Case C, Vasey C, Allen S, Short L, Thomas JD. Prediction of mortality by exercise echocardiography: A strategy of combination with the Duke treadmill score. *Circulation* 2001;**103**:2566–2571.

Marwick TH, Case C, Poldermans D et al. A clinical and echocardiographic score for assigning risk of major events after dobutamine echocardiograms. *J Am Coll Cardiol* 2004;**43**:2102–2107.

Morise AP, Haddad WJ, Beckner D. Development and validation of a clinical score to estimate the probability of coronary artery disease in men and women presenting with suspected coronary disease. *Am J Med* 1997;**102**:350–356.

Wackers F. Customized exercise testing. *J Am Coll Cardiol* 2009;**54**(6):546–548.

Guidelines

Gibbons RJ, Balady GJ, Bricker JT et al. ACC/AHA 2002 guideline update for exercise testing: summary article: a report of the American College of Cardiology/American Association Task Force on Practice Guidelines. *Circulation* 2002;**106**:1883–1892.

Review Articles

Froelicher VF, Myers J. *Manual of Exercise Testing*, 3rd edn. Philadelphia: Saunders-Mosby, 2006.

25 Cardiac MRI and CT

Chandra Katikireddy and Michael V. McConnell

Department of Internal Medicine, Division of Cardiology, Stanford
University School of Medicine, Stanford, CA, USA

Cardiac MRI

Cardiac MRI has become an important part of clinical management as a result
of rapid MR technological advancement as well as clinical validation and
experience. MRI provides superior tissue contrast with high image quality
and resolution from unlimited imaging planes. This has transformed MRI into
a powerful clinical tool to comprehensively assess cardiac anatomy and function; myocardial tissue characterization, viability, and ischemia; and valvular,
pericardial, and congenital heart disease.

MRI Basics

The primary source of the MRI signal is the hydrogen nucleus (proton), which
is abundant in the water and fat of body tissues. Protons become aligned in
the presence of a large magnetic field. A radiofrequency (RF) pulse excites
protons out of alignment and then their signal can be detected with an RF
coil. Gradients in all three directions are used to encode the 3D location of the
signal.

- The typical magnetic field strengths used for cardiac MRI are 1.5 and 3 Tesla
  (T). Higher fields strength can provide greater MRI signal and/or resolution, but may be prone to more artifacts.
- T_1 (longitudinal relaxation time) is the time constant that defines the expo-
  nential recovery rate of longitudinal magnetization. This determines how
  quickly the protons realign with the main magnetic field after excitation,
  and hence the amount of signal available for the next excitation. The T_1 of
  blood is on the order of 1 s at 1.5 T.
- T_2 (transverse relaxation time) is the time constant that defines the expo-
  nential decay rate of transverse magnetization. This determines how

A Practical Approach to Cardiovascular Medicine, First Edition. Edited by Reza Ardehali,
Marco Perez, Paul Wang.
© 2011 Blackwell Publishing Ltd. Published 2011 by Blackwell Publishing Ltd.

quickly the protons get out of phase after excitation, and hence lose signal. The T_2 of blood is on the order of 200 ms at 1.5 T.

- Tissue signal on MRI is proportional to its magnetization. Therefore, tissue with greater proton density will have higher signal. The major tissue contrast, however, comes from difference in T_1 and T_2. A tissue with shorter T_1 will recover its magnetization more quickly on a T_1-weighted image and appear brighter. A tissue with a shorter T_2 will lose its signal more quickly on a T_2-weighted image and will appear darker.
- Values of T_1, T_2, and proton density vary from tissue to tissue and between normal and diseased myocardium. MRI pulse sequences utilize a series of RF excitations, magnetic gradient field switches, and data acquisition methods to weigh the images toward T_1, T_2, or other tissue parameters (e.g. velocity) to aid in distinguishing tissue types and normal versus diseased tissue.
- Gadolinium contrast agents are can be given intravenously to shorten the T1 value of blood or myocardium, which makes it brighter than surrounding tissue.
- On T_1-weighted images, bright regions are typically fat or diseased tissue that has accumulated gadolinium. On T_2-weighted imaging, bright regions are typically edema. Calcium, due to lack of protons in water or fat, typically appears dark on both T_1- and T_2-weighted imaging.

Advantages and Disadvantages
- **Advantages:**
  - Superior tissue contrast and high resolution
  - Not subjected to acoustic window limitation, with the capability of multiplanar imaging of any desired cardiovascular structure
  - Reproducible, quantitative measures
  - No ionizing radiation
  - Most imaging can be done without contrast agents. Gadolinium is noniodinated
- **Disadvantages:**
  - Contraindicated with certain ferromagnetic devices, such as pacemakers, implantable cardioverter defibrillators (ICDs)
  - Image quality can be affected by cardiac arrhythmias
  - Artifacts may result from poor breath holding or respiratory motion

Clinical Indications
- Gold standard test for the assessment of ventricular volumes, mass, and ejection fraction (EF)
- Standard reference test for the assessment of myocardial scar and viability
- Evaluation of the etiology of systolic or diastolic dysfunction, cardiomyopathies, arrhythmias
- Detection of stress-induced myocardial ischemia

- Diagnosis of anomalous coronaries
- Cardiac mass characterization
- Pericardial pathology assessment
- Diagnosis of valvular disease, quantification of valvular regurgitation
- Congenital heart disease diagnosis and postoperative follow-up
- Left atrial and pulmonary vein mapping before or after ablation procedures
- Vascular assessment (aorta, pulmonary, carotid, renal, peripheral)

Planning the Basic Cardiac MRI Views

To understand complex cardiac anatomy and function accurately and thoroughly, it is necessary to scan the heart in multiple imaging planes. Basic cardiac MRI views primarily include axial imaging as well as classic cardiac short- and long-axis planes. Thorough knowledge of the clinical scenario is essential to customize the study protocol on an individual basis according to the clinical question. Ideally, MRI protocols should be dynamic and adaptable to investigate any unexpected findings detected during the examination.

Common Clinical Applications

Ventricular Function and Volumes

- MRI is considered the "gold standard" test to accurately measure ventricular volumes, left ventricular (LV) mass, and EFs.
- Steady-state free procession (SSFP) imaging is typically performed with ECG gating during breath-holding. This provides "bright blood" ciné images with high spatial and temporal resolution and excellent contrast between blood and myocardium.
- In contrast to standard 2D echo, MRI images the entire 3D volume of the heart, so ventricular volumes can be measured directly without relying on geometric assumptions. From the endocardial and epicardial borders defined on the short-axis views of the heart from apex through base, end-systolic and end-diastolic volumes, as well as LV mass can be quantified and stroke volume and EF calculated.
- Myocardial tagging techniques may be helpful to assess regional myocardial function and strain, as well as ventricular dyssynchrony.

Myocardial Scar/Fibrosis Imaging

Gadolinium is predominantly distributed in the extracellular space and cleared from normal myocardium quickly. However, in the event of myocardial cellular injury or fibrosis, gadolinium enters the injured cells or the interstitial space, respectively. This results in both greater gadolinium accumulation and delayed clearance, causing marked difference in gadolinium concentration between normal and injured/scarred myocardium after approximately 10 min. This has been termed late gadolinium enhancement (LGE) or simply delayed enhancement (DE). A T_1-weighted scan is performed

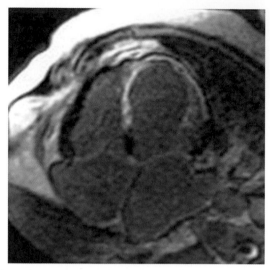

Figure 25.1 MRI four-chamber view. Transmural delayed enhancement is depicted by the bright late-gadolinium enhancement (LGE) signal in the septum, apex, and lateral wall in a patient with ischemic cardiomyopathy

with an inversion pulse timed to null the signal from normal myocardium, resulting in the diseased myocardium appearing bright (Figure 25.1).

- LGE is not specific for myocardial infarction, as the process of myocardial necrosis or fibrosis can be seen in nonischemic states such as myocarditis, nonischemic cardiomyopathy, and myocardial infiltration.
- LGE is more sensitive than SPECT, PET, and dobutamne echo in the detection of myocardial injury or infarction (MI), in particular subendocardial infarcts.
- In general, the LGE pattern of MI (ischemic cardiomyopathy) is either subendocardial or transmural in a coronary artery segmental distribution.
- Typically, in nonischemic myocardial pathology, LGE is seen in a mid-wall or epicardial pattern that does not follow a coronary distribution.
- Extent of transmural LGE of a myocardial segment is inversely proportional to its likelihood of functional recovery following revascularization. In general, myocardial segments with LGE >50% of wall thickness are unlikely to recover contractile function following coronary revascularization.
- Extent of LGE is also an indicator of worse prognosis in acute MI. In severe acute infarcts, there can be a region within the infarct that does not enhance due to microvascular obstruction, which portends the worst prognosis.
- T_2-weighted imaging can detect myocardial edema, which occurs with acute ischemia and can be used to assess the "area at risk" in acute coronary syndromes and may also be present in myocarditis or transplant rejection.
- In nonischemic cardiomyopathies, presence of LGE may be indicative of worse prognosis with increased risk of future cardiovascular events.

Box 25.1 MRI: major cardiomyopathies

Etiology	MR findings	Other remarks
Ischemic cardiomyopathy	Subendocardial or transmural pattern of DE in coronary artery distribution	Accurate assessment of myocardial viability assists in decision making of revascularization
Dilated cardiomyopathy and chronic myocarditis	Mid-wall septal DE pattern seen in 30% of patients.	Presence of DE may increase mortality and future cardiovascular events
Hypertrophic cardiomyopathy (HCM)	More sensitive than echo to estimate segmental wall thickness, LV mass, and volumes Useful in diagnosing apical HCM DE pattern is patchy, focal, mid-myocardial. Most common DE pattern is RV free-wall insertion points to the septum	DE on MRI is associated with increased risk factors for sudden cardiac death; may be predictive of inducible ventricular arrhythmias Useful to assess mitral valve systolic anterior motion (SAM), mitral regurgitation, and left ventricular outflow tract (LVOT) obstruction Efficacy of septal ablation procedure may be assessed by LGE imaging of the postprocedural scar
Inflammatory/infiltrative/ genetic cardiomyopathy (sarcoidosis, Anderson– Fabry's disease, Chagas disease, Duchenne's muscular dystrophy)	Mid-wall or epicardial LGE pattern typically in basal septal and/or inferolateral wall segments	LGE may be seen in asymptomatic patients and carriers of genetic disease

DE, delayed enhancement; LGE, late gadolinium enhancement; LV, left ventricular; RV, right ventricular

Heart Failure

Cardiac MR of a heart failure patient provides comprehensive assessment of function, pathophysiology, and therapeutic guidance (Box 25.1):

- Assessment of regional and global myocardial dysfunction and quantification of systolic dysfunction by measurement of volumes and EF.
- Distinguishing ischemic versus nonischemic cardiomyopathies by the LGE pattern.
- Differentiation of nonischemic cardiomyopathies in selective cases by myocardial tissue characterization (e.g. scar pattern, edema, architecture, iron

or fat deposition). In addition, MR is helpful in diagnosing primary or secondary valve disease and pericardial pathology.
- Measurement of myocardial viability/scar/fibrosis burden to provide therapeutic guidance regarding revascularization as well as prognosis in both ischemic and nonischemic cardiomyopathies.
- Diagnosis of cardiomyopathy-associated thrombi, better sensitivity than echo.
- Measurement of ventricular dyssynchrony related to potential cardiac resynchronization therapy (CRT) therapy.

Other Selective Cardiomyopathies
- **Acute myocarditis:**
  - In a patient with clinical presentation mimicking acute coronary ischemia (ECG changes, elevated cardiac enzymes, and chest pain), MR LGE imaging assists in arriving at the diagnosis of acute myocarditis noninvasively.
  - Subepicardial LGE pattern involving predominantly inferolateral wall or septum in a noncoronary territory distribution is indicative of acute myocarditis in appropriate clinical context.
  - Edema and inflammation appear bright on T_2-weighted imaging
  - Increased yield of myocardial biopsy if guided by MRI findings.
- **Amyloidosis:**
  - Diffuse myocardial LGE is typically seen, which may be erroneously attributed to a technical problem as nulled myocardium may not be seen due to the absence of normal myocardial tissue.
- **Hemochromatosis:**
  - MR is the best noninvasive means of diagnosing presence of myocardial iron. Tissues with iron deposition cause rapid dephasing (T_2^*) of the MRI signal, and thus appear dark
  - In patients with beta-thalassemia and primary hemochromatosis, myocardial iron deposition can be detected quantitatively by measuring T_2^* in a multiecho gradient echo sequence. It is a strong marker of prognosis and can improve with chelation therapy.
- **Arrhythmogenic right ventricular dysplasia (ARVD):**
  - Focal or global RV aneurysms, RV dilatation, and wall motion abnormalities associated with fibrofatty infiltration and delayed enhancement of the RV wall are typical findings (Figure 25.2).
- **Isolated noncompaction of ventricular myocardium:**
  - MRI allows clear visualization of the two-layered myocardium – the inner, highly trabeculated (noncompacted) region and the outer, solid (compacted) region
  - A ratio ≥ 2.3 of noncompacted-to-compacted myocardium at end-diastole is indicative of the disease
  - MRI is also helpful in the assessment of myocardial dysfunction, ventricular thrombi, and LGE. Spin echo "black-blood" imaging may

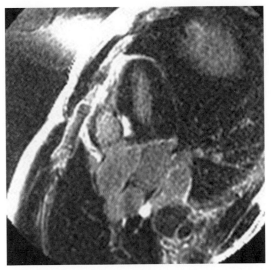

Figure 25.2 Late gadolinium enhancement seen in the right ventricle of a patient with ARVD

demonstrate bright signal in the deep intertrabecular recesses due to stagnant flow.
- **Endomyocardial fibroelastosis:**
  - Diffuse LGE of thick, fibrosed endocardium with associated thrombus may be seen on MRI.

Myocardial Ischemia

Stress-induced myocardial ischemia is detected by MRI in two ways:
- Adenosine-induced perfusion defects
- Dobutamine-induced wall motion abnormalities.

Adenosine Stress Perfusion Test
- A fast T_1-weighted gradient echo sequence is used with gadolinium contrast to image the first-pass myocardial perfusion at rest and with adenosine stress.
- These rest and stress MR perfusion studies are analogous to the rest–stress studies in technetium or thallium nuclear imaging.
- Multiple LV short axis views from base to apex are imaged during breath-holding.
- Subendocardial or transmural perfusion defects inducible with adenosine stress but absent at rest are interpreted as ischemic defects by qualitative analysis.
- In comparison to angiography and radionuclide stress imaging, perfusion MR at rest and with adenosine stress has demonstrated good sensitivity (80–90%) and specificity (75–100%).
- Coronary microvascular disease may show diffuse subendocardial perfusion defects with adenosine stress MR.

Dobutamine Stress Study
- Escalating doses of IV dobutamine infusion are used to detect ischemia-induced wall motion abnormalities.
- This is analogous to dobutamine stress echo.
- Bright blood ciné steady-state free precession (SSFP) sequences are used for short- and long-axis cardiac views.
- Dobutamine stress MRI has more consistent image quality that echo, and thus a higher sensitivity for detecting ischemia.
- In comparison to adenosine stress MR, dobutamine stress MR has shown comparable sensitivity (80%) but higher specificity (>90%) in detecting ischemia.

Evaluation of Pericardial Disease
MRI accurately characterizes pericardial effusion and or thickening, with an added advantage of hemodynamic assessment.

Pericardial Pathology
- T_1-weighted spin echo dark-blood imaging depicts pericardium in between epicardial and pericardial fat. Pericardial thickness is normally $\leq$2 mm; $\geq$4 mm is considered clearly abnormal.
- MR tagging is a technique that places "grid lines" on the image that move with tissue. In the presence of pericardial adhesion, the grid lines remain unbroken across the pericardium, rather than the normal sliding motion which causes the grid lines to separate.
- SSFP ciné imaging can show abnormal septal motion as well as a short, abrupt diastole, so-called "checking," consistent with restricted filling of constriction.
- Real-time MRI can show the effects of inspiration, with a leftward septal shift in constriction or RV indentation/collapse in tamponade.
- LGE imaging may reveal pericardial enhancement, indicative of active acute or chronic inflammatory or infectious pericarditis.
- Phase contrast velocity mapping may be helpful to detect significant respiratory variation of transvalvular flow associated with pericardial pathology.

Cardiac Tumors
Evaluation of a suspected or known cardiac mass is a common indication for cardiac MRI (Box 25.2).

MRI Protocol
Scout images, black blood, and ciné imaging of the heart and surrounding structures provide anatomic information regarding the size, location, extension, morphology (mobility, pedunculated vs sessile), and pericardial involvement of the mass and surrounding structures.

Box 25.2 **MRI: Cardiac mass differential diagnosis**

Cardiac/ pericardial mass	MRI findings	Remarks
Thrombus	Appearance depends on the stage and the imaging sequence used: chronic thrombus appears dark on T1- and T2-weighted imaging; acute thrombus can appear bright There is minimal perfusion or hyperenhancement	MRI is more sensitive in detecting ventricular thrombi compared to echo
Myxoma	Bright on T2-weighted imaging Superficial thrombi and calcifications may alter the picture Increased perfusion with heterogeneous enhancement may be seen	Most common primary benign cardiac tumor; commonly seen in left atrium attached to the interatrial septum
Papillary fibroelastoma	May be difficult to visualize on MR because of small size and rapid motion of valve	Most common tumor originating from the valves
Lipoma (Figure 25.3)	Bright on T1-weighted spin echo sequence	Fat saturation pulse suppresses the signal
Lymphoma	Multiple nodules of varying size involving epicardial, pericardial surfaces with pericardial effusion Hypointense on T1; bright on T2; variable delayed enhancement	B-cell lymphomas; commonly involve right atrium or right ventricle Unlike sarcomas, they are less likely to necrose or infiltrate heart chambers
Angiosarcoma	Typically presents as a large, bulky infiltrating mass with pericardial involvement May be associated with hemorrhage or thrombus Increased perfusion and heterogeneous enhancement with contrast	Most common primary malignancy (40% of cardiac sarcomas) Typically arises from right atrium (unlike other sarcomas)
Metastatic disease	Pericardial involvement with loculated, complex effusions; infiltration of myocardium, valves; increased perfusion and intense hyperenhancement on DE imaging; infiltration of adjacent mediastinal structures	Bright signal on T1 is typical of malignant melanoma

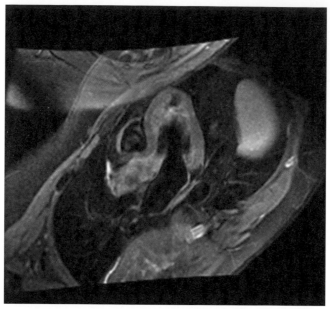

Figure 25.3 Left ventricular apical lipoma with suppressed signal on fat-saturated sequence

- T_1- and T_2-weighted imaging of the mass by spin echo sequences:
  - Fat suppression or water-fat separation sequences can be helpful
  - SSFP ciné sequences may delineate tissue characteristics (mobility, heterogeneity, fluid content, degree of inflammation) to provide additional information.
- Perfusion and LGE imaging are useful to determine the vascularity and nonviable/necrotic or enhancing areas of the mass.

MRI in Coronary Artery Pathology
- MRI is considered a standard approach to assess for anomalous coronary arteries:
  - Typically a 3D bright blood sequence is used to evaluate the origins and proximal course of the coronary arteries
  - It is advantageous, particularly in young patients, as no radiation is involved and it is typically performed without the need for intravenous contrast.
- MRI has also been shown to detect and characterize coronary aneurysms as well as coronary fistulae.
- In experienced centers, MRI can reliably assess the presence of left main or multivessel coronary artery disease (CAD), particularly in evaluating patients with a cardiomyopathy of unknown etiology (where LGE can provide complementary data). It has also been shown to have advantages over CT in evaluating heavily calcified vessels.

- MRI has had good success in determining the patency of saphenous and internal mammary bypass grafts:
  - Sensitivity and specificity in the 90% range
  - Relatively stationary and larger grafts have a straighter and predictable course making MRI suitable for their evaluation
  - However, metallic clips and stents may limit assessment of focal stenoses.

MRI in Vascular Disease

- MRI has been shown to be useful in characterizing disease in vessels outside the heart, including the thoracic and abdominal aorta, carotid and intracranial arteries, renal arteries, and peripheral vascular disease.
- 3D MR angiography sequences with and without gadolinium contrast enhancement are typically used. Additional ciné and T1-, T2-weighted sequences can be used to assess vessel wall pathology including hemorrhage, calcification, lipid, fibrous cap thinning/rupture, and inflammation.

Aortic Disease

As an example, MRI is commonly used to assess aortic pathology (Box 25.3). Noncontrast imaging can be performed in patients with renal dysfunction or other contraindications to contrast CT.

Box 25.3 MRI evaluation of aortic pathology

Pathology	MRI	Remarks
Aortic dissection	Extent of false and true lumen, point of intimal tear, and assessment of pericardial or coronary involvement can be determined	Classified into Stanford type A (ascending aortic involvement) or type B (ascending aorta not involved)
Aortic aneurysm	Aortic dilatation is considered when aortic root diameter is >4 cm or the abdominal aorta is >3 cm	This allows a nonradiation approach to routine follow-up to monitor disease progression
Intramural hematoma	Blood in aortic media with no intimal flap	Differential diagnosis: thrombosed false lumen of dissection
Congenital	Right-sided or double aortic arch, patent ductus arteriosus (PDA), aortic coarctation, and hypoplastic arch can be easily visualized	All congenital aortic lesions should prompt further cardiac imaging to detect associated cardiac abnormalities
Vasculitis	Depicts inflammatory changes and thickening of vessel wall, mural thrombus, focal vascular stenoses and/or dilatation	Particularly useful in large vessel vasculitis (e.g. Takayasu's) Useful for monitoring of disease response to therapy

MRI in Congenital Heart Disease (Box 25.4)

- Accurate evaluation of atrial and ventricular morphology, function, and volumes, with detection of transposition, obstruction, atresia, ASD/VSD, etc.
- Identification of vascular anomalies such as PDA, coarctation of aorta, APVR
- Direct measurement of Qp:Qs, comparable to oximetry calculations from cardiac catheterization
- Quantification of valvular regurgitation and stenosis
- Diagnosis and assessment of postoperative complications, such as baffle obstruction/patch leaks
- Myocardial fibrosis detection (clinical significance in longstanding congenital heard disease is unknown)

MRI in Valvular Disease

MRI can directly measure blood flow velocity, so while echo Doppler is excellent for detecting valvular disease and quantifying stenosis, MRI is superior in quantifying valvular regurgitation. Phase-contrast velocity mapping by MRI can measure flow through valves, shunts, vessels, and conduits.

- Spin echo DIR (black blood) sequence allows morphological assessment of valves
- Stenotic or regurgitant valvular pathology is associated with turbulent flow which typically results in jets of signal loss on ciné SSFP (bright blood) images. Thus, ciné SSFP is helpful in detection of stenosis, regurgitation, as well as abnormal valve motion such as systolic anterior motion (SAM) of mitral valve. However, the size of the jet on SSFP imaging is dependent on multiple factors and is not a reliable indicator of severity.
- Phase-contrast MRI, by comparison, has a very high sensitivity (98%), specificity (95%), and diagnostic accuracy in quantification of valvular regurgitation.
- MRI can helpful in estimating valvular stenosis by measuring valve area by direct planimetry from ciné bright blood imaging and/or by peak velocity by phase contrast. However, MRI typically underestimates peak velocity compared to Doppler.
- Aortic regurgitation (AR) volume can be calculated directly from the phase contrast aortic flow waveform, with the AR regurgitant fraction being the ratio of diastolic regurgitant volume to aortic systolic outflow volume. PR can be quantified in a similar fashion.
- Mitral regurgitation (MR) volume can be calculated directly from measuring flow across the mitral valve (MV), but this is prone to greater error due to eccentric jets and motion of the MV annulus. Thus, MR volume is typically calculated as LV stroke volume (from cardiac ciné images) minus aortic outflow volume, with the MR regurgitant fraction the ratio of MR volume to LV stroke volume. TR is quantified in a similar fashion.

Box 25.4 MRI evaluation of congenital heart disease

Congenital heart disease	MRI evaluation	Other remarks
Atrial septal defect (ASD)	Can identify rarer types: sinus venosus, coronary sinus defects; Qp:Qs Suitability for percutaneous device or surgical repair can be assessed	Anomalous pulmonary venous return should be investigated in patients with sinus venosus ASD
Ventricular septal defect (VSD)	Useful to assess location, size, shunt magnitude, and associated anomalies	Suboptimal echo may miss perimembranous VSD
Anomalous pulmonary venous return (APVR)	Suspect in RV dilatation or failure of unclear etiology; also with sinus venosus ASD	RV dilatation/dysfunction and Qp:Qs >1.5 can indicate need for surgery
Transposition of great vessels (TGV)	In atrial switch (Mustard procedure) postoperative assessment of RV, LV size, function, RV, LV outflow obstruction, tricuspid regurgitation (TR), baffle obstruction or leak In arterial switch procedure, in addition to above, assessment of pulmonic stenosis (PS), aortic regurgitation (AR), and aortic dilatation	Myocardial fibrosis may be assessed Stress MR may be considered in the context of coronary reimplantation in arterial switch procedure
Tetralogy of Fallot (TOF)	Severity of VSD, PS, RV outflow obstruction, RV function and morphology Anomalous origin and course of coronaries should be investigated	Useful to assess postsurgical complications such as pulmonic regurgitation (PR), RV dysfunction, VSD patch leak
Single ventricle physiology with Fontan procedue	Assessment of atrial septum, systemic ventricular outflow, Fontan obstruction, baffle leaks, thrombus formation, LV function, valve regurgitation	Percutaneous endovascular metallic devices (commonly seen in this group) may cause artifacts
Coarctation of aorta	LV function, mass, aortic valve (AV) morphology, aortic arch (elongated and hypoplastic), arch vessels, collaterals, aortic wall complications (dissection and aneurysm)	Assess for the presence of known associated problems; bicuspid AV, mitral valve (MV) disease, VSD, PDA
Patent ductus arteriosus (PDA) (Figure 25.4)	RV, LV failure, pulmonary hypertension (PHTN), PR of unclear etiology should prompt PDA work up	

LV, left ventricular; RV, right ventricular

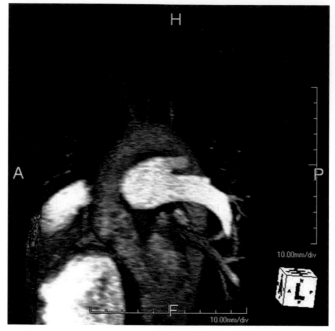

Figure 25.4 MRI reconstruction of a patent ductus arteriosus

- In general, the degree of valvular regurgitation is estimated by regurgitant fraction (RF) as follows:
  - Mild = <20%
  - Moderate = 20–40%
  - Severe = >40%.
- In patients with bicuspid aortic valve, MRI is helpful in screening for the abnormalities of the ascending arch and descending aorta, such as coarctation, PDA, and interrupted arch.

MRI in Right Heart Failure

Two-dimensional (2D) echo is suboptimal for evaluation of the right ventricle due to its complex shape and orientation. The multiplanar imaging capability of MRI allows thorough interrogation of right heart anatomy, function, volumes, and flow, in addition to tissue characterization, which is particularly important in the evaluation of congenital heart disease.

MRI may play a vital role in the evaluation of right heart failure (RHF) secondary to the following clinical entities:
- ARVD: MRI is the imaging modality of choice to demonstrate fibrofatty infiltration, LGE, and abnormal RV structure/function
- CHD with or without left-to-right shunt: TOF, TGV, ASD, VSD, PDA, APVR
- RV morphology and function in PHTN.

CLINICAL PEARLS

- MRI is the standard reference for the assessment of myocardial viability, ventricular morphology, volumes, and function.
- Subendocardial or transmural LGE pattern is indicative of ischemic cardiomyopathy; subepicardial, mid-wall, or noncoronary-distribution LGE pattern is suggestive of nonischemic cardiomyopathy.
- Presence and extent of myocardial LGE has prognostic importance in ischemic and nonischemic disease.
- MRI can characterize cardiac masses based on multiple signal characteristics and contrast enhancement.
- MRI provides both anatomic as well as physiologic information in the assessment of pericardial pathology.
- MR is the noninvasive imaging test of choice to detect and quantify myocardial iron in hemochromatosis.
- Valvular regurgitation is better quantified by MRI in comparison to echo.
- MRI is a superior imaging modality to evaluate complex congenital heart disease and postoperative follow-up of cardiac structure, function, and complications.
- Anomalous coronary artery assessment is a Class I indication for MRI.

Cardiac CT

CT has seen major technical improvements, which have allowed increased utility for the evaluation of cardiac pathology, particularly CAD. Rapid multi-detector row technology enables capture of the entire beating heart and rapidly moving coronaries with very high spatial resolution.

Cardiac CT Basics

The signal intensity on CT relates to the penetration of X-rays from an X-ray source, through tissue, to a detector. "Harder" tissues, such as calcium and bone, do not allow as much X-ray penetration and are typically displayed as bright on CT images. In CT, the source and detector are typically rotated around the patient to reconstruct a 2D tomographic image, which becomes a 3D image dataset when the patient is moved through the scanner.

- Most widespread CT technology in use is multidetector row CT (MDCT), where there are multiple detectors (64–320) to allow imaging of a larger volume of tissue with each rotation.
- Spatial resolution is of the order of 0.5 mm in x, y, and z (i.e. isotropic).
- Rapid 3D imaging is typically performed by continuously rotating the source/detector while the patient constantly moves through the scanner (i.e. spiral or helical scanning). A 320-row scanner can cover the whole heart in a single rotation without moving the patient.
- Iodinated contrast is used to distinguish blood (which becomes brighter with contrast) from the coronary wall and myocardium.

- Signal intensity is measured in Hounsfield units, named after an inventor of CT.

Patient Preparation

- Most scanning protocols still favor beta-blockers (oral or IV) given prior to scanning to achieve a heart rate of <65 bpm, which lengthens diastole and improves image quality.
- Sublingual nitroglycerin is typically given immediately prior to scanning to cause coronary vasodilatation and improve image quality.
- As ECG gating (scanning is synchronous with the cardiac cycle) is an essential component of cardiac CT, arrhythmia should be avoided.

Imaging Steps

- Initial scout imaging defines the basic volume and boundaries of the heart and aorta.
- Noncontrast, ECG-gated study for coronary calcium scoring.
- Either a test bolus (to measure peak time for ascending aorta enhancement) or bolus tracking (real-time tracking of the ascending aorta to trigger scan at the time of enhancement) can be used to determine scan timing to optimize contrast enhancement.
- Contrast-enhanced, ECG-gated imaging of the whole heart in a single breath hold. Saline or lower-concentration contrast is commonly timed to enter the right heart during coronary angiography to minimize artifacts near the right coronary artery.

Data Acquisition and Reconstruction

- **ECG gating:**
  - Prospective gating:
    - Imaging data are collected only during the desired phase (typically diastole) of the cardiac cycle
    - Complete anatomic data of heart and coronaries in a pre-prescribed cardiac phase is collected in a sequential fashion as the table moves forward ("step and shoot")
    - This limits radiation exposure but is more dependent on a slow, stable rhythm.
  - Retrospective gating:
    - Data are collected continuously (X-ray source on) throughout the cardiac cycle.
    - Image reconstruction of any desired cardiac phase can then provide optimal visualization of coronaries.
    - Data redundancy can allow removal of irregular beats.
    - Having data for the entire cardiac cycle allows assessment of cardiac function, similar to cardiac MRI.
    - There is greater radiation exposure due to continuous, overlapping scanning.

- **MDCT:** increasing the number of detector rows increases the volume acquired per rotation, reducing scan time.
- **Multisegmented reconstruction:** temporal resolution of a cardiac phase can be improved by reconstructing the phase from multiple, sequential segments of different cardiac cycles.
- Most scanners have a single X-ray source, which can provide a temporal resolution of the order of 150 ms.
- A dual-source scanner has two X-ray tubes arranged at 90° to each other, so it only has to rotate half the amount of a single-source scanner to generate an image. This improves temporal resolution to approximately 80 ms and has been shown to minimize the need for preprocedure beta blockers.

Data Post-Processing

In general, the axial source images are the primary diagnostic information. However, advanced reformatting protocols and visualization modes facilitate reaching an accurate diagnosis in complex, challenging cases.

Standard workstations usually have the following advanced reformatting and visualization tools to interactively manipulate and visualize large 3D dataset:

- **Multiplanar reformatting (MPR):**
  - 2D image display of the targeted area helps in detailed plaque characterization
  - Multiplanar capabilities of the workstation allow manual rotation and visualization of any anatomic structure in any desired plane and axis.
- **Curved MPR:**
  - Allows sampling of volume along the center line of a predefined curved structure (e.g. coronary artery).
- **3D Volume rendering** (Figure 25.5):
  - Whole dataset is displayed with a 3D depth
  - Useful for an overall assessment of cardiac and coronary anatomy, anomalous coronaries, and other anatomic variants.
- **Maximum intensity projection (MIP):**
  - Visualization tool where only the high-attenuation pixels (i.e. vasculature and cavities filled with contrast) are displayed
  - Stenoses may be overestimated as it displays stenotic lesions and calcifications prominently, but helpful for rapid initial assessment.

Advantages and Disadvantages

- **Advantages**
  - Very high, isotropic spatial resolution
  - Rapid volumetric coverage
  - Safe to image with pacemakers, ICDs, though may cause artifacts.
  - Superior 3D visualization software for postscanning analysis
- **Disadvantages**
  - Radiation.
  - Coronary CT angiography requires iodinated contrast

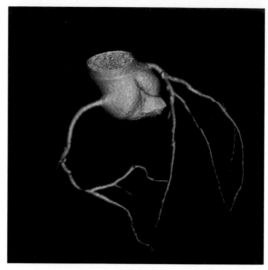

Figure 25.5 3D Volume rendering of the aortic root and coronary arteries

---

Box 25.5   Coronary artery calcification (CAC) score

- CAC is an independent predictor of CAD
- In asymptomatic patients at intermediate risk (by Framingham risk score) for CAD, CAC may be helpful in further modification of risk prediction and selection of therapeutic strategy
- CAC on CT has a high sensitivity (>95%) for obstructive CAD but lacks specificity
- Absence of calcium on CT (score = 0) has a high NPV (>95%) for obstructive CAD
- CAC grading:
  - 0: None
  - 1–100: mild
  - 101–300: moderate
  - >300: severe

- Temporal resolution suboptimal, requiring preprocedure beta-blockade
- Susceptible to arrhythmia

Clinical Indications
- Calculation of coronary artery calcium score (Box 25.5) for risk stratification and therapeutic management (Figure 25.6).
- Noninvasive coronary angiography to detect obstructive CAD in intermediate-risk patients with equivocal stress testing.
- Triaging acute chest pain patients in emergency department: the high negative predictive value (NPV) of coronary CT angiography (CTA) can rapidly

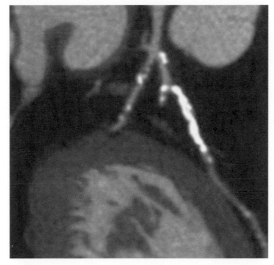

Figure 25.6 Coronary CT angiography (curved MPR) depicting coronary artery calcification

exclude CAD in low-to-intermediate risk patients and avoid delays and costs from further observation and testing.

- Assessment of grafts in symptomatic patients after coronary artery bypass grafting (CABG).
- Detection of coronary anomalies, fistulae.
- Evaluation of in-stent restenosis or occlusion: diagnostic results primarily in large stents (≥3.5 mm) in proximal vessels.
- Pericardial disease (thickening, calcification).
- Pulmonary venous mapping prior to and/or after atrial fibrillation ablation.
- Vascular angiography.

Contraindications
- Iodinated contrast hypersensitivity (may consider premedication)
- Relative:
  - Cardiac arrhythmias, morbid obesity, poor breath holding, metallic stents and excessive coronary calcium may cause artifacts resulting in poor image quality
  - Young/female – most radiosensitive

Noninvasive Coronary Angiography
- CT can image the entire coronary tree.
- Image quality depends on minimizing cardiac and respiratory motion.
- Heavy calcification "blooms" to appear larger than it actually is, appearing to show greater luminal stenosis.

- Contrast dose/timing and patient body habitus can adversely affect signal-to-noise ratio (SNR)
- Obstructive CAD is typically defined as >50% or >70% luminal narrowing, depending on the study (some studies assess the accuracy of both criteria).
- Three large multicenter trials to date have evaluated coronary CT in patients referred for invasive X-ray angiography:
  - Sensitivities ranged from 85–99%, specificities from 64–90%
  - Most showed a high NPV, but the positive predictive value (PPV) was quite variable, particularly when lower-risk patients were studied.
- Coronary CTA can detect noncalcified plaques. The assessment of coronary plaque and coronary stenosis by CTA was more predictive of prognosis than coronary calcium scoring.
- Several studies of acute chest pain patients showed rapid triage by CTA in a majority of patients with excellent short-term prognosis with a negative scan.
- Coronary anomalies are readily detected by coronary CT.
- Incidental extracardiac findings are common (20–50% of studies), with the majority pulmonary nodules.

Coronary Plaques

Coronary CT readily sees coronary plaque in addition to luminal stensoses (Figure 25.7), which has prognostic value. In a manner similar to intravascular ultrasound, investigators have used CT to try to estimate the characteristics of atherosclerotic plaque based on Hounsfield Units (HU).

- CT density increases when moving from lipid-rich, soft plaque to fibrous to calcified plaque.
  - Proposed CT density of plaque components:
    - Soft: $<50 \pm 70$ HU
    - Fibrous: 100 ± 80 HU
    - Fibrocalcific: 300 ± 100 HU
    - Calcific: 400 ± 200 HU
- Higher-risk plaques are thought to be more lipid-rich and are also associated with speckled calcification and positive arterial remodeling.
- However, the spatial resolution is suboptimal to reliably separate plaque components and the presence of contrast (particularly in the adjacent lumen) can alter the measured HU of the plaques.
- Most reliable distinction is between calcified and noncalcified plaque.

Radiation in Cardiac CT

Typical radiation exposure from coronary CTA is variable and ranges from 2 to 30 mSv, depending on the scanner and the scanning protocol.

Radiation exposure can be reduced during coronary CTA by adopting the following methods:

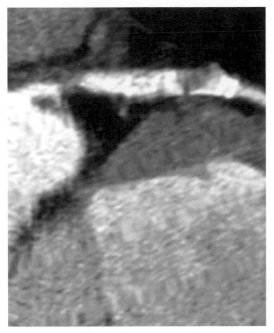

Figure 25.7 CTA depicting a soft plaque in the coronary artery

- Comparative radiation dose:
  - Annual ambient radiation exposure in US: 3 mSv
  - Chest X-ray: 0.1 mSv
  - Coronary calcium scoring: 1 mSv
  - Diagnostic X-ray angiogram: 7 mSv
  - Nuclear stress test: 10–30 mSv.
- Estimated added lifetime fatal cancer risk from a 10 mSv cardiac CT scan: 0.05–0.08%.
- X-ray dose, coverage: decreasing the volume of coverage and the tube current/voltage will decrease radiation dose.
- Pitch: pitch indicates the amount of scanner table advancement with each rotation of the X-ray tube, which determines the extent of spatial overlap. Radiation exposure is reduced by using higher pitch.
- Dose modulation: for retrospective ECG gating protocols, the dose of the rotating X-ray source can be kept high only during diastole and reduced during the rest of the cardiac cycle.
- Prospective ECG gating: This "step and shoot" axial imaging approach only images in diastole and also avoids the redundant spatial coverage of spiral/helical scanning, both of which can reduce radiation dose to 2–3 mSv.

> ## CLINICAL PEARLS
>
> - 64-slice MDCT can achieve a spatial resolution of 0.4 × 0.4 × 0.6 mm, with temporal resolution of approximately 150 ms (80 ms with a dual-source scanner).
> - 256- and 320-slice MDCT scanners can cover the heart in 1–2 heart beats.
> - Coronary CTA has very high NPV. This can allow effective diagnostic accuracy in higher-risk stable chest pain patients, but the PPV is suboptimal when applied to lower-risk patients.
> - Extensive coronary calcification, as well as fast or irregular heart rhythm, will limit image quality and diagnostic accuracy.
> - Coronary calcium scoring provides prognostic value for future cardiac events beyond the Framingham risk score. Coronary plaque characterization by CT is still investigational.
> - Coronary CT is promising for rapid triage of acute chest pain patient in the emergency department.
> - Coronary CT can also assess coronary anomalies and map the coronary venous anatomy for cardiac resynchronization therapy.
> - Radiation exposure of cardiac CT is decreasing, primarily with the advent of prospective ECG gating and aggressive X-ray dose modulation. Radiation levels of the order of the annual ambient exposure in the US (i.e. 3 mSv) are now achievable.

Recommended Reading

Clinical Trials and Meta-Analyses

Polonsky TS, McClelland RL, Jorgensen NW et al. Coronary artery calcium score and risk classification for coronary heart disease prediction. *JAMA* 2010;**303**(16):1610–1616.

Guidelines

American College of Cardiology Foundation Task Force on Expert Consensus Documents, Hundley WG, Bluemke DA, Finn JP et al. ACCF/ACR/AHA/NASCI/SCMR 2010 Expert Consensus Document on Cardiovascular Magnetic Resonance: A Report of the American College of Cardiology Foundation Task Force on Expert Consensus Documents. *J Am Coll Cardiol* 2010;**55**:2614–2662.

American College of Cardiology Foundation Task Force on Expert Consensus Documents, Mark DB, Berman DS, Budoff MJ et al. ACCF/ACR/AHA/NASCI/SAIP/SCAI/SCCT 2010 Expert Consensus Document on Coronary Computed Tomographic Angiography: A Report of the American College of Cardiology Foundation Task Force on Expert Consensus Documents. *J Am Coll Cardiol* 2010;**55**:2663–2699.

Hendel RC, Patel MR, Kramer CM et al.; ACCF/ACR/SCCT/SCMR/ASNC/NASCI/ SCAI/SIR 2006 appropriateness criteria for cardiac computed tomography and cardiac magnetic resonance imaging. *J Am Coll Cardiol* 2006;**48**(7):1475–1497.

Hundley WG, Bluemke D, Bogaert JG et al. Society for Cardiovascular Magnetic Resonance guidelines for reporting cardiovascular magnetic resonance examinations. *J Cardiovasc Magn Reson* 2009;**11**(1):5.

Kramer CM, Barkhausen J, Flamm SD, Kim RJ, Nagel E; Standardized cardiovascular magnetic resonance imaging (CMR) protocols, Society for Cardiovascular Magnetic Resonance. *J Cardiovasc Magn Reson* 2008;**10**(1):35.

Review Articles

Sundaram B, Patel S, Bogot N, Kazerooni EA. Anatomy and terminology for the interpretation and reporting of cardiac MDCT: part 1, Structured report, coronary calcium screening, and coronary artery anatomy. *AJR Am J Roentgenol* 2009;**192**(3):574–583.

Sundaram B, Patel S, Agarwal P, Kazerooni EA. Anatomy and terminology for the interpretation and reporting of cardiac MDCT: part 2, CT angiography, cardiac function assessment, and noncoronary and extracardiac findings. *AJR Am J Roentgenol* 2009;**192**(3):584–598.

26 Clinical Cardiac Hemodynamics

Shirley Park and Euan Ashley

Department of Internal Medicine, Division of Cardiology, Stanford University School of Medicine, Stanford, CA, USA

Cardiac hemodynamics refers to the measurement of pressures, flow, and resistance within the cardiovascular system. Here the most clinically relevant hemodynamic parameters in cardiology are discussed, and how they are measured and interpreted.

Pulmonary Artery Catheter

The pulmonary artery (PA) catheter is the tool necessary to make the majority of measurements that are discussed in this chapter. A PA catheter should be placed in patients where cardiac output or vascular resistance could be helpful in management:
- Differentiate cardiogenic versus distributive shock in hypotensive patients
- Differentiate cardiogenic versus noncardiogenic pulmonary edema.
- Manage unstable patients with decompensated heart failure
- Diagnose shunting in patient with hypoxemia
- Evaluation for transplant candidacy
- Perioperative hemodynamic management.

Patients with a permanent pacemaker PPM or implantable cardioverter device (ICD) leads, particularly recently (<3 months) implanted, should have a PA catheter placed under fluoroscopy. In patients with left bundle branch block (LBBB), transvenous pacing should be readily available since the right bundle can become quiescent. These patients should also be considered for fluoroscopic placement.

A Practical Approach to Cardiovascular Medicine, First Edition. Edited by Reza Ardehali, Marco Perez, Paul Wang.
© 2011 Blackwell Publishing Ltd. Published 2011 by Blackwell Publishing Ltd.

Insertion

- Vascular access:
  - Generally with 7F sheath via the right internal jugular (IJ) or left subclavian veins, which provide routes to the PA that are most compatible with the natural curve of the PA catheter
  - A femoral vein approach is possible but is usually performed under fluoroscopy.
- Flush all ports of the PA catheter and connect the distal port to the pressure transducer.
- Zero the catheter by opening the system to air to establish atmospheric pressure as zero at the level of the mid-right atrium.
- Prior to inserting the catheter, inflate the balloon under water to check for air leaks.
- Advance the catheter through the sheath to 15–20 cm before inflating the balloon to ensure that it has cleared the tip of the sheath. Do *not* advance the catheter if there is resistance.
- Use approximate distance (Table 26.1) and the pressure waveform (Figure 26.1) to determine the position of the catheter tip:
  - Advance to the pulmonary wedge position and deflate the balloon to record the PA pressure.
  - The catheter can then be withdrawn to the right ventricle (RV) and right atrium (RA).
  - Make sure the balloon is deflated if the catheter is to remain in the PA or is being withdrawn.

Table 26.1 Distances from access sites to cardiac structures

Access site	Distance to (cm)		
	RA	RV	PA
Internal jugular	15–20	15–20	45
Subclavian	30	30	55
Femoral	40	40	65
Brachial	40(R), 50(L)	50(R), 60(L)	60(R), 70(L)

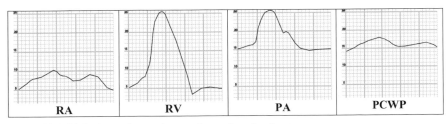

Figure 26.1 Distinct waveforms at separate cardiac structures

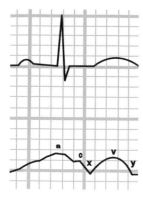

Figure 26.2 Components of the waveform. a, atrial contraction; c, tricuspid valve closure; v, atrial filling during ventricular contraction; x, descent: atrial relaxation; y, descent: atrial emptying. Note the V-wave occurs after the QRS complex on the ECG

Pressure Tracings

Pressures normally fall during inspiration and rise during expiration. Mean pressures must be documented during end of expiration, when intrathoracic pressures are closest to atmospheric pressure.

- **Right atrium** (RA; 2–8 mmHg):
  - Components of the waveform are shown in Figure 26.2.
  - Abnormal atrial waveform patterns:
    - Loss of A-waves: atrial fibrillation
    - Sawtooth F-waves: atrial flutter
    - Prominent A-waves: tricuspid stenosis, pulmonary stenosis
    - Cannon A-waves: AV dissociation [ventricular tachycardia (VT), V-pacing, complete AV block]
    - Prominent V-waves: tricuspid regurgitation (TR)
    - Prominent y-descent: restriction or pericardial constriction.
- **Right ventricle** (RV; 15–30/2–8 mmHg): diastolic pressure should equal RA pressure.
- **Pulmonary artery** (PA; 15–30/8–15 mmHg): diastolic pressure should equal pulmonary capillary wedge pressure (PCWP).
- **PCWP**: 8–15 mmHg: take a mean of the waveform.

Troubleshooting

- **Unable to advance into PA:**
  - In patients with particularly large RVs, floating into the PA can be difficult
  - Fluoroscopy may be necessary.
- **Ventricular arrhythmias:**
  - Present in about half of insertions, usually nonsustained
  - Withdraw the catheter and, if hemodynamically stable, readvance.
- **Complete heart block:**
  - Quickly withdraw the PA catheter and advance a balloon-tipped temporary transvenous pacing catheter through the same sheath.

- **Underdamping:**
  - High-frequency oscillations causing falsely high peak systolic pressures
  - Check for small air bubbles in the pressure line rapidly accelerating and decelerating
  - This is also seen with excessive tube length, tachycardia, and high output states.
- **Overdamping:**
  - A blunted and delayed pressure transmission
  - This is commonly due to a large air bubble or blood in the pressure line, or "overwedging" where the catheter is advanced too distally
  - Solution is to flush the lines or pull back on the catheter.

Hemodynamic Measurements

Cardiac Output
Cardiac output (CO) is the measurement of blood flow that the heart is able to generate in liters/minute. Cardiac index, which is simply CO divided by body surface area (BSA), is normally 2.4–4.0. CO is the principle measurement of heart function and can help guide management in critically ill patients. In essence:

$$CO = SV \times HR$$

where SV is stroke volume, or the amount of blood pumped out of the heart with every beat, and HR is the heart rate.

Although there are a few noninvasive methods of calculating CO, more accurate means require the use of a PA catheter.

Fick Method
The underlying assumption is that at equilibrium, the amount of oxygen used by the body is equal to the amount of oxygen consumed, which is equal to the flow rate of blood times the amount of oxygen extracted by the body. The higher the flow rates, the less time the body has to extract oxygen from the blood. With high CO, blood returns to the heart with higher oxygen concentration. Rearranged, the formula becomes:

$$CO \, (l \, blood / min) = \frac{Oxygen \; consumption \; (mL \; oxygen / min)}{Oxygen \; extracted \; (mL \; oxygen / L \; blood)}$$

Oxygen extraction can be calculated by measuring arterial oxygen saturation and oxygen saturation in the blood before it enters the lungs:

Oxygen extracted =

(Arterial − Venous O_2 saturation)(Hb g / dL)(1.36 mL O_2 / g Hb) × 10

Arterial O_2 saturation can be measured from any arterial source, usually radial or femoral artery, and venous saturation is ideally measured from the PA, after mixing of blood from the superior and inferior vena cava (SVC and IVC).

Oxygen consumption is generally constant and can be estimated with various formulas accounting for age and sex. Most patients at rest will consume $125\,mL\ O_2/min$ for every square meter of BSA. In patients with sepsis or other metabolic demands, consumption can be measured more accurately with a spirometer.

Simplified, the formula becomes:

$$CO = \frac{125 \times BSA}{(Arterial - Venous\ O_2\ sat) \times Hb \times 13.6}$$

Dilution Methods

These measurements are based on the concept that when a substance is injected into the RA, it will mix in the RV and emerge diluted in the PA. At high COs, the distal concentration measured will rise and fall quickly. The CO can be estimated by integrating rates of change in concentration:

$$CO = \frac{I}{\int C\,dt}$$

where I is the amount of the substance and C is the concentration.

Saline at room temperature is commonly used (thermodilution). A thermister at the tip of the PA catheter can measure temperature changes and CO can be calculated using the same principles. Modern hemodynamic monitoring equipment will have these features incorporated and will automate these measurements.

Choice of Method

There are advantages and disadvantages to each method. The Fick method requires an arterial blood sample and assumes no left-to-right shunting of blood. The dilution method performs poorly in very low CO states or atrial fibrillation and assumes absence of TR or shunting.

Filling Pressures

Given that CO is a function of SV and HR, estimating SV is useful in the management of patients with heart failure. SV itself is a function of left ventricular end-diastolic volume (LVEDV) via the Frank–Starling relationship (Figure 26.3).

In general, there are no accurate methods of measuring volume in real-time, even by echo or other noninvasive modalities. The following assumption is therefore relied upon:

$$LVEDV \ \alpha \ LVEDP \approx LAP \approx PCWP$$

LVEDV is proportional to LV end-diastolic pressure (LVEDP), which is approximately equal to left atrial pressure (LAP) and PCWP. PCWP can be measured with a PA catheter, which will in turn be proportional to LVEDV. These assumptions hold true in most patients, but can be inaccurate in the presence of mitral stenosis or regurgitation.

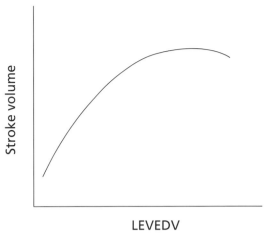

Figure 26.3 Frank–Starling curve

SV and CO can therefore be optimized by adjusting the filling pressures via diuresis in the case of volume overload, or volume infusion in the case of volume depletion.

Vascular Resistance

The formulas for measuring vascular resistance parallel those of Ohm's law and assume that vascular flow is proportional to difference in pressures and inversely proportional to resistance. Rearranged, the generic formula becomes:

$$\text{Vascular resistance} = \frac{\text{Pressure difference}}{\text{Cardiac output}}$$

Systemic vascular resistance (SVR) helps in titrating afterload reduction in patients with decompensated heart failure. It is calculated as:

$$\text{SVR} = \frac{\text{Mean arterial pressure} - \text{Mean RA pressure}}{\text{Cardiac output}}$$

Pulmonary vascular resistance (PVR) helps in estimating the severity of pulmonary vascular disease in transplant candidates and candidates for congenital corrections. It is calculated as:

$$\text{PVR} = \frac{\text{Mean PA pressure} - \text{PCWP}}{\text{Cardiac output}}$$

As a reminder:

$$\text{Mean pressure} = \frac{(2 \times \text{diastolic pressure}) + \text{Systolic pressure}}{3}$$

PVR is usually reported in Woods Units, which are mmHg/(L/min). Patients with PVR >4 Woods Units are usually poor candidates for heart transplantation. In patients being considered for atrial septal defect (ASD) closure, the goal PVR is <15 Woods Units.

SVR is usually reported in dyne/s/cm^5, which are equivalent to Woods Units x 80. The goal SVR in patients with decompensated heart failure is usually <1000 dyne/s/cm^5. SVR 600<dyne/s/cm^5 usually indicates distributive shock (ex. sepsis) or excessive afterload reduction.

Valve Stenoses

Pressure Gradients

The most accurate way to measure the gradient across a valve is to transduce simultaneous pressures from either side of the valve, e.g. a gradient across the aortic valve can be measured by simultaneous pressure measurements of the LV and aorta (for mitral stenosis, the LA and LV). Catheter-based assessment of severity is indicated only if the clinical findings (physical exam, symptoms) are inconsistent with Doppler findings.

- **Aortic valve (AV) gradient:** Can be measured in multiple ways:
  - Dual arterial punctures with one catheter in the LV and one in the ascending aorta
  - Single arterial puncture with a double-lumen pigtail catheter transducing the LV and aortic pressure simultaneously
  - Single arterial puncture with a pigtail catheter transducing LV pressure, and the side arm of the sheath transducing femoral artery pressure as a surrogate for central aortic pressure:
    - Peak femoral artery pressure is usually higher than peak central aortic pressure secondary to reflected pressure waves in the periphery. This leads to an underestimation of mean gradient
    - Can partially correct for this by subtracting the difference between peripheral and aortic pressure measurements.
    - Alignment mismatch: simultaneous tracings of the LV and femoral artery are not aligned due to the time delay of the pulse wave to travel from the LV to the femoral artery. The tracings should be realigned prior to measuring the mean pressure gradient by shifting the femoral artery tracing leftward until the upstroke coincides with the LV upstroke
  - Pull back method: pullback of catheter from LV to aorta with continuous pressure wave monitoring:
    - Can obtain a peak-to-peak gradient between the maximum aortic and LV pressures; however, this only gives an estimate of mean gradient because the peaks are occurring at different times
    - Pullback hemodynamics: in severe aortic stenosis, a 7 or 8F catheter across the AV may occupy a significant amount of the orifice area and increase the severity of stenosis. If there is a peripheral systolic pressure rise of >5 mmHg with LV catheter pullback, this is about 80% sensitive for a valve area ≤0.5 cm^2.

- **Mitral valve (MV) gradient:**
  - Simultaneous pressure measurements of the LA (via PCWP) and LV (via pigtail catheter):
    - Alignment mismatch: simultaneous pressure tracings of the LA/LV are not aligned because there is a time delay in the transmission of LA pressure back via the pulmonary veins
    - PCWP should be realigned with the LV pressure by shifting leftward 50–70 ms such that the V-wave peaks immediately before the downstroke of the LV (V-wave should be bisected by the rapid LV pressure decline).

Calculating Valve Orifice Area

Gorlin Formula
Derived from Torricelli's law describing flow across a round orifice:

$$F = AVC_c$$

where F = flow (L/s), A = orifice area (cm²), V = velocity of flow, and C_c = coefficient of orifice contraction (correction factor for area of stream flowing through orifice being less than true orifice area).

Expressing velocity in terms of pressure gradient, the formula can be rearranged as:

$$A = \frac{F}{(C)(44.3)\sqrt{h}}$$

where C = empiric constant and h = pressure gradient (mmHg).

Flow can also be expressed as:

$$A = \frac{\text{Cardiac output (L/min)}}{\text{Duration of forward flow across valve (s/beat)} \times \text{HR(beats/min)}}$$

Duration of forward flow =

$$\frac{\text{SEP (systolic ejection period) across the aortic valve}}{\text{DFP (diastolic filling period) across the mitral valve}}$$

Thus, the orifice area is:

$$A = \frac{\text{Cardiac output (L/min)}}{(C)(44.3)\sqrt{h}*(\text{SEP or DFP})(\text{HR})}$$

*This is based on the observation that (C)(44.3)(SEP or DFP)(HR) is close to 1.0 for most patients with hemodynamics measured in the resting state.

Hakki Formula
A simplified formula which can be used if the HR is within normal range. This formula is more commonly used because of its simplicity:

$$A = \frac{\text{Cardiac output (L/min)}}{\sqrt{h}}$$

Intraventricular Pressure Gradients (Hypertrophic Cardiomyopathy)

In hypertrophic cardiomyopathy (HCM) with an LV outflow tract obstruction (LVOT), the gradient lies below the aortic valve, is dynamic, and there may be little or no resting gradient.

- There are a number of ways to distinguish an LVOT gradient from aortic stenosis:
  - During the LV pullback, there should be a gradient detected from the LV apex to the LVOT, but not through the aortic valve
  - Upstroke of the aortic pressure waveform is nearly vertical compared with the delayed and slow upstroke seen in aortic stenosis
  - Highest pressure gradient occurs in mid-systole compared with aortic stenosis, where the largest gradient usually occurs in early systole.
- Methods for provoking intracavitary pressure gradient:
  - Decrease ventricular end diastolic volume: Valsalva maneuver, nitroglycerin, isoproterenol (to induce tachycardia and decrease diastolic filling time)
  - Increasing force or duration of ventricular contraction: isoproterenol, post-extrasystolic potentiation:
    - Brockenbrough–Braunwald sign: after a premature ventricular contraction (PVC), the LV systolic pressure and LV/aortic pressure gradient increase, while the aortic systolic pressure and aortic pulse pressure decrease in patients with HCM (Figure 26.4)
  - Decreasing aortic outflow resistance: nitroglycerin, any vasodilator therapy.

Pericardial Compressive Hemodynamics (Box 26.1)

Cardiac Tamponade

Hemodynamic findings:

- Equalization of diastolic pressures between the RA, RV diastolic, PA diastolic, and PCWP.
- Response to pericardiocentesis -
  - Phase I: intrapericardial pressure (IP) < RA and PCWP (LV):
    - Pericardiocentesis → ↓IP and ↓RA pressures, no change in PCWP, pulsus paradoxus, or CO
  - Phase II: IP = RA but <PCWP:
    - Pericardiocentesis → ↓IP and ↓RA pressures, ↓PCWP (somewhat), ↓pulsus paradoxus, modest ↑CO
  - Phase III: IP = RA = PCWP:
    - Pericardiocentesis → ↓IP, ↓RA, and ↓PCWP, ↓pulsus paradoxus, ↑CO.

Constrictive Physiology

Hemodynamic findings from scarring/thickening of the pericardial sac and loss of elasticity:

- Equalization of diastolic pressures between the RA, RV, PA, and PCWP:
  - This may not be present if patient has been on diuretics leading to a low or normal RA pressure

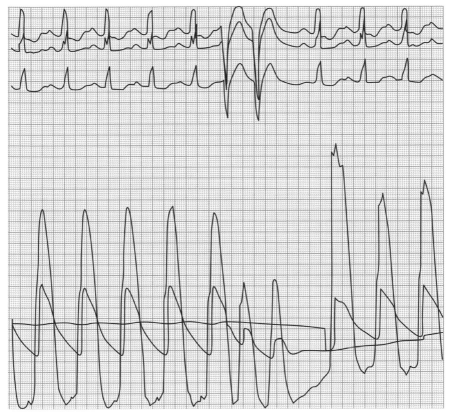

Figure 26.4 Brockenbrough–Braunwald sign

Box 26.1 Summary of pericardial compressive haemodynamics

	Equalization of diastolic pressure	"Dip and plateau" ventricular morphology	"M" or "W" atrial morphology	Discordance of LV/ RV pressures through respiratory cycle
Tamponade	Yes	No	No	No
Constriction	Yes	Yes	Yes	Yes
Restriction	Yes	Yes	Yes	No

- Fluid loading during catheterization is needed to detect constriction in this case.
- "Dip and plateau" configuration of ventricular pressure (Figure 26.5):
  - Caused by rapid early diastolic ventricular filling followed by abrupt cessation due to pericardial restraint.
- "M" or "W" configuration of right atrial pressure:

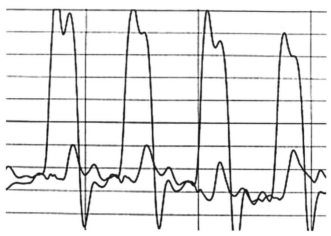

Figure 26.5 Dip and plateau configuration

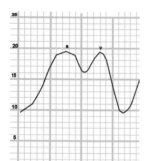

Figure 26.6 "M" configuration

- Due to the effects of attenuated diastolic filling on atrial pressure
- Attenuated X descent and prominent Y descent (representing rapid atrial emptying during diastole; Figure 26.6).

Restrictive Physiology
- Results from a rigid, nondilated ventricle leading to severe restrictive filling and diastolic dysfunction.
- Hemodynamic findings include:
  - Equalization of diastolic pressures
  - "Dip and plateau" ventricular morphology
  - Atrial "M" or "W" morphology.

Constrictive Versus Restrictive Physiology
Differentiating constrictive versus restrictive physiology can be challenging as both have similar hemodynamic findings. The key distinction is the difference in response to breathing and changes in intrathoracic pressures. Changes in LV and RV pressures must therefore be observed during the respiratory cycle.

- In constrictive pericarditis, the ventricles are shielded from transmission of intrathoracic pressures by the thickened and scarred pericardium
- There is also enhanced ventricular interaction as the septum can move normally in the setting of LV/RV free-wall constriction
- During inspiration, negative intrathoracic pressure results in a decrease in PCWP. However, the LV is shielded from this negative pressure and the LV diastolic pressure does not fall. This leads to a decrease in LA–LV pressure gradient, less LV filling, and a fall in LV systolic pressure.
- Because of the enhanced ventricular interaction due to normal septal motion, a decrease in LV filling leads to an increase in RV filling and a rise in RV systolic pressure.
- In restrictive physiology, intrathoracic pressure is transmitted normally to the myocardium. During inspiration, PCW and LV diastolic pressures fall equally, with the LA–LV pressure gradient, and thus LV filling, remaining unchanged. This is seen as a concordance of LV and RV pressures throughout the respiratory cycle.

Left-to-Right Shunt

Left-to-right shunting should be suspected when the CO is much higher than anticipated based on the patient's functional status or degree of heart failure. The degree of shunting can be calculated from an oximetry run.

Oximetry Run

- Oxygen content is measured in blood samples from the PA, RV, RA, SVC, and IVC. The right atrium receives more blood from the SVC than the IVC in a 3:1 ratio.
- A left-to-right shunt can be detected and localized by the finding of a significant "step-up" in oxygen saturation from one chamber to the next that exceeds normal variability (Table 26.2).
- Once a "step-up" is identified, additional blood samples can be taken in the chamber of interest to better define the location of rise in oxygen saturation.

Calculation of Shunt Fraction

The shunt fraction quantifies the degree of shunting by calculating the ratio of pulmonary to systemic blood flow (Q_p/Q_s). The greater the degree of left-to-right shunting, the greater the Q_p/Q_s, while a ratio of 1 indicates no shunting.

Table 26.2 Detection and localization of left-to-right shunts

Level of shunt	Change in oxygen saturation
SVC/IVC to RA	≥7%
RA to RV	≥5%
RV to PA	≥5%
SVC to PA (any point)	≥7%

Blood flow is calculated using the standard Fick equation:

$$Q_p = \frac{\text{Oxygen consumption (mL/min)}}{(1.36)(\text{Hb}) \times \text{PV O}_2 \text{ content} - \text{PA O}_2 \text{ content (mL/L)}}$$

$$Q_s = \frac{\text{Oxygen consumption (mL/min)}}{(1.36)(\text{Hb}) \times \text{SA O}_2 \text{ content} - \text{MV O}_2 \text{ content (mL/L)}}$$

where PV = pulmonary venous, PA = pulmonary arterial, SA = systemic arterial, and MV = mixed venous

If a pulmonary vein has not been accessed, systemic arterial O_2 content can be substituted for PV O_2 content if O_2 saturation is ≥95% (right-to-left shunt unlikely in this setting).

The mixed venous sample must be measured in the chamber immediately proximal to the shunt (Table 26.3).

Thus:

$$Q_p/Q_s = \frac{\text{SA O}_2 \text{ content} - \text{MV O}_2 \text{ content}}{\text{PV O}_2 \text{ content} - \text{PA O}_2 \text{ content}}$$

Table 26.4 gives the severity of shunt for different values of Q_p/Q_s.

Table 26.3 Mixed venous sample according to level of shunt

Level of shunt	Site of mixed venous sample
PA (e.g. patent ductus)	Average of RV oximetry samples
RV (e.g. VSD)	Average of RA oximetry samples
RA (e.g. ASD)	[3(SVC) + 1(IVC)]/4 at rest
	or
	[1(SVC) + 2(IVC)]/3 during exercise

Table 26.4 Severity of shunt

Q_p/Q_s	Severity of shunt
<1.5	Small
1.5–2.0	Moderate
>2.0	Large

CLINICAL PEARLS

- Most patients in heart failure can be managed without a PA catheter. Changes in CO in response to therapy can often be measured by other means, such as changes in creatinine. However, if noncardiogenic edema or distributive shock are suspected, or if the degree of cardiac compromise cannot be otherwise estimated in hypotensive patients, a PA catheter can be helpful.

- In aortic stenosis, catheter-based assessment of severity is indicated if the physical exam or clinical symptoms are not consistent with echo measurements.
- The key difference when distinguishing constrictive versus restrictive pericarditis hemodynamically is discordance of LV/RV pressures through the respiratory cycle.
- A high CO in the setting of decompensated heart failure should raise suspicion for a left-to-right shunt.

Recommended Reading

Clinical Trials and Meta-Analyses

Reddy PS, Curtiss EI, Uretsky BF. Spectrum of hemodynamic changes in cardiac tamponade. *Am J Cardiol* 1990;**66**:1487–1491.

Guidelines

American College of Cardiology/American Heart Association Task Force on Practice Guidelines; Society of Cardiovascular Anesthesiologists; Society for Cardiovascular Angiography and Interventions; Society of Thoracic Surgeons, Bonow RO, Carabello BA, Kanu C et al. ACC/AHA 2006 guidelines for the management of patients with valvular heart disease. *Circulation* 2006;**114**(5):e84–231.

Hakki AH, Iskandrian AS, Bemis CE et al. A simplified valve formula for the calculation of stenotic cardiac valve areas. *Circulation* 1981;**63**(5):1050–1055.

Review Articles

Bain DS, Grossman W. *Grossman's Cardiac Catheterization, Angiography, and Intervention*, 6th edn. Philadelphia: Williams & Wilkins, 2000.

Kern MJ. *Hemodynamic Rounds: Interpretation of Cardiac Pathophysiology from Pressure Waveform Analysis*. New York: Wiley-Liss, Inc, 1993.

27 | Percutaneous Interventions

Aiden O'Loughlin and Alan Yeung
Department of Internal Medicine, Division of Cardiology, Stanford
University School of Medicine, Stanford, CA, USA

Coronary angiography remains the gold standard in the diagnosis of coronary artery disease (CAD). Although noninvasive imaging modalities are gaining ground, angiography is still best suited to differentiating calcification and other artifacts from true luminal stenosis. Section II gives a thorough discussion on the management of patients with CAD and indications for coronary angiography. Here the focus is the technical aspects of the coronary angiogram and available percutaneous interventions (PCIs).

Preparing a Patient for Angiography

History and Examination

A complete medical history and physical examination should be performed. However, in situations where time is limited [e.g. the patient requires primary angioplasty for an ST segment elevation myocardial infarction (MI)] a focused history and examination is more appropriate. Items of particular interest are:
- Detailed history of the present illness.
- Current medications:
  - **Metformin:**
    - Carries a small risk of lactic acidosis, which usually occurs in patients with renal insufficiency
    - Common recommendations include stopping metformin 48 h before and recommencing it 48 h following the procedure (if there is no evidence of acute renal failure)
  - **Coumadin:**
    - Should be stopped 4–5 days before intervention
    - Goal INR is operator-dependent, but an INR <1.5 is preferred
    - Patients at high risk of cardiovascular accident (CVA) should be bridged with low-molecular-weight heparin (LMWH) before and after

A Practical Approach to Cardiovascular Medicine, First Edition. Edited by Reza Ardehali, Marco Perez, Paul Wang.
© 2011 Blackwell Publishing Ltd. Published 2011 by Blackwell Publishing Ltd.

procedure, but LMWH should be held the night before and morning of the procedure

- **Heparin:** for patients receiving heparin for other indications (atrial fibrillation), heparin infusions should be held approximately 4 h before procedure.
- Past medical history, focusing on:
  - Detailed history of CAD:
    - Previous angiograms, PCI, coronary artery bypass grafting (CABG)
    - Previous angiographic images should be obtained and operative reports of CABG should be documented
  - Recent stress imaging with distribution of wall motion abnormalities
  - Risk factors for CAD and their management
  - Peripheral vascular disease
  - Renal disease
  - Bleeding risk.
- Assess for contraindications: fever, anemia, hypokalemia, severe renal dysfunction, other acute illnesses.
- History of medication, iodine, and shellfish allergies.
- Cardiovascular examination:
  - Check peripheral (femoral, dorsalis pedis, and posterior tibialis) pulses
  - Check for pre-existing femoral lumps and bruits
  - If radial access is planned, perform an Allen test: patient makes a fist, then compress ulnar and radial nerves, ask patient to open fist, release pressure on ulnar side. The hand should turn pink in a few seconds, unless there is radial artery disease
- Baseline electrocardiogram (ECG): note distribution of ST elevations (if any) and Q-waves.

Consent

Consent for coronary angiography, angioplasty and stenting, and emergency bypass surgery should be obtained in all patients. Consent for adjunctive devices such as intra-aortic balloon pump, intravascular ultrasound or rotablator should be obtained in advance if their use is planned. The procedure should be explained in simple terms but with sufficient detail.

- **Major complications:**
  - Death (0.1%)
  - Major MI (0.5%)
  - Stroke (0.7%)
  - Major vascular complications, such as pseudoaneurysms, thrombosis and bleeding requiring transfusion occur at a rate of <1%
  - When combined with other major complications such as ventricular arrhythmias, perforation, and significant contrast allergy, the total risk of a major complication is <2%
  - Risk obviously depends on the patient population.

- **Minor complications:**
  - Isolated CK-MB rise
  - Transient ischemic attack
  - Transient renal insufficiency
  - Infection
  - Vascular complications that can be managed conservatively
  - Minor contrast allergies
  - Atrial arrhythmias
  - Together these carry a risk close to 4–5%
  - Risks of restenosis and in-stent thrombosis should be mentioned and are dependent on a number of factors including:
    – Vessel diameter
    – Treatment length
    – Lesion at the site of vessel bifurcation
    – Type of stent used.

Prevention of Contrast Nephropathy

The risk of contrast nephropathy is dependent on a number of factors, including baseline renal function and the amount of contrast used in the procedure.

- **IV fluids:**
  - Normal saline or sodium bicarbonate infusions are commonly given before and after the procedure to hydrate the patient
  - Care should be taken if patient has heart failure.
- **N-acetyl-cysteine (Parvolex, Mucomyst):**
  - Can be given orally in patients with pre-existing renal failure
  - Usual dose is 600 mg orally bid with two doses before and two following the procedure, or as an IV infusion.

Blood Tests

- A complete blood count, electrolytes, creatinine, PT, and blood for type and screen are commonly tested prior to an interventional procedure.
- A beta-hCG is obtained in all women of reproductive age to exclude pregnancy.

Contrast Allergies

Patients who report prior allergies to contrast, iodine or shellfish should receive preprocedure treatment with steroids, antihistamines and, optionally, H_2 blockers. Several pretreatment strategies are available. The authors prefer:

- Prednisone 50 mg orally the night before and on the morning of the procedure and diphenhydramine 25–50 mg orally on the morning of the procedure.

Antiplatelet Agents

- **Aspirin:** 75–325 mg daily should be given prior to and on the day of the procedure. This should be continued long-term following the procedure.

- **Clopidogrel:** The clinical situation and operator preference will determine whether the patient is preloaded (300–600 mg) before the procedure or if the loading dose is given following coronary intervention.

Other Preparatory Steps

- **Groin shave:** bilateral groin shaves should be performed if femoral access is to be obtained.
- **Intravenous access:** peripheral intravenous access should be obtained prior to the procedure to allow for the rapid administration of fluid and medications if necessary during the procedure.
- **Fast:**
  - Patient should fast for at least 4–6 h prior to the procedure
  - Oral medications can be given during this period.
- **Pre-procedure sedation:** depends on operator preference:
  - Benzodiazepines such as diazepam 2.5–10 mg are commonly given with care taken not to over-sedate the patient with possible respiratory depression or arrest
  - Diphenhydramine 12.5–50 mg before a procedure can help prevent contrast reactions and provide sedative effects.
  - Note that consent should be obtained *prior* to sedative administration.

Procedure

Arterial Access

Operators should be carefully trained in proper arterial access techniques as this can significantly impact rates of complications and influence patient comfort.

- Majority of coronary angiograms are performed using a femoral arterial approach.
- In patients with difficult femoral access, such as those with extensive lower extremity vascular disease, morbid obesity or significant scarring, a radial or brachial arterial approach is an option.
- Some centers routinely perform upper extremity access which allows for quicker recovery times, but can be more technically challenging.
  The goal in obtaining proper femoral access is to minimize subsequent vascular complications.
- Ideal site of entry into the femoral artery is at the mid-point of the femoral head, superior to the bifurcation of the femoral profundus:
  - This allows for proper compression of the artery after sheaths are pulled and leaves the option for use of closure devices.
- Anatomically, the ideal site of skin entry is two finger-breaths below the inguinal ligament, which can be identified by a line that connects the iliac crest and the pubis.
  - Note that the superficial inguinal crease can be misleading and should not be used as a reference, particularly in obese patients.
  - If doubt remains, fluoroscopy can be used to locate the femoral head.

- Skin can be then be anesthetized with 1% lidocaine or other local anesthetic.
- Depending on operator preference, a small skin incision can be made before or after insertion of the needle.
- A subcutaneous tunnel can then be created using Kelly forceps to allow easier sheath insertion.
- A modified Seldinger technique, where only the anterior arterial wall is penetrated, is preferred when inserting the needle (without an obturator) at a 30–45° angle over the femoral pulse.
- Once pulsatile flow is obtained, a guidewire is inserted, the needle is removed, and a sheath is introduced.

Coronary Artery Cannulation
- Preshaped guiding catheters are used to cannulate the coronary arteries.
- These catheters should be inserted over a guidewire to avoid shearing of the arterial wall.
- A number of catheters are available with varying sizes and shapes, including Judkins and Amplatz right and left catheters
  - Specialized catheters designed for facilitated access of the internal mammary arteries and venous grafts are available
  - 6F guide catheters are used for the majority of procedures
  - 7 and 8F guide catheters may be required if kissing balloons/stents or adjunctive devices such as the larger rotablator burr sizes will be used.
- Special care should be taken when cannulating the left main coronary artery:
  - Pressure dampening upon cannulation usually indicates osteal disease and prolonged occlusion can lead to MI and cardiac arrest.

Coronary Angiography
A grasp of the three-dimensional anatomy of the heart is necessary to properly image and interpret the coronary arteries. In addition, each heart carries varying degrees of lateral and vertical rotation. There are, however, a handful of standard views that are used to image the left and right coronary arteries. Deviations from the standard views are often necessary to obtain better appreciation of areas of interest.

Left Coronary Arteries
- **Left anterior oblique (LAO) view** (Figure 27.1):
  - Place the septum down the middle of the heart
  - Left anterior descending artery (LAD) will run down the line of the septum, while the left circumflex (LCx) will head towards the right of the screen
  - Cranial angulation allows for easier view of the LAD, with the diagonal arteries branching off the LAD

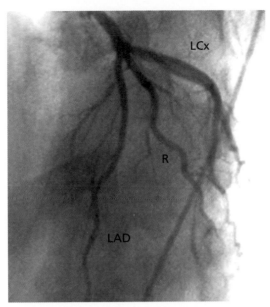

Figure 27.1 LAO cranial: left anterior descending artery (LAD) runs down the middle of the image. Ramus (R) arises between the LAD and the left circumflex (LCx). Note the diagonal arteries are not prominent, likely because of the large Ramus, which could actually be a "high diagonal"

- A Ramus can sometimes be seen trifurcating between the LAD and the LCx
- Caudal angulation ("spider" view) allows for a better appreciation of the left main artery.
- **Right anterior oblique (RAO) view** (Figure 27.2):
  - Place the anterior wall of the heart at the top of the screen, while the inferior wall of the heart is at the bottom of the screen and the apex is on the right
  - LAD will therefore be at the top of the screen, while the LCx penetrates "into the screen," comes down around the atrioventricular (AV) groove and then "towards" the screen
  - Obtuse marginal arteries are seen branching off the LCx towards the right of the screen
  - Septal perforators can also be seen branching downwards off the LAD in this view
  - Caudal angulation best separates the LCx and LAD.

Right Coronary Arteries
- **RAO view:**
  - Right coronary artery (RCA) comes "towards" the screen, heads down along the AV groove, and then goes "into" the screen

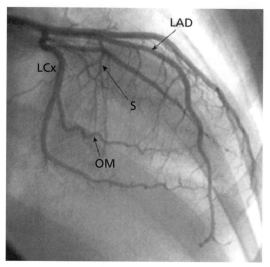

Figure 27.2 RAO caudal: left anterior descending artery (LAD) runs along the anterior aspect of the heart down to the apex and can be further identified as the artery that gives off the septal (S) perforators. Obtuse marginals (OM) are branches of the left circumflex (LCx)

- Posterior descending artery (PDA) and posterolateral left ventricular (PLV) artery can be seen branching off the RCA towards the right of the screen, along the inferior wall of the heart
- **LAO view** (Figure 27.3):
  - "Opens" the body of the RCA for a better appreciation of the vessel
  - Cranial angulation allows a better view of the PDA and PLV:
    - If the RCA supplies both the PDA and the PLV, then the anatomy is "right-dominant" (60%)
    - If the RCA supplies the PDA but not the PLV, then there is "codominance" (25%)
    - If the LCx supplies both these arteries, then the anatomy is "left-dominant" (15%).

Coronary Intervention
- Decision to intervene on a stenosis depends on multiple clinical factors.
- Principal question is whether or not the stenosis is severe enough to cause flow limitation that leads to ischemia:
  - Once a stenosis of >50% of the luminal diameter is identified, intervention may be considered if the lesion is presumed to be causing chest pain or cardiac enzyme elevation, particularly if there are associated areas of ischemia on stress testing.
- If doubt remains as to which lesion is the culprit, fractional flow reserve (FFR) can be used to assess the flow limitation caused by the stenosis:
  - An FFR <0.75 would warrant intervention.

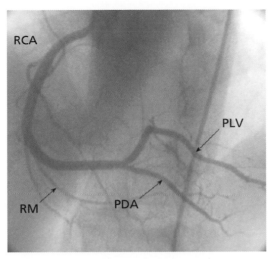

Figure 27.3 LAO cranial. Body of the right coronary artery (RCA) is seen running along the AV groove. There are small right marginal (RM) branches. This is a right-dominant system with the RCA giving rise to both the posterior descending artery (PDA) and the posterolateral left ventricular (PLV) artery. Note that the ascending catheter remains on the right side of the screen in the LAO view (the catheter will be on the left side of the screen in the RAO view)

- Plain old balloon angioplasty (POBA) is rarely performed given the high rates of restenosis.
- Bare metal stents (BMS) reduce the rates of restenosis dramatically and drug-eluting stents (DESs) virtually eliminate the risk:
  - However, because of the higher risk of in-stent thrombosis and the need for long-term clopidogrel with DESs, BMSs are still used when stenting large vessels or if urgent surgery is anticipated.

Coronary Wires
- Coronary interventions are performed with 0.014" wires:
  - Comprise an inner core wire and an outer spring tip
  - Tip can be shaped (usually with a J-tip), which allows the wire to be steered down the vessel.
- There are numerous 0.014" wires available and selection will depend on lesion location and characteristics, and operator preference:
  - Simpler cases are usually performed with an operator's "workhorse" wire, e.g. BMW and floppy wires
  - Hydrophilic wires are sometimes used for more distal lesions in tortuous vessels, e.g. Prowater and Pilot wires
  - Supportive wires may be required to advance balloons and stents through tortuous or calcified arteries, e.g. Ironman and Wiggle wires
  - Specialized wires are often required to cross chronic total occlusions, e.g. Miracle brothers and Confianza wires

Coronary Balloon Catheters

- The most commonly used balloons are on rapid-exchange (monorail) catheters:
  - These catheters have only a 30–40 cm length of lumen for the wire at the distal tip of the catheter
  - This enables a shorter (190 cm) coronary wire to be used when compared to an over-the-wire catheter
  - The lumen for the wire in the over-the-wire catheters runs the full length of the catheter, which requires a long (300 cm) coronary wire to be used.
- Balloon catheters are also classified into compliant and noncompliant balloons dependent on the stiffness of the inflatable material of the balloon:
  - *Compliant* balloons are more malleable to the shape of the artery and are generally used for lesions predilatation
  - *Noncompliant* balloons will hold their shape better and are usually used for stent postdilatation:
    - Can also be used for predilatation of heavily calcified lesions that will not dilate with a compliant balloon
    - Carry with this an increased risk of vessel dissection or perforation.
- Length and size of the balloon chosen is determined by the lesion length and vessel size.
- **Lesion predilatation:**
  - Balloon is undersized to the vessel diameter
  - Vessel diameter is usually estimated visually by comparison with the size of the guiding catheter (6F = 2 mm; 7F = 2.31 mm; 8F = 2.64 mm).
  - Low-pressure inflations (<10–12 atm) are usually used
  - Careful observation that the lesion dilates with the balloon (with loss of the balloon's "waist" during inflation) confirms that a stent will be able to be expanded in this location.
  - Re-estimation of vessel (and subsequent stent) sizing can also be performed by comparing the vessel size with that of the known size of the inflated balloon (by use of the balloon sizing chart)
  - Distal vessel will often vasodilate following predilatation (with or without the administration of 100–200 µg of intracoronary glyceryl trinitrate), requiring further recalibration of vessel diameter.
- **Stent postdilatation**:
  - Usually performed with a noncompliant balloon
  - Length of the balloon chosen is shorter than the stent to ensure that the balloon does not overhang from the ends of the stent with potential dissection or intimal damage to the adjacent vessel
  - Higher pressures (14–20 atm) are usually used
- Balloon catheters are prepared following removal from their packaging by aspiration of any residual air in the balloon lumen using a leuer-lock syringe, usually filled with a 50:50 combination of contrast and saline.

Indeflator

- Balloons (with or without stents) are inflated and deflated using an inflation–deflation device usually filled with a 50:50 mixture of contrast and saline.
- Air is removed from the indeflator prior to attachment to the balloon lumen.
- Negative pressure is then usually applied to the indeflator.
- When the balloon is in position for inflation, the negative pressure is released and the balloon is inflated by clockwise rotation of the indeflator handle.
- A manometer on the indeflator indicates the pressure in atmospheres within the balloon.
- Duration of balloon inflation is usually <60 s.
- Balloon deflation is aided by application of negative pressure with the indeflator.

Coronary Stents

- BMSs and DESs are available in a variety of diameters and lengths.
- Selection of stent type will depend on lesion size and characteristics, risk of subsequent restenosis, operator preference, and patient factors:
  - Predictors of restenosis: previous restenosis, vessel size, and lesion length.
  - Patient factors: compliance with antiplatelet therapy, the need for elective surgery following revascularization, and bleeding risk with antiplatelet therapy.

Anticoagulation

There are a number of different anticoagulant and antiplatelet treatment strategies available during and after the procedure to minimize restenosis and thrombosis with PCI.

- **Unfractionated heparin:**
  - A bolus dose is typically given prior to commencing coronary intervention
  - Common dosing schedules are:
    - 100 U/kg if heparin is used alone
    - 70 U/kg if used in conjunction with a IIb/IIIa inhibitor
  - Activated clotting time (ACT) can be used during the procedure to monitor heparin therapy:
    - HemoChron ACT of 300–350 s or HemoTec ACT of 250–300 s are commonly used if heparin is being used alone
    - ACT of >200 is sufficient if a GP IIb/IIIa inhibitor is also being used
  - Heparin is not routinely continued following the procedure.
- **Low molecular weight heparin:**
  - Dose will depend on the agent used and whether it will be given in conjunction with a IIb/IIIa inhibitor. Commonly used agent is enoxaparin.
  - If the patient has *not* been given enoxaparin in the previous 12 h:
    - Bolus dose of 1.0 mg/kg is given without a GP IIb/IIIa inhibitor, or
    - 0.5–0.75 mg/kg is given in conjunction with a GP IIb/IIIa inhibitor

- If the patient has been given a dose 8–12 h before, a supplemental dose of 0.3 mg/kg is given.
- **GP IIb/IIIa inhibitors**
  - **Eptifibatide:**
    - Two boluses of 180 µg/kg (maximum dose 22.5 mg for a 125-kg person) given over 1–2 min IV 10 min apart, followed by a 2 µg/kg/min infusion (maximum dose of 15 mg/h for a 125-kg person) for 12–24 h
    - If creatinine clearance is <50 mL/min, same boluses given followed by a 1 µg/kg/min infusion.
  - **Tirofiban:**
    - Single bolus of 0.4 µg/kg/min over 30 min or 25 µg/kg over 3 min is given, followed by an infusion of 0.15 µg/kg/min for 12–24 h
    - If the creatinine clearance is <30 mL/min, give half the bolus dose and half the infusion.
  - **Abciximab:**
    - Bolus of 0.25 mg/kg IV followed by an infusion of 0.125 µg/kg/min (maximum dose of 10 µg/min) for 12 h.
- **Bivalirudin:**
  - Direct thrombin inhibitor
  - Bolus of 0.75 mg/kg followed by an infusion of 1.75 mg/kg/h during and/or up to 4 h following the procedure
  - If creatinine clearance is <30 mL/min, the same bolus is given but the infusion is reduced to 1 mL/kg/h
  - If the patient is on dialysis, the same bolus is given but the infusion rate is reduced to 0.25 mg/kg/h.

EVIDENCE-BASED PRACTICE

BRIEF-PCI Trial

Context: Ideal duration of a GP IIb/IIIa inhibitor infusion following PCI was not well established.

Goal: To compare prolonged infusion versus shorter infusion of eptifibatide following PCI.

Method: Randomized patients after successful PCI with stent to either an 18-h infusion or an under-2-h infusion of eptifibatide. The primary end-point was the incidence of periprocedural ischemic myocardial injury within 24 h.

Results: Primary end-point present in 30.1% of the under-2-h infusion group, compared with 28.3% of those in the standard 18-h group (p < .012 for noninferiority). There was no difference in the secondary endpoints which included 30-day incidence of MI and the rate of urgent target vessel revascularization (TVR). Postprocedural major bleeding was less frequent in the under-2-h group (1.0% versus 4.2%).

Take-home message: Duration of infusion of a GP IIb/IIIa inhibitor can be significantly shortened following PCI.

EVIDENCE-BASED PRACTICE

HORIZONS AMI Trial

Context: Role of bivalirudin in patients with STEMI was unclear.

Goal: To compare infusion of bivalirudin with unfractionated heparin plus a GP IIa/IIIb inhibitor prior to PCI.

Method: Randomized patients with STEMI to either bivalirudin with provisional GP IIb/IIIa inhibitor use or unfractionated heparin and GP IIb/IIIa inhibitor prior to primary PCI.

Results: At 30 days, there was no difference (5.4% versus 5.5%) in the rate of major adverse cardiac events (all-cause death, reinfarction, ischemic TVR, or stroke). There was a significant 40% reduction (4.9% versus 8.3%) in major bleeding. However, the acute (<24h) stent thrombosis rate was 1.3% for the bivalirudin-treated patients versus 0.3% for the heparin/GP IIb/IIIa inhibitor-treated patients.

Take-home message: Bivalirudin may provide lower rates of major bleeding with comparable major cardiac events.

Postprocedure Care

- Patient should be monitored closely following the procedure:
  - Telemetry, regular vital signs, and access site and relevant peripheral pulses should be observed.
- Intravenous hydration should be given to reduce the risk of contrast nephropathy.
- Antiplatelet therapy should be administered if this has not already been done.

Sheath Removal

- Arterial sheaths should be removed once the ACT has fallen below 180s:
  - Protamine (30mg reverses 10000U of heparin) can be given to expedite the process and should be infused slowly, over 5min
  - Shaking, flushing, back pain and hypotension may signal a protamine reaction which is managed supportively with IV fluids, vasopressors, diphenhydramine and sedatives as necessary.
- After removal of the sheaths:
  - Manual pressure must be applied over the artery, against the femoral head, for 20–30min depending on whether or not antiplatelet therapy was used.
  - Near-occlusive pressure of the femoral artery for 5min, followed by gradual relaxation of pressure to 25–50% should be administered directly over the femoral pulse.
  - In obese patients, it is critical to assess that pressure is indeed being held over the femoral pulse, which can be difficult to find.

- External compression devices (Femo-Stop) can be used to apply arterial pressure; these devices must be placed by well-trained staff and must be checked frequently for proper hemostasis
- Several arterial closure devices (Angio-Seal, Perclose) are available and can reduce the amount of bed rest required (usually 6h for a 6F sheath); however, each device carries a small risk of complications and failure.

Common Complications
- **Arterial bleeding:**
  - Suspect if there is evidence of expanding hematoma, swelling, pain, or hypotension
  - Retroperitoneal bleeding:
    - Can present as back pain or hypotension in the absence of visible hematoma
    - Vagal response (bradycardia) is often seen
    - Pelvic CT should be performed if suspected
  - Manual pressure remains the key to obtaining adequate hemostasis in the event of arterial bleeding:
    - Arterial puncture site(s) are usually 1–2cm above the skin incision (depending on the angle of entry of the introducer needle)
  - Rapid intravascular volume resuscitation is crucial to the management of patients with hemodynamic compromise due to bleeding.
  - Protamine administration should be considered if the patient is in the catheter laboratory or has recently returned to the recovery ward to reverse the residual effects of the heparin that has been given:
    - A total empiric dose of up to 50mg can be given by slow IV injection over 10min
  - Less serious local bleeding is common and can be managed with manual pressure:
    - If prolonged pressure is needed, a FemoStop femoral artery compression device, a sandbag, or a hemostasis pad (such as a Chito-Seal pad) can be used
    - Superficial skin and tract bleeding is sometimes managed with local infiltration of epinephrine-containing lidocaine
  - CBC is routinely measured the following morning.
- **Arterial occlusion:**
  - Rare but limb-threatening complication
  - A pale and pulseless limb results
  - Emergent vascular surgical review with a view to arterial exploration and repair is required.
- **Pseudoaneurysms and aortovenous fistulas:**
  - Suspect in the presence of expanding hematoma, excessive groin pain, and development of bruits.
  - Femoral arterial ultrasound is the diagnostic test of choice.

- **Coronary artery**
  - **Dissection:** usually treated with stent placement due to the risk of thrombus formation and abrupt vessel closure.
  - **Perforation:** N
    - Nearly always evident during the procedure
    - Depending on the severity of the perforation, treatment options include conservative management, reversal of anticoagulation, balloon occlusion of the vessel, covered stent placement, pericardiocentesis, and emergency surgical repair.
  - **No reflow:**
    - Thought to be due to occlusion of the microvasculature with debris comprised of thrombus and plaque
    - Manifests as minimal or absent flow in the vessel being treated
    - Management options include intracoronary nitroglycerine, adenosine, and verapamil.
  - **In-stent thrombosis:**
    - Can occur acutely or several months post-implant, usually in patients with DESs who have stopped taking clopidogrel
    - Due to thrombus formation within the stent, and usually presents with the acute onset of symptoms, ischemic changes on ECG
    - Best managed by prompt return to the laboratory for percutaneous intervention.
  - **CK-MB rise:**
    - Cardiac enzymes are routinely measured on the following morning bloods in a number of centers
    - Their elevation has been correlated with a greater risk for late mortality
    - Management is tailored to the clinical situation.
  - **Restenosis:**
    - Gradual renarrowing of the treated vessel segment with representation with myocardial ischemia usually within 6 months of the intervention
    - DESs minimize the risk of restenosis.
- **Renal failure:**
  - Electrolytes and creatinine levels are routinely measured the following morning
  - Peak creatinine level in patients who develop contrast nephropathy is usually seen 48–72 h following the procedure
  - Usually be managed with fluid administration, but occasionally requires transient hemodialysis.
- **Contrast reactions/anaphylaxis:**
  - Can manifest as urticaria/pruritis, bronchospasm, facial and laryngeal edema, or hypotension/shock
  - Treatment should be tailored to the clinical situation

- Treatment options include:
  - Diphenhydramine 25–50 mg orally/IV
  - Cimetidine 300 mg or ranitidine 50 mg in 20 mL of normal saline IV over 15 min
  - Hydrocortisone 200–400 mg IV
  - Epinephrine 10 µg boluses q1min or infusion of 1–4 µg/min
  - Supplemental oxygen, airway protection, or intubation.

Discharge Medications

Care should be taken to ensure that patients are aware of any alterations to their medical therapy, especially the addition of antiplatelet therapy (Aspirin, clopidogrel). The importance of dual antiplatelet therapy in preventing stent thrombosis should be highlighted to patients following stent implantation.

The long-term prognosis of patients can be significantly improved by optimizing the management of the major risk factors for atherosclerosis. Their hospitalization for coronary intervention should be seen as an opportunity to optimize their risk factor profile, which may include initiation of antihyperlipidemia therapy, smoking cessation, and optimized diabetic control.

Intra-Aortic Balloon Pump (IABP) Counterpulsation

The purpose of the IABP is to support hemodynamic function in decompensated heart failure and to improve coronary perfusion.

- **Principal indications:**
  - Cardiogenic shock refractory to noninvasive inotropic support
  - Refractory unstable angina
  - High-risk PCI
  - Bridge to transplant
  - Decompensated aortic stenosis
  - Refractory ventricular arrhythmias
- **Clear-cut contraindications:**
  - Aortic insufficiency
  - Aortic dissection
  - Abdominal or thoracic aneurysms
  - Severe peripheral vascular disease.

Procedure

The IABP is placed in the descending aorta, inflates during diastole and deflates during systole, thereby providing negative pressure during systole, which decreases afterload, and positive pressure during diastole, which improves coronary perfusion.

- The balloon is most commonly introduced by the femoral artery approach using standard techniques and the equipment provided with the IABP to ensure compatibility of wire (usually 0.025″) and central lumen.

- Central lumen is used for pressure monitoring and advancement during insertion over a guidewire:
  - Tip of the balloon catheter has a radio-opaque marker and is placed 1–2 cm distal to the left subclavian artery.
- A second lumen is used for inflation and deflation of the balloon.
  - A negative vacuum using a one-way valve and syringe are applied to the balloon through this lumen prior to removal from the packaging.
- Balloon volume is selected based on patient height.
- A sheathless or sheathed approach can be used.
- The central lumen is connected to pressure tubing with aspiration and flushing.
  - A stylet within the balloon lumen often requires removal to allow connection of this lumen to the balloon pump tubing.
- Intravenous heparin is usually administered during balloon pump therapy. However, the risk of bleeding requires assessment and commonly negates the use of heparin in settings such as immediately following cardiothoracic surgery.
- ECG triggering is the most common mode of triggering used for balloon deflation and inflation; however, pressure triggering can also be used:
  - The balloon pump software usually optimizes the timing of deflation and inflation of the balloon, although settings can be manually adjusted.
  - Ideal inflation occurs just before the dicrotic notch on the aortic pressure wave (Figure 27.4).

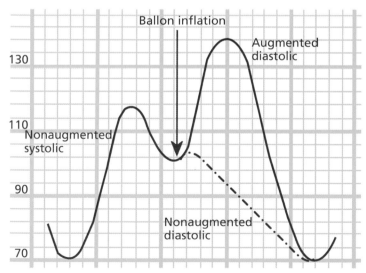

Figure 27.4 Balloon inflation. A single cardiac cycle depicting intra-aortic pressure with balloon inflation, which should occur at the time when the dicrotic notch is typically seen. The dashed line represents aortic pressure without balloon inflation. Improperly timed balloon inflation can lead to suboptimal pressure augmentation

Complications
- Limb ischemia, infection, balloon rupture leading to thrombus formation and embolism, hemolysis and thrombocytopenia (cellular shear stress), and occlusion of the renal and mesenteric arteries.
- CBC and creatinine must be followed carefully.
- Daily chest X-ray should be performed to ensure that the balloon has not migrated.

Weaning
- Usually performed by gradually reducing the rate of inflation/deflation cycles (from 1:1 to 1:8) and ensuring maintenance of an adequate hemodynamic state prior to proceeding to removal.
- Balloon can often be removed through the sheath (if present) but preparations should be in place for the possibility that the sheath requires removal concomitantly (heparin discontinued prior to removal).

Peripheral Interventions

There are a number of similarities between coronary and peripheral interventions. However, there are also important differences. One of these is the use of digital subtraction angiography for most peripheral interventional procedures. Some of the other differences will be briefly highlighted.
- **Carotid interventions:**
  - **Antiplatelet therapy:** Aspirin and clopidogrel
  - **Anticoagulation:** heparin 70–100 U/kg alone with boluses to maintain a target ACT ≥250 or 300 is the most commonly used anticoagulation strategy.
  - **Antihypertensive medications:** usually omitted on the day of the procedure due to hypotension that commonly results from local pressure on the carotid body.
  - **Minimal sedation:** allows for neurologic assessment of the patient during the procedure.
  - **Aortogram:** usually performed to assess the anatomy of the aortic arch and its major branches.
  - **Diagnostic angiography:** a number of different diagnostic catheters (JR4, H1, JB1, IMA, Berenstein, Simmons, Headhunter, or Vitek) are used to account for the array of different innominate or carotid take-offs encountered
  - **Guide sheaths/catheters:**
    - Commonly a 6F shuttle sheath or an 8F coronary guide catheter is used
    - A "telescoping" technique is used to advance this into the common carotid artery (CCA)
    - A diagnostic catheter is used to engage the innominate or left CCA

- A 0.035″ guidewire is advanced into the distal common carotid or external carotid artery
- Diagnostic catheter is advanced over the wire
- Shuttle sheath or coronary guide catheter is advanced over the diagnostic catheter to the mid-to-distal portion of the CCA
- **Wire/distal protection device (DPD):**
  - Lesion is crossed with a 0.014″ wire and DPD
  - Some distal protection devices are attached directly to the wire whilst others have a monorail system, allowing delivery following first crossing the lesion with a wire alone
  - DPD examples are the Accunet, Emboshield, Angioguard, FilterWire, and Spider devices
- **Atropine/phenylephrine:**
  - Local pressure on the carotid body often results in bradycardia and hypotension.
  - Premedication with atropine 0.5 mg and phenylephrine 25–50 μg is often given prior to balloon inflations and stent deployment
  - Infusions of these medications following the procedure are sometimes required for persistent hypotension or bradycardia
  - A temporary wire is rarely needed
- **Intravenous fluid:** often administered for hypotension.
- **Predilatation:** stenosis is commonly predilated with an undersized (relative to the vessel) compliant balloon.
- **Stent:** tapered or nontapered self-expanding nitinol stents (e.g. Acculink, Xact, Precise, and NexStent) are used.
- **Postdilation:** stent is postdilated with an aim for a residual stenosis ≤30%
- **DPD retrieval** is then performed.
- **Complications:**
  - Stroke (embolic or hemorrhagic)
  - Dissection (due to balloon, stent or sheath)
  - Perforation
  - Acute or subacute thrombosis
  - Arterial spasm (treated with nitroglycerine)
  - Hypotension (commonly due to carotid body pressure but also can be due to retroperitoneal hemorrhage or contrast reaction)
  - No reflow [due to spasm or a full DPD (managed with an extraction catheter or device retrieval)]
  - Hyperperfusion syndrome (presenting as confusion with or without localizing symptoms). CT is useful to confirm the diagnosis and to exclude intracranial hemorrhage. Managed with control of SBP to <160 mmHg)
  - Contrast encephalopathy
  - Restenosis.

- **Renal interventions:**
  - **Antiplatelet therapy:** Aspirin and clopidogrel.
  - **Access:** usually a retrograde femoral approach is adequate; occasionally an arm approach is required.
  - **Aortogram/selective diagnostic angiography:**
    - Aortogram is frequently performed initially
    - Selective angiography is then commonly performed
    - Diagnostic catheters include JR4, IMA, Hockey Stick guide, or RDC1 catheters
  - **Heparin:** is given prior to intervention
  - **Guide catheters:**
    - 6–8F guide catheters are used depending on compatibility with the likely stent size to be used
    - Guide catheters include JR4, short IMA, Hockey Stick, renal double curve, SOS II and III
  - **Wires:**
    - Usually a 0.014″ wire is sufficient; however, 0.018 or 0.035″ guidewires can be used
    - Careful consideration of the location of the wire tip is important to reduce the risk of renal perforation
  - **Angioplasty:** alone is the recommended therapy for fibromuscular dysplasia
  - **Stents:** balloon-expandable stents are recommended for the more common atherosclerotic lesions.
- **Lower limb interventions:**
  - Inflow disease is usually treated before more distal disease
  - Antiplatelet and heparin are administered prior to intervention
  - **Iliac interventions:**
    - Usually performed using an ipsilateral common femoral artery approach (unless the stenosis is in the distal external iliac artery)
    - A 7F system is usually adequate for intervention
    - 0.035″ guidewires are commonly used.
    - Guide catheters are not usually required
    - Balloon-expandable stents are usually used for common iliac lesions
    - Self-expanding nitinol stents are commonly used for external iliac lesions.
  - **Superficial femoral artery interventions:**
    - May be performed with a contralateral leg or arm approach, or with an ipsilateral antegrade approach
    - Angioplasty alone, stenting, cryoplasty, mechanical or laser atherectomy are common treatment options
  - **Below-knee interventions:**
    - Ipsilateral antegrade approach is preferred if possible
    - Angioplasty alone is the most common strategy with bailout stenting for suboptimal results.

CLINICAL PEARLS

- Arterial access should not be rushed. Proper access techniques will avoid future complications.
- Hypotension during or immediately following coronary angiography should prompt assessment of: arterial bleeding, including retroperitoneal blood loss; contrast dye anaphylaxis; myocardial perforation; protamine reaction.
- Difficult cannulation of a coronary artery or bypass graft often requires use of alternative catheters.
- Knowing a particular patient's indications for coronary angiography will help with management of specific lesions (distribution of regional perfusion defects, presence of angina, etc.).
- Not all vessels require use of DESs. Consider BMSs in large vessels.
- Worsening anemia or thrombocytopenia in a patient with a balloon pump can be due to mechanical hemolysis. Consider heparin-induced thrombocytopenia (HIT) if patient is on heparin.
- Acute drop in urine output or rise in creatinine should prompt assessment of IABP migration as this can be due to occlusion of the renal arteries.

Recommended Reading

Clinical Trials and Meta-Analyses

Mahmud E, Prasad A. Optimal platelet therapy during coronary interventions includes glycoprotein IIb/IIIa inhibitors eliminate the infusion. *J Am Coll Cardiol* 2009;**53**:846–848.

Moliterno DJ, Yakubov SJ, DiBattiste PM et al.; TARGET investigators. Outcomes at 6 months for the direct comparison of tirofibran and abciximab during percutaneous coronary revascularization with stent placement: the TARGET follow-up study. *Lancet* 2002;**360**: 355–360.

Stone GW, Witzenbichler B, Guagliumi G et al., HORIZONS-AMI Trial Investigators. Bivalirudin during primary PCI in acute myocardial infarction. *N Engl J Med* 2008;**358**: 2218–2230.

Review Articles

Baim DS. *Grossman's Cardiac Catheterization, Angiography and Intervention*, 7th edn. Philadelphia: Lippincott Williams & Wilkins, 2005.

28 Pacemakers and ICD Troubleshooting

Marco Perez and Paul Wang

Department of Internal Medicine, Division of Cardiology, Stanford University School of Medicine, Stanford, CA, USA

The complexity of pacemakers and defibrillators continues to grow rapidly. Urgent interrogation and evaluation, often by general cardiologists and internists, is commonly requested when a pacemaker seems to be malfunctioning, a shock episode has occurred, or a patient with a device is symptomatic.

This chapter will review the fundamentals of pacemakers and implantable cardioverter defibrillators (ICDs), cover troubleshooting the most common problems encountered, and outline how to interrogate a device to make sure leads and the device are working appropriately.

Pacemaker Fundamentals

The vast majority of pacemakers are used for sinus node and/or atrioventricular (AV) node malfunction. Patients have either a single pacemaker lead system (RV or RA) or a dual lead system (RV + RA). The pacemaker is programmed with a specific set of rules or instructions on how to pace. The basic pacing instructions, or mode, are abbreviated with four letters, e.g.:

D D D R

- First letter: chamber paced, A = atrium, V = ventricle, D = dual (both chambers)
- Second letter: chamber sensed, A = atrium, V = ventricle, D = dual (both chambers).
- Third letter: response to sensing:
  - I = inhibit. If an event is sensed, no pacing will occur in the same chamber
  - T = trigger: After an event is sensed, pacing occurs in the chamber being paced.
  - D = Dual. If an atrial event is sensed, a ventricular paced event will occur after the programmed AV delay unless a ventricular event is sensed. If

A Practical Approach to Cardiovascular Medicine, First Edition. Edited by Reza Ardehali, Marco Perez, Paul Wang.

a ventricular event is sensed, ventricular pacing is inhibited and atrial pacing is inhibited until an atrial escape interval elapses.
- Fourth letter: R = rate adaptation or modulation. The rate adjusts to a sensor to respond to a need for a more rapid rate.

Common Pacing Modes and Their Uses
- **VVI:** –
  - Single-chamber ventricular mode
  - Pacemaker will simply wait for a ventricular impulse, and if one is not sensed within the lower rate interval, it will pace in the ventricle regardless of what is happening in the atrium
  - Often used in patients with atrial arrhythmias
  - If the patient is in sinus, however, AV synchrony will not occur.
- **DDD:**
  - Most common mode used with dual-chamber devices
  - After the last ventricular event, the pacemaker waits for an atrial signal; if one is not sensed within the programmed interval, it will pace the atrium
  - After the sensed or paced atrial event, the pacemaker waits for a ventricular signal and, if one is not sensed within the programmed AV interval, it will pace the ventricle.
- **AAI:**
  - Used in patients who may have sinus node disease, but intact AV node conduction
  - In patients with dual-chamber devices, this mode can be used to help avoid ventricular pacing
  - In some devices algorithms that switch the mode from AAI to DDD can be programmed to occur if AV conduction fails.
- **DDDR/VVIR/AAIR:**
  - "R" stands for rate adaption or modulation
  - When sensor activity is detected, the lower rate is increased proportionally to the measured sensor values
  - Common sensors include accelerometers and minute ventilation.
- **VOO:**
  - "O" stands for "none"
  - Will pace the ventricle asynchronously
  - Often used in patients who are pacemaker-dependent and are undergoing surgical intervention involving electrocautery, which can inhibit pacing.
- **ODO:** turns off all pacing.

Timing Cycles
To understand normal and abnormal pacemaker function, the pacemaker timing cycles must be understood (Figure 28.1). These are a series of blanking and refractory zones around the atrial and ventricular events which are designed to minimize problems inherent in pacing. "Events" refers to either an intrinsic beat, or a paced beat.

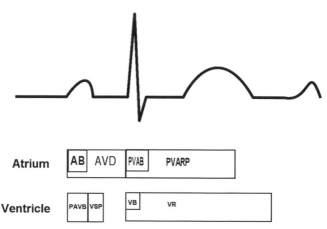

Figure 28.1 Pacemaker timing cycles (see text for explanation of acronyms)

- **Blanking periods**:
  - Periods during which the pacemaker does not "see" any events
    - Atrial blanking (AB; atrial blanking after atrial event)
    - Postatrial ventricular blanking (PAVB; V blanking after atrial event)
    - Postventricular atrial blanking (PVAB; A blanking after ventricular event)
    - Ventricular blanking (VB; V blanking after ventricular event)
  - Designed primarily to prevent sensing lead polarization following pacing or sensing activity in the opposite channel, called crosstalk or far-field sensing.
- **Refractory periods**:
  - Periods during which the pacemaker "sees" events and records them, but does not use them to reset the timing cycle
    - Postventricular atrial refractory period (PVARP): programmed time after a ventricular event during which the atrium is not sensed or tracked in a dual chamber mode. Designed primarily to prevent pacemaker-mediated tachycardia (PMT) (see below)
    - Atrial refractory period: time after an atrial event that the atrium is not sensed
    - Ventricular refractory (VR) period: time after a ventricular event that ventricular activity is not sensed
    - AV interval or AV delay (AVI or AVD): maximum time between an atrial paced or sensed event and a paced ventricular event.
- **Safety pacing:**
  - Ventricular safety pacing (VSP):
    - After an atrial paced event, a ventricular event sensed in the crosstalk safety window will result in a ventricular paced event called a ventricular safety paced beat, at an AV interval of 80–130 ms
    - Prevents inhibition of the ventricular channel by an atrial paced event.

Pacemaker Troubleshooting

The intrinsic hardware of a pacemaker rarely malfunctions. Problems more commonly arise because of nonoptimal pacing settings, battery depletion, or lead abnormalities (see Boxes 28.1 and 28.2 below).

Box 28.1 Urgent pacemaker and ICD interrogation checklist

When called to interrogate a pacemaker, besides assessing for the above problems, an assessment of the battery, leads and recorded events should be documented and will often help with troubleshooting. A suggested checklist is given below.

1. Determine type of device: number of leads, make and model of pacemaker
2. Assess battery life: a very low battery life can affect pacing function
3. Underlying rhythm: if unclear, temporarily set device to pace at VVI 40 or 30 bpm (if tolerated) and assess for intrinsic sinus rates and AV nodal conduction
4. Check atrial and ventricular sensing: by measuring the amplitude of the atrial and ventricular signals either through the pacemaker programmer or by measuring the amplitude on the recorded electrogram:
   - In the VVI mode, the rate is lowered to evaluate sensing
   - In the DDD mode, ventricular sensing may be assessed by lengthening the AV delay until sensing occurs or, if there is long AV conduction, by changing to VVI at a slow rate.
   - Atrial sensing may be assessed in the DDD mode by lowering the lower rate limit
   - Atrial sensing should be evaluated in the AAI mode only when AV conduction is intact
5. Check atrial and ventricular thresholds:
   - Lower the output until loss of capture is noted
   - Ventricular thresholds may be checked in the VVI mode at a rate faster than the intrinsic ventricular rate or in the DDD mode, and shortening the AV interval if AV conduction is present
   - When AV conduction is normal, atrial thresholds may be checked in the AAI mode at a rate faster than the sinus rate
     When AV conduction is not intact, atrial thresholds are performed in the DDD mode by increasing the lower rate limit. Monitoring the intracardiac atrial electrogram may be particularly helpful to assess capture. In some cases, a surface ECG may be required
6. Check lead impedance:
   - An elevated impedance implies a lead fracture
   - A low impedance implies an lead insulation break
   - If there is an abnormal impedance, the device may be manipulated and the arm moved while examining ECGs and/or while repeating lead impedance measurements

(Continued)

7. Review the EGMs from recorded atrial or ventricular tachycardia events.
   - Note number of events, duration, atrial and ventricular rates
   - Assess if there are events consistent with atrial arrhythmias or ventricular arrhythmias
8. Review any alerts or remarks about lead abnormalities. Note percentage of atrial and ventricular pacing and the rate distribution

Specific steps to evaluate ICDs

9. Review all ventricular tachyarrhythmia events for which therapy has been given (shock and ATP events):
   - Determine the rhythm for which therapy has been given
   - Determine if it is appropriate or inappropriate
10. Examine lead impedances:
    - Determine if there are any short intervals, which may represent signs of lead abnormalities, oversensing sinus rhythm or ventricular tachyarrhythmias
11. Assess if detection zones are appropriate. Assess if VT was quickly sensed.
12. Assess if therapy is appropriate:
    - If antitachycardia pacing has been successful, keep it programmed on
    - If antitachycardia therapy is unsuccessful, adjust it to be more aggressive or if acceleration has occurred frequently, remove antitachycardia pacing
    - Examine if shock therapy has been successful:
      - If it has not, increase the energy delivered
      - If it is maximum energy, testing such as defibrillation threshold testing may be needed
13. Evaluate for undersensing:
    - Measured R-waves usually should be 4 or 5 mV or greater
    - Examine episodes for which tachyarrhythmia therapy has been delivered to find evidence of undersensing
    - Undersensing may require programming to a more sensitive setting, or if the R-waves are small, a new lead may need to be inserted
14. Evaluate for oversensing

Oversensing (Figure 28.2)

- Occurs when a signal not representing true myocardial depolarization (atrial or ventricular)is sensed.
- Ventricular oversensing, particularly in pacemaker-dependent individuals, can lead to a dangerous lack of ventricular pacing.
- Commonly due to cross-talk, electromagnetic interference, myopotentials, T-waves, and noise from lead fractures.

Undersensing (Figure 28.3)

- Failure to sense myocardial depolarization.
- Ventricular undersensing usually leads to pacing when it is not necessary and atrial undersensing in the DDD mode results in failure to track.

Box 28.2 Special considerations for biventricular pacing

- If phrenic nerve stimulation is present:
  - Program left ventricular output just above the threshold
  - Also try additional pacing configurations if available
  - Examine chest X-ray to evaluate for dislodgment
- Program left ventricular output with a lower safety margin to save battery
- Examine the chest X-ray to assess if the lead appears to be in the proper location (posterior toward the spine on the lateral view) and usually lateral
- Consider using algorithms to set AV and VV intervals
- If the patient does show a clinical response to biventricular pacing, consider echocardiographic guidance to select AV and VV intervals:
  - In selecting AV interval, start by evaluating intervals that avoid truncation of the A-wave but not so long as to cause diastolic mitral regurgitation
  - VV intervals may be assessed using the velocity time integral

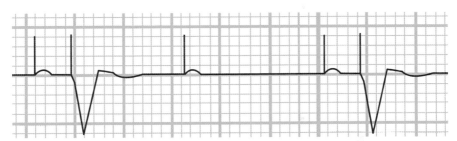

Figure 28.2 Oversensing. The second beat has an atrial stimulus followed by a P-wave, but there is no ventricular stimulus, likely due to intermittent inappropriate ventricular sensing of the atrial stimulus (crosstalk). Ventricular safety pacing would prevent asystole in this situation

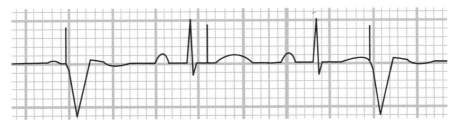

Figure 28.3 Ventricular undersensing. The first QRS complex is paced. The second QRS complex, which is an intrinsic ventricular event, was not sensed and a ventricular stimulus was delivered during the refractory period of the myocardial tissue. The third QRS complex was also not sensed, and a ventricular stimulus was then delivered and captured since it occurred longer after the previous ventricular depolarization

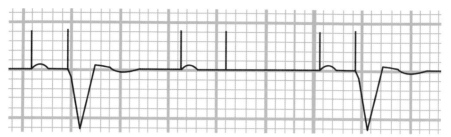

Figure 28.4 Ventricular failure to capture. The second beat has a ventricular spike that was appropriately timed, but ventricular depolarization (capture) did not occur

Most common causes are small intrinsic signals, lead dislodgement, poor lead positioning, and lead abnormalities.

Failure to Capture (Figure 28.4)
- Occurs when there is an appropriate pacing stimulus, but there is no evidence of depolarization.
- Commonly caused by elevated pacing thresholds often due to excessive fibrosis at the lead tip, lead dislodgement, lead abnormalities, such as insulation break or lead fracture, and metabolic abnormalities (hyperkalemia).
- If a pacing stimulus occurs when the myocardial tissue is in the refractory period, myocardial depolarization will not occur; often called functional failure to capture.

Upper Rate Behavior
Dual chamber devices in the DDD mode will track intrinsic atrial events up to a programmed rate, called the upper rate limit or upper tracking rate. Of note, upper rate behavior will not be seen when AV conduction is intact.
- **Pacemaker Wenckebach:**
  - When the intrinsic atrial rate exceeds the upper tracking rate, ventricular pacing no longer occurs with each atrial beat.
  - In order not to violate the upper tracking rate, the ventricular stimulus must be delayed, resulting in a longer than programmed AV interval.
  - The sensed atrial event to ventricular paced event interval will progressively lengthen until the next atrial sensed event occurs within the PVARP.
  - This atrial sensed event will not be tracked and the next event will be either the next sensed atrial event or a paced atrial event.
  - This repetitive pattern is called pacemaker pseudoWenckebach.
- **Pacemaker 2:1 AV block:**
  - When the atrial cycle length increases to the point that it equals the sum of the AV interval and the PVARP [called the total atrial refractory period (TARP)], every other sensed atrial event will be followed by a ventricular event.

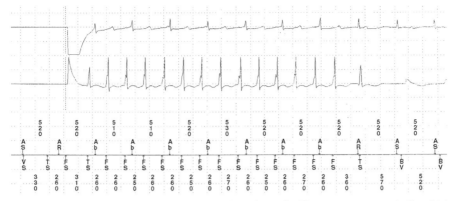

Figure 28.5 Intracardiac electrogram of ventricular tachycardia. The top row represents the atrial intracardiac electrogram (EGM), second row represents the ventricular EGM. The bottom row is how the device interprets the EGMs. Different devices use different codes. In this example, AS is A sensed, Ab is A blanking, VS is V sensed, FS is a V sense that is fast enough to be considered a ventricular tachyarrhythmia, and BV is biventricular pacing. Note the 2:1 relationship of ventricular to atrial events

Evaluating Tachycardia in Pacemakers or ICDs

A common request for urgent interrogation of a device is to help diagnose tachyarrhythmias. The pacemaker or ICD can provide intracardiac electrograms that can be used to diagnose arrhythmias:

- Most diagnostic situation is when there are more "V" sensed events than "A" sensed events, which is most consistent with VT (Figure 28.5).
- When there are more "A" than "V" sensed events there may be:
  - An atrial tachyarrhythmia, or
  - An atrial tachyarrhythmia and a ventricular arrhythmia, a so-called double tachycardia
  - Comparing the intrinsic ventricular electrogram morphology at baseline with that during the tachyarrhythmia will help distinguish these two possibilities.
- Very fast, highly irregular atrial events suggest atrial fibrillation (AF).
- When there is a 1:1 relationship, it is more difficult to distinguish the etiology of the tachycardia, and again examining the morphology may help make the diagnosis.
- When the patient has an A-sensed, V-paced tachycardia, the differential includes sinus tachycardia, an atrial tachyarrhythmia, or pacemaker-mediated tachycardia (PMT).
  - PMT occurs when there is a ventricular paced beat, followed by retrograde atrial depolarization, which is then "sensed" on the atrial channel and tracked.
  - The subsequent ventricular paced beat again is retrogradely conducted to the atrium.
  - This pattern continues as PMT.

- PMTs are often initiated by premature ventricular beats with retrograde conduction.
- Preventing PMT usually requires the PVARP to be lengthened. Excessively 0long PVARPs will limit the upper tracking rate and may cause 2:1 tracking to occur.

CLINICAL PEARLS

- Ventricular rates that are slower than expected are usually due to ventricular oversensing.
- Too much pacing is usually due to ventricular undersensing.
- Avoid ventricular pacing by programming long AV delay in DDD mode or a mode such as managed ventricular pacing that provides ventricular pacing only when AV conduction worsens.
- Program on features such as safety pacing, mode switching.
- Magnet response for a pacemaker results in asynchronous pacing. Magnet application will stop PMT and may prevent tracking of atrial fibrillation in pacemakers

---

ICD Function

ICD Detection Zones
- One, two, or three detection zones may be created for ventricular tachycardia (VT) (first one or two zones) and ventricular fibrillation (VF, last zone).
- Slowest VT zone should be at least 10 bpm slower than the slowest suspected VT (slower if drug therapy is initiated).
- It is important to determine if the VT or VF zone is fast enough to decrease likelihood of sensing sinus tachycardia or atrial fibrillation.
- If there is nonsustained VT or increased likelihood of rapidly conducted atrial fibrillation, consider lengthening the detection time.

ICD Therapy
- Consists of antitachycardia pacing or shock therapy.
- Antitachycardia pacing:
  - May be delivered as a series of beats in a row, usually 8 or 10 or more.
  - Rate of antitachycardia pacing is usually selected to be 75–90% of the VT cycle length.
  - There may be multiple trains, usually 2–4, with each successive train being more aggressive than the previous train by 10 ms or so.
  - Ramp pacing, in which each beat in the train has a progressively shorter interval, may also be used.
- Output of the first shock may be at the maximum or it may be lower, particularly in the VT zone for slower VTs.

ICD Discrimination Algorithms

- In order to prevent the ICD from detecting supraventricular arrhythmias as VT, it is important to program on discrimination algorithms.
- "Stability" indicates the variability from beat-to-beat and an increased variability usually is used to detect AF.
- "Sudden onset" acts to identify the rapid onset of a tachycardia arrhythmia and is useful in avoiding detection of sinus tachycardia.
- Many devices utilize a counter that compares the number of ventricular and atrial events:
- If there are more ventricular events than atrial events, VT will be detected.
- Some devices utilize a morphology or timing algorithm that accounts for differences in ventricular activation patterns in AV conduction and ventricular arrhythmias.
- There are also some algorithms that examine beat-to-beat AV relationships.

ICD Indications

- Sustained VT or VF
- Syncope and inducible VT
- Nonsustained VT, coronary artery disease (CAD), and inducible VT
- Ejection fraction (EF) <30%, CAD
- EF <35%, Class II or III heart failure
- Selected patients with hypertrophic cardiomyopathy, arrhythmogenic right ventricular dysplasia/cardiomyopathy, cardiac sarcoidosis, long QT syndrome

---

CLINICAL PEARLS

- Program on SVT discrimination algorithms
- Magnet application on ICD will usually suspend tachyarrhythmia therapies, as long as it is held over the device, but does not affect pacing function. In selected cases, magnet response may be turned off or magnet application may be used to activate or inactivate tachyarrhythmia therapy.
- Program on antitachycardia pacing in most cases
- Program tachycardia rate cut-off slower than slowest VT

Recommended Reading

Guidelines

ACC/AHA/HRS 2008 Guidelines for Device-Based Therapy of Cardiac Rhythm Abnormalities. *Heart Rhythm* 2008;5:e1–e62.

29 Introduction to Electrophysiology Studies

Ronald Lo and Henry Hsia

Department of Internal Medicine, Division of Cardiology, Stanford University School of Medicine, Stanford, CA, USA

An electrophysiology (EP) study is a procedure designed to evaluate cardiac arrhythmias. A typical diagnostic EP study (Figure 29.1) includes:

- Placement of a catheter with multiple electrodes into the high right atrium (RA), His position, and right ventricular (RV) apex via access through the femoral and internal jugular veins.
- A multielectrode catheter may also be placed into the coronary sinus (CS), which then reaches to the left side of the heart and can record left atrial electrical activity.

The poles on these catheters can record *local* electrical activity as intracardiac electrograms (EGMs) and can deliver pacing stimuli in different locations throughout the heart.

Unlike the surface ECG, where the focus is the morphology of the waveform, in the EGM the focus is the activation patterns and timing of the local deflections. By establishing the position of the catheters with fluoroscopy or three-dimensional technologies, the information needed to diagnose conduction system disease or arrhythmia is ascertained. For example:

- Interval between the atrial signal and the His deflection (AH) on the His catheter is an estimate of AV nodal conduction.
- Interval between the His deflection and earliest ventricular activation is a close approximation of His–Purkinje conduction time (HV).

Other important electrophysiologic properties that can be measured are effective refractory periods (ERPs) and nodal recovery periods. The ERP is the interval at which a stimulus is no longer able to depolarize myocardial or nodal tissue because these tissues have not yet repolarized.

The basic EP study comprises the following:

- Measurement of baseline conduction intervals, including AH and HV
- Measurement of refractory periods in the atrium, ventricle and AV node

A Practical Approach to Cardiovascular Medicine, First Edition. Edited by Reza Ardehali, Marco Perez, Paul Wang.

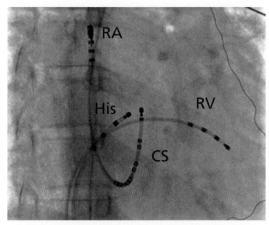

Figure 29.1 RAO view of the typical diagnostic catheters. RA: right atrium, usually placed high in the atrium. RV: right ventricular, typically placed near the apex. His: usually located in the anteroseptal aspect of the tricuspid valve. CS: coronary sinus osteum, usually just posterior to the base of the tricuspid valve. The CS catheter runs perpendicular to the RV catheter

- Atrial pacing:
  - Sinus node function
  - AV nodal and His–Purkinje function
  - Induction of atrial arrhythmias
- Ventricular pacing:
  - Retrograde AV nodal function
  - Induction of ventricular arrhythmias

Abbreviations
- BCL: baseline cycle length in milliseconds
- CL: cycle length in milliseconds; calculated as 60000/bpm
- CSNRT: corrected sinus node recovery time
- SNRT: sinus node recovery time
- S1: pacing train cycle length
- S2: first extra stimulus
- S3: second extra stimulus
- S4: third extra stimuli
- AERP: atrial effective refractory period
- VERP: ventricular effective refractory period
- AVNERP: AV nodal effective refractory period

Normal Intervals
- AH interval: 65–135 ms
- HV interval: 35–55 ms
- AERP: 170–300 ms
- AVNERP: 230–430 ms
- VERP: 170–290 ms

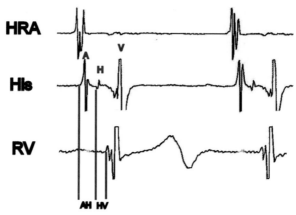

Figure 29.2 Normal intracardiac EGMs with a high right atrial (HRA), His bundle recording, and right ventricular apex (RV) recording. The lines indicate how the AH and HV intervals are measured

Measurement of Baseline Conduction Intervals

With the basic catheter position in the high RA, His bundle, and RV, the baseline intervals are measured (Figure 29.2). Because the majority of intervals are very short, these are measured and reported in milliseconds. To convert milliseconds to beats/min, 60000 is divided by the number of milliseconds. The baseline rhythm is noted and confirmed based on the activation pattern of the catheters. Sinus rhythm, for example, should start high in the atrium, then proceed down to the lower atrium and then through the AV node. The AH and HV intervals are measured on the His bundle EGM. Care must be taken to measure the HV from a more "proximal" His position, as measuring from a catheter too far into the RV may result in the measurement of a right bundle potential.

Sinus Node Function

The EP study can be used to assess the function of the sinus node by a phenomenon known as overdrive suppression.
- Rapid pacing of an automatic focus such as the sinus node causes overdrive suppression of the sinoatrial (SA) node, and upon cessation of pacing, there will be a pause before resumption of normal automaticity (Figure 29.3).
- A diseased SA node will exhibit a longer pause (Box 29.1).
- Typical protocols involve atrial pacing at a site in the high RA near the sinus node at 600, 500, 400, and 300 ms for 30 s, and measuring the time it takes for the sinus node to generate an impulse.
- As there is significant variability in sinus node function secondary to autonomic tone, often the corrected sinus node recovery time (CSNRT) is used.

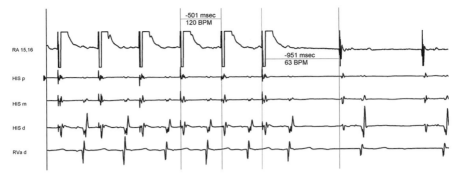

Figure 29.3 Normal SNRT at 950 ms. Note that the four electrical poles on the His catheter are used to divide the signals into a proximal, mid, and distal set of poles and are labeled as His p, m, and d respectively. This is done to better assess the often elusive His signal

---

Box 29.1 Abnormal sinus node recovery times

SNRT > 1500 ms
CSNRT > 550 ms
CSNRT = SNRT – BCL
SNRT/BCL > 160%

Sinoatrial Conduction Times

The SA conduction time (SACT) was designed to evaluate the conduction from the SA node to the surrounding tissue.

Return interval = BCL + 2 SACT

If the SACT is elevated (normal SACT = 50 – 125 ms), there is thought to be a predisposition to develop sinus node exit block.

To measure the SACT, a catheter is placed in the high RA near the sinus node and atrial pacing is performed just above the basic cycle length, and the return beat is measured.

Two methods have been developed to measure the SACT:
- Strauss method uses a single premature atrial contraction to ensure no overdrive suppression.
- Narula method uses a short pacing train barely faster than the sinus rate.

Both methods are essentially the same, with the goal of no overdrive suppression.

Intrinsic Heart Rate

The sinus node is sensitive to changes in the sympathetic and parasympathetic influences. In conditions such as neurocardiogenic syncope and athletes with high vagal tone with sinus bradycardia, they are the result of parasympathetic tone and *not* of sinus node dysfunction. It is useful to determine if sinus node "dysfunction" is due to external sources such as parasympathetic tone or to intrinsic sinus node disease. Total autonomic blockade is performed by giving large doses of propanolol and atropine and observing the intrinsic heart rate (IHR).

$$IHR = 117.2 - (0.53 \times age)$$

Patients with normal IHRs are considered to have normal sinus node function, whereas patients with depressed IHRs are considered to have sinus node dysfunction.

AV Node Function

AV conduction problems are fairly common, particularly as fibrosis develops with age. When AV conduction block is observed:
- Determination of the site of the block along the AVN to His–Purkinje system is important, as block in the AV node carries a more benign prognosis, whereas block below the His is more dangerous (Box 29.2).
- Block located in the AV node is most often benign and asymptomatic as there are subsidiary pacemakers that have an escape in the 40–55 bpm range.
- Block located below the His often leads to escape rhythms in the 20–40 bpm range and are unreliable.
- **First-degree AV block:**
  - A misnomer, as there is no real block present.
  - There is delayed conduction from the atrium to the ventricle, manifested as a PR interval of > 200 ms on the surface electrocardiogram and an AH interval > 135 ms (Figure 29.4).
- **Second-degree AV block:**
  - Defined as intermittent conduction from the atrium to the ventricle.
  - Often divided into two types:
    – Type I or Wenckebach manifests as gradual prolongation of the PR interval followed by a blocked beat (Figure 29.5). Typically the beat following the dropped beat has a shorter PR interval than the beat preceding the blocked beat.
    – Type II is defined as intermittent block where an atrial beat suddenly fails to conduct to the ventricle (Figure 29.6). There is no gradual pro-

---

Box 29.2 Noninvasive differentiation of AV nodal block and infranodal block

	AV nodal	Infranodal
Exercise/isoproterenol	Improves	Conduction ratio may worsen
Atropine	Improves	Conduction ratio may worsen
Vagal maneuvers	Worsens	Conduction ratio may improve
Beta-blockers	Worsens	Conduction ratio may improve

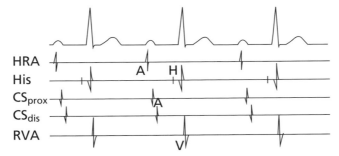

Figure 29.4 Intracardiac recordings with a prolonged AH interval. Note that the HV interval is normal, with the delay primarily between the A and the H

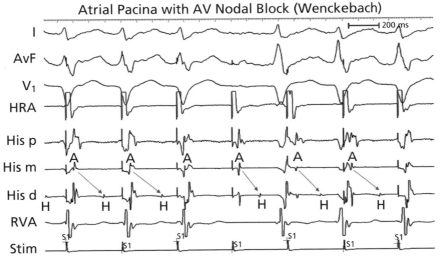

Figure 29.5 Intracardiac recordings during atrial pacing with progressive prolongation of AH intervals with a nonconducted atrial beat typical of Wenckebach phenomenon

longation of the PR interval preceding the dropped beat. This typically implies infranodal block.

- **Third-degree AV block:**
  - Defined as complete block of conduction from the atrium to the ventricle (Figure 29.7).
  - There is AV dissociation with the atrium and ventricle going at separate and unrelated rates.
  - Often the sinus rate will be higher in an attempt to compensate for the slow ventricular rate.

Atrial Programmed Stimulation

Atrial Pacing
Atrial pacing can be used to evaluate the AV nodal conduction system. Typically, atrial pacing is begun at a cycle length faster than the baseline cycle

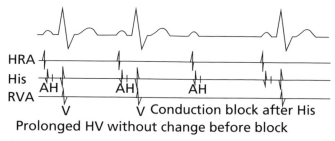

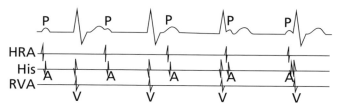

Figure 29.6 Mobitz II second-degree AV block. Intracardiac recording with consistent AH intervals with a sudden nonconducted beat to the ventricle. Note there is a His EGM in the third complex without a ventricular EGM. The QRS is often wide due to His–Purkinje system disease

Figure 29.7 Intracardiac recording of complete heart block. The atrial and ventricular signals are dissociated

length and gradually increased. The normal response of atrial ramp pacing is that the AH interval will gradually prolong and ultimately a beat will not conduct to the ventricle. The cycle length at which this occurs is often called the AV Wenckebach cycle length (AVW).

Atrial Extrastimuli

Programmed atrial stimulation is also used to evaluate the AV node. Typically there is an 8 beat drive cycle (S1), typically started at 600 ms, followed by a single extrastimulus (S2) at 400 ms.

The A2H2 interval is the AH interval following the S2 stimulus:
- Normal AV node should result in a gradual increase in the A2H2 interval as the S2 is delivered earlier and earlier
- A sudden increase in the A2H2 interval of > 50 ms with a 10 ms decrement in S2 signifies block in the fast pathway (FP) of the AV node and transition to the slow pathway of the AV node.

The S2 decrement is usually continued until there is block in the slow pathway and hence, the entire AV node:
- S2 interval at which this occurs is termed the AV node ERP.
- Presence of a "jump" signifies the existence of a slow and fast pathway in the AVN, which is a prerequisite for AV nodal re-entry tachycardia, but does not necessarily mean that this arrhythmia will be clinically present.

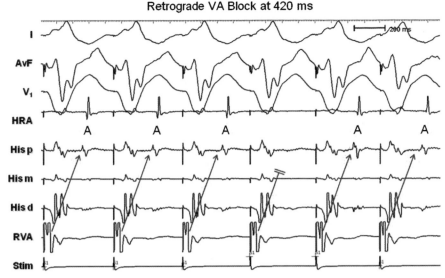

Figure 29.8 Intracardiac recording during ventricular pacing. Ventriculoatrial (VA) block was observed

Atrial extrastimulation can be continued down to where the S2 fails to capture the atrium. This is useful to characterize the atrial effective refractory period (AERP).

Ventricular Programmed Stimulation

Ventricular Pacing

Ventricular pacing is often used to assess the retrograde properties of the AV node (Figure 29.8):

- In most patients, retrograde conduction through the AVN is present, with a wide heterogeneity in the differences between antegrade, or forward, conduction compared to retrograde conduction.
- Approximately 60% of patients have slower retrograde conduction and 15% have better retrograde conduction.
- The retrograde activation sequence in the atrium is important to note, especially with a coronary sinus catheter in place:
  - Normal retrograde activation sequence should be midline up the AVN with earliest atrial activation in the His.
  - Alternative sites of earliest activation may indicate presence of a bypass tract.

Straight ventricular pacing with decreasing cycle lengths is performed while measurements of the VH intervals, or the VA intervals if the His cannot be clearly demarcated, are made. The cycle length at which the ventricle fails to consistently conduct to the atrium is termed the VA Wenckebach (VAW) cycle length.

Single ventricular extrastimulation with a ventricular paced drive train (S1) usually of 8 beats and a premature ventricular stimulus (S2) is initially performed with the right ventricular apex catheter. The first interval that fails to conduct to the atrium is referred to as the retrograde VA ERP.

Single extrastimuli can be continued until the S2 fails to capture the ventricle; this interval is termed the ventricular effective refractory period (VERP).

Induction of Arrhythimas

The ability to induce, analyze, and terminate atrial and ventricular tachyarrhythmias has become the most powerful feature of the EP study. Diagnosis and treatment of tachycardia is now the most common indication for the procedure. At the time of the EP study, depending on the arrhythmia diagnosed, radiofrequency energy (or alternative energy sources) can provide definitive treatment of the tachycardia.

As discussed in Chapter 14, the predominant mechanisms behind tachyarrhythmias include re-entry, automaticity, and triggered activity. Re-entry tachycardias are most easily induced with programmed atrial or ventricular stimulation (PES). Rapid burst pacing or multiple extrastimuli can be delivered as well as medications, such as isoproterenol, to help bring out these tachycardias.

Once induced, the activation patterns can help differentiate between the different tachycardias (Figures 29.9–29.11). In addition, observing how the tachycardia was induced, how it terminates, and how it responds to overdrive pacing and other pacing maneuvers can help more firmly establish the diagnosis. Ablative energy can be delivered at the source of an automatic tachycardia or in a critical limb of the circuit in re-entry tachycardia.

CLINICAL PEARLS

- HV interval > 60 ms with syncope or block below the AV node would warrant pacemaker implantation. However, most patients with sinus or AV nodal disease meet other criteria for pacemaker implantation and can usually bypass the EP study altogether.
- EP study is performed in cases where the patient is symptomatic (syncope) but, although suspected, no clear-cut evidence of conduction system disease has been established with the surface ECG.
- Similarly, most patients with cardiomyopathy who are considered for implantable cardioverter defibrillator (ICD) implantation for primary prevention meet other clinical criteria. EP study to establish risk of sudden cardiac death (by attempting to induce VT with programmed stimulation) is still used in some patients with borderline ejection fraction (30–40%) and equivocal symptoms/syncope or NSVT.
- Supraventricular tachycardia refractory to medical intervention is an indication for EP study and possible ablation. Many patients, however, prefer to undergo EP study and attempt at ablation rather than life-long drug therapy.

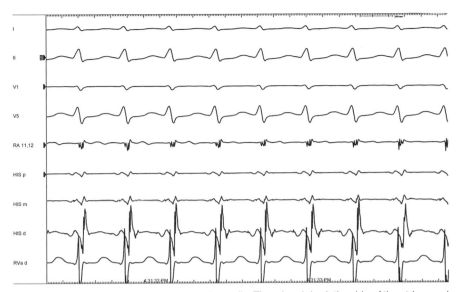

Figure 29.9 Typical AV nodal re-entrant tachycardia. There is a 1:1 relationship of the atrium and the ventricle. Note there is almost simultaneous activation of both the atrium and ventricle. Also note how the surface ECG is displayed in this view. Analyzing the surface ECG and the intracardiac EGMs simultaneously is often necessary to make the correct diagnosis

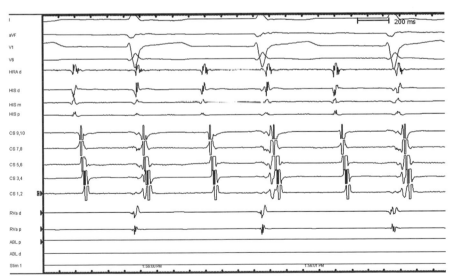

Figure 29.10 Atrial tachycardia. Note there are clearly more atrial signals than ventricular signals and there is 2:1 conduction to the ventricle. Also note the activation pattern of the CS catheter. CS 9,10 refers to the proximal poles of the CS, closest to the osteum of the CS, while CS 1,2 refers to the more distal poles. This atrial tachycardia likely begins somewhere in the lower RA, near the His and then travels towards the RA and left lateral atrium. Finer mapping would be necessary to better identify the source

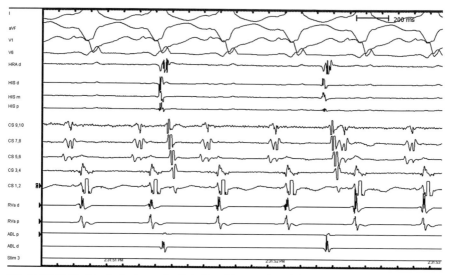

Figure 29.11 Ventricular tachycardia. Note the wide complex ECG and that there are clearly more ventricular signals than atrial signals. The atrial and ventricular EGMs are dissociated

Recommended Reading

Guidelines

ACC/AHA/NASPE 2002 Guideline Update for Implantation of Cardiac Pacemakers and Antiarrhythmia Devices: Summary Article. *Circulation* 2002;**106**:2145–2161.

Guidelines for Clinical Intracardiac Electrophysiological and Catheter Ablation Procedures. A report of the American College of Cardiology/American Heart Association Task Force on practice guidelines. (Committee on Clinical Intracardiac Electrophysiologic and Catheter Ablation Procedures). Developed in collaboration with the North American Society of Pacing and Electrophysiology. *Circulation* 1995;**92**(3):673–691.

Review Articles

Josephson ME. *Clinical Cardiac Electrophysiology: Techniques and Interpretation*, 3rd edn. Philadelphia: Lippincott, Williams & Wilkins, 2001.

Index

Page numbers in *italics* denote figures, those in **bold** denote tables.

A Practical Approach to Cardiovascular Medicine, First Edition. Edited by Reza Ardehali,
Marco Perez, Paul Wang.
© 2011 Blackwell Publishing Ltd. Published 2011 by Blackwell Publishing Ltd.